Sensors-Based Healthcare Diagnostics, Monitoring and Medical Devices

Sensors-Based Healthcare Diagnostics, Monitoring and Medical Devices

Guest Editors

Shih-Lin Wu
Jen-Jee Chen

MDPI

Basel • Beijing • Wuhan • Barcelona • Belgrade • Novi Sad • Cluj • Manchester

Guest Editors
Shih-Lin Wu
Department of Computer Science and Information Engineering
Chang Gung University
Taoyuan City
Taiwan

Jen-Jee Chen
College of Artificial Intelligence
National Yang Ming Chiao Tung University
Hsinchu
Taiwan

Editorial Office
MDPI AG
Grosspeteranlage 5
4052 Basel, Switzerland

This is a reprint of the Special Issue, published open access by the journal *Sensors* (ISSN 1424-8220), freely accessible at: https://www.mdpi.com/journal/sensors/special_issues/937CD9TI03.

For citation purposes, cite each article independently as indicated on the article page online and as indicated below:

Lastname, A.A.; Lastname, B.B. Article Title. *Journal Name* **Year**, *Volume Number*, Page Range.

ISBN 978-3-7258-7941-0 (Hbk)
ISBN 978-3-7258-7942-7 (PDF)
https://doi.org/10.3390/books978-3-7258-7942-7

Contents

About the Editors

Shih-Lin Wu

Shih-Lin Wu received his Ph.D. degree in Computer Science and Information Engineering from National Central University, Taiwan, in 2001. He is currently a Professor with the Department of Computer Science and Information Engineering at Chang Gung University. He served as the Chair of the department from 2007 to 2011 and from 2015 to 2018, and as the Director of the AI Innovation Center at Chang Gung University from 2018 to 2020. His research interests include next-generation wireless mobile networks, wireless sensor networks, the Internet of Things (IoT), localization technologies, and artificial intelligence applications in medical imaging, healthcare, home health monitoring, and industrial systems. Prof. Wu has published numerous papers in high-quality SCI-indexed journals and international conferences, and several of his papers have received best/selected/distinguished paper awards. His publications have been cited several thousand times. His research team actively collaborates with industry to develop practical application systems and has completed multiple research projects, including healthcare technology programs funded by the Ministry of Economic Affairs. The team has also conducted extensive industry–academia collaborations with companies such as Microsoft, TECO Electric & Machinery, Chang Gung Memorial Hospital, and enterprises within the Formosa Plastics Group. These collaborations have resulted in several patents and successful technology transfers to industry. Prof. Wu has served in numerous leadership roles for international conferences, including Program Chair, General Chair, and Track Chair positions. Most recently, he served as the Track Chair of "Medical Image Processing and Analysis" at the ACM International Conference on Image, Video and Signal Processing. He currently serves as a member of the editorial boards of *Telecommunication Systems* and the *International Journal of Ad Hoc and Ubiquitous Computing*.

Jen-Jee Chen

Jen-Jee Chen received his B.S. and M.S. degrees in computer science and information engineering and his Ph.D. degree in computer science from National Chiao Tung University (NCTU). He has an extensive academic background, including being a Visiting Scholar with the University of Illinois at Urbana–Champaign, and a Postdoctoral Research Fellow with the Department of Electrical Engineering, NCTU. He is currently an Associate Professor and the Director of the Institute of Smart Industry and Green Energy, College of Artificial Intelligence, National Yang-Ming Chiao Tung University (NYCU), Taiwan. Prior to joining NYCU, he was with the Department of Electrical Engineering, National University of Tainan, Taiwan. His research interests include AI, 5G V2X, and IoT, robotics and assistive applications, and AI Medical Health. Dr. Chen is a member of IEEE and the Phi Tau Phi Society. Throughout his career, he has been a reviewer for numerous computer and communication journals and has been a technical program committee (TPC) member for various computer and communication conferences. He received several awards, including best paper awards from APNOMS, MC, WASN, and ITAOI, and the Best Poster Award from MC.

sensors

MDPI

Article

Identification of Comorbidities in Obstructive Sleep Apnea Using Diverse Data and a One-Dimensional Convolutional Neural Network

Kristina Zovko [1,*], Ljiljana Šerić [1], Toni Perković [1], Ivana Pavlinac Dodig [2], Renata Pecotić [2], Zoran Đogaš [2] and Petar Šolić [1]

1 Faculty of Electrical Engineering, Mechanical Engineering and Naval Architecture, University of Split, 21000 Split, Croatia; ljiljana@fesb.hr
2 Department of Neuroscience, School of Medicine, Sleep Medicine Center, University of Split, 21000 Split, Croatia; ivana.pavlinac@mefst.hr
* Correspondence: kzovko00@fesb.hr

Abstract

Recent advances in deep learning (DL) have enabled the integration of diverse biomedical data for disease prediction and risk stratification. Building on this progress, the overall objective of this study was to develop and evaluate a multimodal DL framework for robust multi-label classification (MLC) of major comorbidities in patients with obstructive sleep apnea (OSA) using physiological time series signals and clinical data. This study proposes a robust framework for multi-label classification (MLC) of comorbidities in patients with OSA using diverse physiological and clinical data sources. We conducted a retrospective observational study including a convenience sample of 144 patients referred for overnight polysomnography at the Sleep Medicine Center (SleepLab Split), University Hospital Centre Split (KBC Split), Split, Croatia. Patients were selected based on predefined inclusion criteria and data availability. A one-dimensional Convolutional Neural Network (1D-CNN) was developed to process and fuse time series signals, oxygen saturation (SpO_2), derived SpO_2 features, and nasal airflow (FP0), with demographic and physiological parameters, enabling the identification of key comorbidities such as arterial hypertension, diabetes mellitus, and asthma/COPD. The instruments included polysomnography-derived signals (SpO_2 and FP0 airflow) and structured demographic/physiological parameters. Signals were preprocessed and used as inputs to the proposed fusion model. The proposed model was trained and fine-tuned using the Optuna hyperparameter optimization framework, addressing class imbalance through weighted loss adjustments. Its performance was comprehensively assessed using multi-label evaluation metrics, including macro/micro F1-score, AUC-ROC, AUC-PR, subset and partial accuracy, Hamming loss, and multi-label confusion matrix (MLCM). The study protocol was approved by the Ethics Committee of the School of Medicine, University of Split (Approval No. 003-08/23-03/0015, Date: 17 October 2023). The 1D-CNN achieved superior predictive performance compared to traditional machine learning (ML) classifiers with macro AUC-ROC = 0.731 and AUC-PR = 0.750. The model demonstrated consistent behavior across age, gender, and BMI groups, indicating strong generalization and minimal demographic bias. In conclusion, the results confirm that SpO_2 and airflow signals inherently encode comorbidity-specific physiological patterns, enabling efficient and scalable screening of OSA-related comorbidities without the need for full polysomnography. Although the study is limited by data set size, it provides a methodological basis for the application of multi-label DL models in clinical

 https://doi.org/10.3390/s26031056

decision support systems. Future research should focus on the expansion of multi-center datasets, thereby improving model interpretability and potential clinical adoption.

Keywords: obstructive sleep apnea (OSA); deep learning (DL); 1D-CNN; multi label classification (MLC); multi label confusion matrix (MLCM); sleep medicine; polysomnography

1. Introduction

Obstructive sleep apnea (OSA) is one of the most common sleep-related breathing disorders and affects a large portion of the global population. Current estimates suggest that nearly one billion individuals have some degree of OSA, which highlights its significance as a major public health concern [1,2]. OSA is characterized by repeated pauses or reductions in airflow during sleep due to upper airway obstruction. These events cause oxygen desaturation, fragmented sleep, and increased physiological stress. When these disturbances occur chronically, they can lead to serious long-term cardiovascular, metabolic, and respiratory consequences [3,4].

Thus, extensive research has shown that OSA is strongly associated with several important comorbidities, including hypertension [5], type 2 diabetes mellitus [6], and chronic respiratory diseases such as asthma or chronic obstructive pulmonary disease (COPD) [7,8]. The likelihood of developing these conditions increases with OSA severity. In addition, demographic and clinical factors such as age, body mass index (BMI), metabolic irregularities, and inflammatory processes further influence the interaction between OSA and its comorbidities [9,10]. Detecting these comorbidities early is essential for preventing complications and improving patient outcomes.

Polysomnography (PSG) remains the clinical gold standard for OSA diagnosis. PSG includes continuous monitoring of several physiological signals, such as oxygen saturation (SpO_2), airflow, heart activity, brain waves, and muscle tone. Although PSG is highly reliable, it is resource intensive, costly, and time consuming. The interpretation of PSG data typically requires manual scoring performed by trained clinicians, which can introduce variability, slow down the diagnostic process, and limit scalability [11–14]. As the volume and complexity of biomedical data continue to grow, traditional manual analysis becomes increasingly challenging.

Advances in machine learning (ML) and deep learning (DL) have opened new possibilities for improving diagnostic support in sleep medicine. DL models are capable of automatically learning patterns from physiological time series data and often achieve higher performance than traditional analytic methods. Convolutional Neural Networks (CNNs) are particularly effective for analyzing biomedical signals such as SpO_2 and nasal airflow $FP0$ because they can extract meaningful temporal features directly from raw input data [14]. These advantages make DL promising for building automated systems aimed at identifying OSA-related health risks.

Most existing research focuses primarily on detecting, monitoring, or classifying the severity of OSA itself, without addressing the broader clinical presentation in which multiple health conditions often occur together [15]. Studies in this field mainly concentrate on identifying apnea and hypopnea events or estimating OSA severity levels, while very few investigate the prediction or classification of comorbidities associated with OSA [16,17]. To the best of current knowledge, only one study highlights the importance of identifying comorbidities in this patient population, and no DL approaches have been developed specifically for multi-label classification (MLC) comorbidity. This gap indicates a clear

 https://doi.org/10.3390/s26031056

need for models that can analyze diverse physiological and clinical features in order to detect several coexisting conditions more accurately. The aim of this study is to develop a Deep Neural Network (DNN)-based approach for multi-label classification of OSA-related comorbidities using different types of data, including PSG signals, clinical variables, and signal-derived features.

In this study, a DL-based method using PSG signals and additional clinical information is explored to identify several comorbidities associated with OSA. In the next sections of this paper, the dataset and preprocessing steps applied to the physiological signals will be described. The extraction and preparation of clinical and signal-derived features will be explained. The architecture of the proposed one-dimensional Convolutional Neural Network (1D-CNN) for MLC will be presented, the evaluation metrics and comparison procedures will be outlined, and the experimental results and interpretation of model performance will be discussed. This structure provides a complete overview of how DL can support more accurate and efficient identification of comorbidities in patients with OSA. The general objective of this study is to develop and evaluate a multimodal DL framework for multi-label identification of major comorbidities in patients with obstructive sleep apnea by integrating SpO_2, nasal airflow (FP0), and structured clinical parameters. The specific objectives are to preprocess physiological signals and derive representative features, design a fusio-based 1D-CNN for multi-label prediction, evaluate performance using established multi-label metrics in comparison with baseline approaches, and assess robustness across demographic subgroups. We hypothesize that multimodal fusion of SpO_2, FP0, and clinical features improves multi-label comorbidity identification compared with single modality inputs and traditional baseline models, particularly in threshold independent metrics under class imbalance.

2. Related Work

Artificial intelligence (AI) techniques are increasingly used in medicine as the availability of large and diverse datasets grows and as clinical practice demands faster and more accessible diagnostic solutions. Different biomedical modalities, including physiological signals, medical imaging, wearable sensor data, and electronic health records, require analytical methods capable of capturing their temporal, spatial, and structural patterns. While traditional ML approaches remain valuable for structured and interpretable data, modern DL architectures such as CNNs, RNNs, LSTMs, and Transformers dominate contemporary research due to their ability to model complex patterns in signals, images, and multimodal inputs [18]. Nevertheless, despite these advances, many existing AI studies remain largely monomodal, and relatively few address the prediction or identification of OSA-related comorbidities. In the domain of physiological time series, common approaches include RNNs, LSTMs, GRUs, 1D-CNNs, and ensemble methods such as RF and XGBoost [19], as well as multimodal architectures combining CNN and LSTM models on EEG, ECG, SpO_2, and airflow signals [20]. More advanced systems integrate physiological signals and EHR data through hybrid DL/ML frameworks [21], while GAN-based models have been explored for enhancing minority classes in SpO_2 or airflow datasets [22,23]. Other studies fuse physiological signals with CT imaging or EHR data using CNN–Transformer pipelines [24,25]. Similar methodological diversity is observed in EHR, questionnaire, and population-based clinical research, where Transformers, Graph Neural Networks (GNNs), and hybrid architectures are commonly applied [26–28]. In medical imaging, CNNs continue to serve as the foundation, with increasing adoption of Transformers, 3D-CNNs, and hybrid systems that integrate images with physiological or behavioral signals [29–31]. Such multimodal solutions often rely on CNN, GNN, and U-Net-based components or combine multiple

 https://doi.org/10.3390/s26031056

sensor types through CNN–Transformer frameworks [32–35]. A separate line of work has investigated multi-label classification with combinations of ECG, EEG, EMG, MRI, CT, and wearable sensor data using SVM, GAN, or reinforcement learning approaches [36–38]. AI has also become increasingly prominent in sleep medicine, particularly for automated detection of OSA. Early studies relied on handcrafted features extracted from SpO_2 or ECG signals processed with Fully Connected Neural Networks (FCNNs) or classical ML methods [39,40]. More recent research employs ResNet models, contrastive learning, multiscale architectures, and attention mechanisms to detect apnea events or estimate AHI directly from physiological signals [41–43]. EEG-based and multimodal systems combine wavelet-based features, CNNs, BiLSTMs, and attention models to improve event detection and sleep staging [44–49]. Additional OSA-related work integrates anatomical imaging, acoustic data, or thermal and depth information using CNN-based architectures [50–53]. Clinical variable models using logistic regression (LR), XGBoost, SVM, and RF also remain widely used [54–56], together with an increasing emphasis on explainable AI (XAI) for improved clinical trust [57]. Within this broader landscape, prior work specifically targeting OSA comorbidity prediction has mostly focused on predicting individual comorbid conditions or clinically relevant outcomes using ML models trained on demographic, clinical, and sleep-derived descriptors. For instance, ref. [58] addressed OSA-related hypertension prediction by benchmarking multiple ML classifiers, including LR, gradient boosting-based methods (e.g., GBM/XGBoost), ensemble techniques, and a multilayer perceptron, in a cohort of 1493 OSA patients, and further interpreted the best-performing models using permutation importance and SHAP to highlight the relevance of demographic characteristics (e.g., age, BMI) and oxygenation-related measures (e.g., minimum SpO_2, time below 90%). Their best-performing model, GBM, achieved strong discrimination (AUC-ROC = 0.873) and identified key contributors such as family history of hypertension and the percentage of time with $SaO_2 < 90\%$. Ref. [59] extended comorbidity prediction beyond cardiometabolic risk by developing depression risk models in OSA-Hypopnea Syndrome patients, comparing traditional approaches such as LR and Least Absolute Shrinkage and Selection Operator (LASSO) regularization with tree-based models (Random Forest (RF)), demonstrating that the combination of clinical factors and lifestyle variables can improve stratification of mental health comorbidity. In addition, ref. [60] proposed an ML-enhanced framework for predicting incident atrial fibrillation in patients with concurrent type 2 diabetes and OSA syndrome, integrating ML-based risk modeling with clinical predictors and showing that metabolic indices alongside sleep-disordered breathing severity contribute to cardiovascular comorbidity development. Finally, ref. [61] demonstrated the applicability of ML to long-term prognostic modeling by using an RF predictor with feature selection to estimate 10-year cardiovascular disease-related mortality risk in an OSA cohort, illustrating how data-driven models can capture clinically meaningful outcome risk beyond cross-sectional comorbidity status.

Overall, most existing studies address single comorbidities or long-term outcomes using predominantly tabular predictors, whereas fewer works explore multi-label prediction across multiple comorbidities simultaneously. Moreover, despite rapid progress in AI for sleep medicine, OSA-related research still mainly focuses on estimating AHI, detecting apnea and hypopnea events, or assessing disease severity. As a result, the systematic classification of OSA-related comorbidities remains largely underexplored, and many proposed solutions rely on a single data modality, whether imaging, physiological time series, or clinical metadata, thereby overlooking important cross-modal relationships and interactions. In contrast, the proposed approach formulates comorbidity identification as a multi-label task and integrates signal-derived representations with additional clinical

https://doi.org/10.3390/s26031056

parameters, enabling direct assessment of the contribution of non-signal features through comparison with a signal-only baseline model. This combination addresses a clear methodological gap by moving beyond monomodal, single-outcome modeling toward clinically relevant multi-label comorbidity prediction in OSA.

3. Data Description and Preprocessing

3.1. Dataset Description

This study was designed as a retrospective observational analysis conducted at the SleepLab, KBC Split, Croatia. The study protocol was approved by the Ethics Committee of the School of Medicine, University of Split (Approval No. 003-08/23-03/0015; Date: 17 October 2023). No a priori sample size calculation was performed, as this study represents an exploratory DL model development and evaluation. Therefore, the final sample size was determined by data availability and predefined inclusion and exclusion criteria. A non-probabilistic purposive (criterion-based) sampling approach was applied by first selecting eligible patients with complete physiological recordings and available clinical information required for multi-label comorbidity annotation. When multiple patients met the same eligibility criteria, a random selection was performed to obtain sufficient representation of each target comorbidity for model training.

The dataset used in this study consists of 144 patients who underwent standard overnight polysomnography (PSG) at the SleepLab Split. All recordings were acquired in clinically supervised conditions using full PSG systems, and the data were exported in European data format (.edf) [62]. For the purpose of this study, two physiological signals were selected due to their strong relevance for respiratory analysis: oxygen saturation (SpO_2) measured via pulse oximetry and nasal airflow (FP0) recorded using a nasal pressure transducer. Both signals capture essential information about respiratory disturbances during sleep. SpO_2 reflects blood oxygen fluctuations associated with apnea and hypopnea events, whereas FP0 reflects airflow amplitude and respiratory cycles. Alongside the time series signals, the dataset includes clinical and demographic information, such as age, gender, BMI, heart rate (HR), and Apnea–Hypopnea Index (AHI). A set of signal-derived features was also computed to describe the timing and severity of respiratory events, including the duration of airflow cessation, desaturation duration, the delay between airflow loss and oxygen decline, and slope-based markers reflecting the dynamics of oxygen drops and recovery.

The dataset used in this study consists of 144 patients who underwent standard overnight polysomnography (PSG) at the SleepLab Split. All recordings were acquired in clinically supervised conditions using a full PSG system (ALICE 6 Diagnostic System [63]), and the data were exported in European data format (.edf) [62]. In addition, standardized questionnaires were administered as part of the clinical assessment, including STOP Bang, the Berlin Questionnaire, the Pittsburgh Sleep Quality Index (PSQI), and the Epworth Sleepiness Scale (ESS). All PSG recordings and clinical data were de-identified prior to analysis by removing direct personal identifiers. The dataset was stored on secure institutional systems with access restricted to authorized research personnel, and the analyses were performed in compliance with applicable data protection regulations. Due to patient privacy and ethical restrictions, the raw data are not publicly available. For the purpose of this study, two physiological signals were selected due to their strong relevance for respiratory analysis: oxygen saturation (SpO_2) measured via pulse oximetry and nasal airflow (FP0) recorded using a nasal pressure transducer. Both signals capture essential information about respiratory disturbances during sleep. SpO_2 reflects blood oxygen fluctuations associated with apnea and hypopnea events, whereas FP0 reflects airflow amplitude and respiratory cycles. Alongside the time series signals, the dataset includes clinical and

https://doi.org/10.3390/s26031056

demographic information, such as age, gender, BMI, heart rate (HR), and Apnea–Hypopnea Index (AHI). A set of signal-derived features was also computed to describe the timing and severity of respiratory events, including the duration of airflow cessation, desaturation duration, the delay between airflow loss and oxygen decline, and slope-based markers reflecting the dynamics of oxygen drops and recovery.

This multimodal structure provides a comprehensive representation of each patient's physiological and clinical profile. An illustration of the whole process in the 1D CNN model is illustrated in Figure 1.

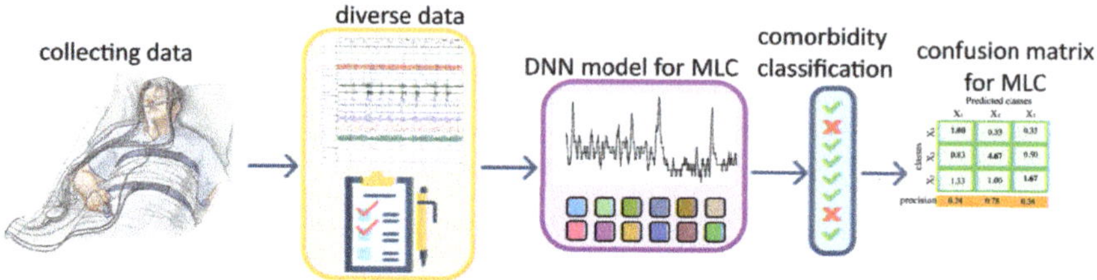

Figure 1. Conceptual workflow of the proposed multi-label comorbidity classification framework in OSA patients. First, overnight PSG data are collected and exported in EDF format. Next, key signals (SpO_2 and FP0 airflow), derived signal features, and structured clinical parameters are prepared. These multimodal inputs are fused in a multi branch 1D-CNN to simultaneously predict three comorbidities (hypertension, diabetes mellitus, and asthma/COPD). Finally, the model is evaluated using multi-label metrics and the MLCM. (Adapted from [64]).

3.2. Signal Preprocessing

The PSG recordings contained noise, artifacts, and varying sampling rates depending on the recording system. Because .edf files occupy a large amount of memory, the SpO_2 and FP0 channels were extracted from the original PSG recordings and stored in the Feather format to enable faster and more efficient processing [65]. To ensure reliable analysis and allow uniform model input, the signals underwent a structured preprocessing procedure. The original recordings had sampling rates that were much higher than required for analyzing slow respiratory processes. Figure 2 shows SpO_2 and FP0 signals of one patient during the night before artifact removal and filtering.

Therefore, both SpO_2 and $FP0$ signals were resampled to a uniform sampling rate of 5 Hz. This rate is widely used in respiratory signal analysis because it preserves the essential shape of desaturation and airflow events while significantly reducing data volume and computational complexity. The raw signals included invalid values caused by sensor displacement, signal loss, saturation clipping, or patient movement. Such artifacts were detected and corrected using interpolation for short missing segments, replacement of physiologically impossible values, smoothing of extreme spikes, and correction of baseline drift in airflow signals. These steps ensure that only physiologically meaningful patterns remain available for feature extraction and model training. A combination of filtering methods was applied to improve signal smoothness and suppress high-frequency noise: low-pass filtering to preserve slow respiratory components [66], moving average smoothing to stabilize short-term fluctuations [67], and Savitzky–Golay filtering before computing derivatives. These filters help reveal true desaturation patterns and airflow changes while avoiding distortion of clinically relevant events.

After cleaning and filtering, both signals were divided into fixed-length windows covering short time intervals. Windowing allows the model to learn local temporal patterns such as apnea onset, airflow reduction, and the progression of oxygen decline. It also allows the dataset to be converted into multiple training samples per patient, improving

https://doi.org/10.3390/s26031056

model robustness. Figure 3 shows the SpO_2 and FP0 signals of one patient during the night after artifact and outlier removal.

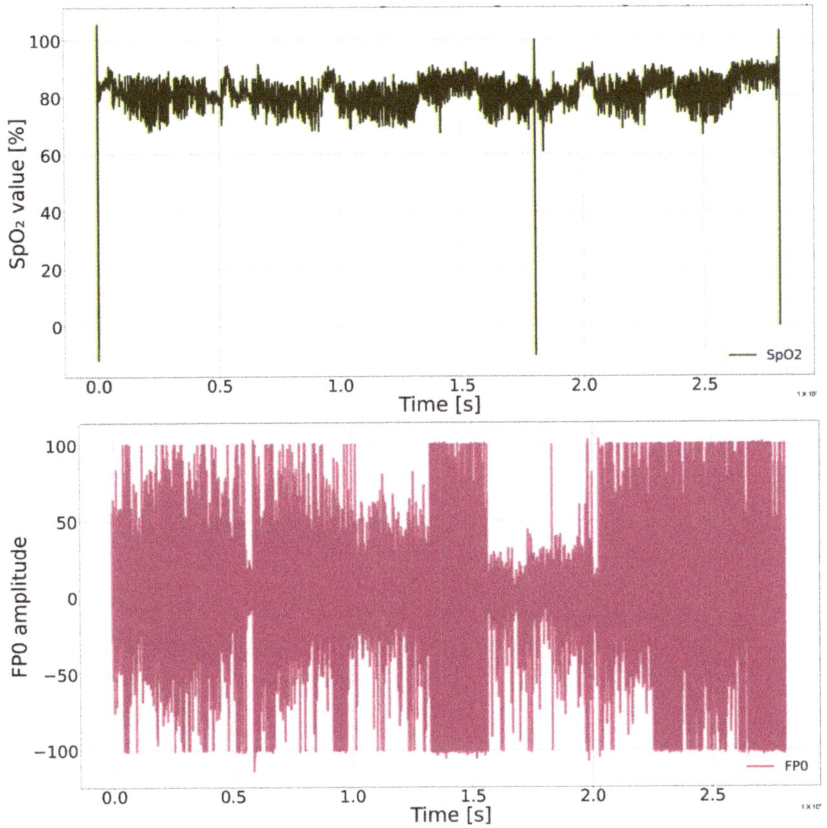

Figure 2. SpO_2 and FP0 signals of the patient before preprocessing procedure.

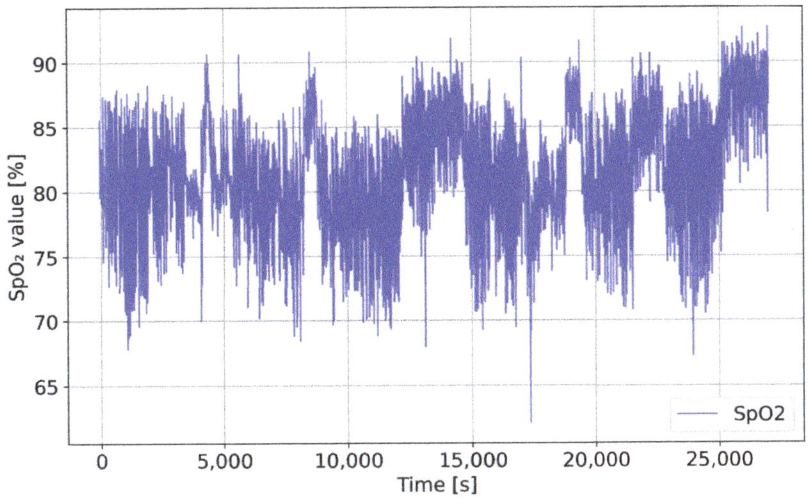

https://doi.org/10.3390/s26031056

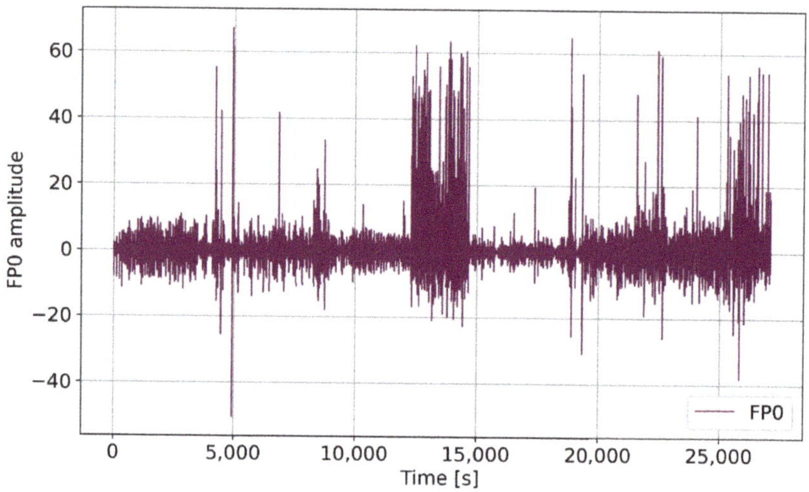

Figure 3. SpO_2 and FP0 signals after artifact removal and filtering.

3.3. Feature Engineering

To complement the raw physiological signals, a set of features was engineered to quantify specific aspects of abnormal breathing events. Desaturation events were identified in the SpO_2 waveform using thresholds related to amplitude drop and minimum event duration. Airflow cessation events were identified in the FP0 signal and paired with corresponding SpO_2 desaturations to ensure that extracted events were clinically meaningful. From each matched event pair, the following temporal and morphological parameters were calculated:

- t3–t1 mean: Defined as the average delay between the onset of FP0 cessation (t1) and the beginning of oxygen desaturation (t3). This parameter quantifies the latency between respiratory obstruction and its physiological manifestation in blood SpO_2.
- t4–t2 mean: Defined as the average delay between the resumption of FP0 (t2) and the start of oxygen recovery (t4). This reflects the time needed for SpO_2 to normalize once breathing resumes.
- *delta_t_FP0_mean*: The mean duration of FP0 cessation episodes, computed directly from the FP0 signal between markers t1 (start of apnea) and t2 (end of apnea). This value represents the average length of respiratory arrest events.
- *delta_t_SpO_2_mean*: The mean duration of oxygen desaturation episodes, calculated as the time interval between t3 (start of desaturation) and t4 (end of desaturation). It provides a measure of how long SpO_2 remains depressed during events.
- *mean_delta_SpO_2*: The average desaturation difference, i.e., the difference between the initial SpO_2 value and the minimum value reached during all detected desaturation events throughout the night. This quantifies the drop in oxygen during the night.
- mean slope: The average slope of the desaturation curves, calculated as $\Delta SpO_2/\Delta t$ during the fall phase of all events. It describes the rate of decline in SpO_2, distinguishing between abrupt and gradual desaturations.

In addition to the above signal-derived features, standard clinical parameters were included: age, gender (female: 1, male: 0), BMI, AHI, and heart rate. All features were then integrated into a feature matrix, where each row represents a patient and each column a clinical or derived feature, shown in Table 1. The additional parameters are shown in Table 2, along with their measurement units and clinical lower limits.

https://doi.org/10.3390/s26031056

Table 1. Example of structured clinical and engineered features used as additional inputs to the proposed model alongside the SpO_2 and FP0 time series signals. Each row corresponds to one patient.

Age	Gender	BMI	AHI	HeartRate	t3_t1_mean	t4_t2_mean	delta_t_FP0_mean	delta_t_SpO2_mean	mean_delta_SpO2	mean_slope
58	1	29.30	2.2	90.0	7.82	7.04	38.76	32.22	4.70	0.18
63	1	44.59	77.2	72.0	20.71	14.14	37.73	18.16	9.99	0.62
68	0	33.95	122.5	90.0	16.72	13.04	38.83	18.70	7.20	0.45
68	0	29.05	72.0	58.0	13.26	10.42	47.03	30.94	7.15	0.24
54	0	29.01	18.7	62.0	8.43	9.73	45.42	36.03	5.04	0.15
...	...	...	...	...	...	...	...	...	...	...
61	1	37.00	35.1	81.4	12.85	11.85	49.09	28.38	4.87	0.21
48	0	45.00	39.9	79.5	11.55	9.60	50.50	36.75	4.10	0.11
70	0	38.00	61.3	39.6	23.70	15.56	57.59	38.40	18.98	0.42
64	0	31.60	41.8	67.2	9.77	12.35	48.95	29.53	4.33	0.16
66	1	30.00	33.9	57.8	6.87	8.03	46.79	35.63	6.43	0.19

Table 2. Additional physiological parameters used in the study with their measurement units and typical clinical ranges.

Parameter	Unit	Lower Bound (Clinical Minimum)
Age	years	18–90
Gender	female = 1, male = 0	0–1
BMI	kg/m^2	18–60
AHI	events/hour	0–120
Heart rate	beats/min	40–120
$t_3 - t_1$ mean	seconds	>3–5%
$t_4 - t_2$ mean	seconds	>3–5%
Δt_{FP0} mean	seconds	≥10
Δt_{SpO_2} mean	seconds	≥10
Mean ΔSpO_2	%	≥3%
Mean slope	%	≥0.02–0.05%

These features describe the physiological relationship between airflow changes and oxygen regulation, capturing clinically relevant respiratory patterns that may reflect underlying comorbidities Figure 4. All extracted features, along with demographic and clinical variables, were normalized to ensure consistent scaling across patients. The final dataset integrates three types of information: preprocessed SpO_2 and FP0 time series windows, computed temporal and morphological features, and clinical and demographic variables. This structure enables the DL model to simultaneously analyze short-term respiratory dynamics and longer-term patient characteristics.

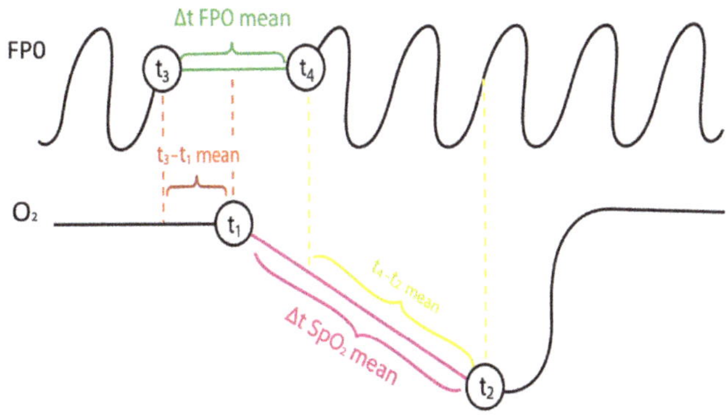

Figure 4. SpO_2 and FP0 signals with defined markers; illustration.

https://doi.org/10.3390/s26031056

3.4. Analysis of Data

To provide clinical context for the dataset, baseline characteristics were analyzed across patient subgroups defined by the presence of comorbidities (hypertension, diabetes mellitus, asthma/COPD), as well as an overall disease/no disease split. This analysis summarizes how demographic, clinical, and signal-derived parameters vary between groups and supports the interpretation of the extracted features used in subsequent modeling.

Table 3 compares patients without comorbidities (NO: $n = 24$) and those with at least one comorbidity (YES: $n = 120$). For each comparison (no comorbidity vs. comorbidity and for each individual comorbidity subgroup), both p-values and an effect size were reported. In addition to p-values, effect sizes were reported using Cohen's d (absolute values) [68], computed as the standardized difference between group means using the pooled standard deviation. Although small numerical differences are observed in several variables, BMI shows the most pronounced separation ($p < 0.01$), with higher mean values in patients with comorbidities. In contrast, AHI values remain similar across groups. Figure 5 visualizes the distributions of selected parameters and illustrates substantial overlap between the two populations. Similar comparisons are reported for the individual comorbidity subgroups (Table 4 (YES: $n = 79$), Table 5 (YES: $n = 65$), and Table 6 (YES: $n = 65$)), highlighting patterns associated with each diagnosis.

Table 3. Comparison of variables between patients without and with any comorbidity (NO: $n = 24$, YES: $n = 120$).

Additional Parameters	NO (Mean ± SD)	YES (Mean ± SD)	p Value	Effect Size (d)
Age	54.08 (±11.82)	58.33 (±10.89)	0.060	0.383
Gender [F = 1, M = 0]	0.38 (±0.48)	0.43 (±0.49)	0.327	0.102
BMI	29.19 (±4.47)	32.37 (±6.04)	0.003	0.545
AHI	32.15 (±27.66)	32.34 (±25.79)	0.488	0.007
Heart Rate	74.43 (±21.39)	67.09 (±14.44)	0.063	0.464
$t_3 - t_1$ mean	15.67 (±5.65)	14.61 (±5.27)	0.207	0.198
$t_4 - t_2$ mean	14.77 (±4.93)	13.07 (±4.78)	0.069	0.353
Δt_{FP0} mean	51.73 (±8.77)	50.01 (±10.01)	0.204	0.175
Δt_{SpO_2} mean	33.02 (±4.98)	32.96 (±5.25)	0.479	0.011
Mean ΔSpO_2	6.93 (±4.11)	6.45 (±2.99)	0.296	0.150
Mean slope	0.24 (±0.15)	0.23 (±0.12)	0.381	0.080

Note: female = 1 (F), male = 0 (M). Effect size is reported as Cohen's d (absolute values), computed using the pooled standard deviation.

Table 4. Comparison of variables between groups with and without hypertension (NO: $n = 65$, YES: $n = 79$).

Additional Parameters	NO (Mean ± SD)	YES (Mean ± SD)	p Value	Effect Size (d)
Age	53.96 (±10.95)	60.65 (±10.40)	0.000	0.626
Gender [F = 1, M = 0]	0.40 (±0.49)	0.43 (±0.50)	0.357	0.060
BMI	30.12 (±5.76)	33.26 (±5.70)	0.001	0.546
AHI	26.96 (±25.70)	36.70 (±25.63)	0.013	0.378
Heart Rate	70.52 (±17.25)	66.50 (±14.74)	0.072	0.252
t3_t1_mean	14.19 (±5.44)	15.29 (±5.22)	0.112	0.206
t4_t2_mean	12.89 (±4.84)	13.73 (±4.82)	0.151	0.173
delta_t_FP0_mean	49.70 (±8.82)	50.80 (±10.57)	0.248	0.112
delta_t_SpO_2_mean	32.75 (±4.80)	33.16 (±5.51)	0.320	0.079
mean_delta_SpO_2	6.32 (±3.48)	6.70 (±2.95)	0.248	0.118
mean_slope	0.23 (±0.13)	0.24 (±0.13)	0.395	0.077

Note: female = 1 (F), male = 0 (M). Effect size is reported as Cohen's d (absolute values), computed using the pooled standard deviation.

https://doi.org/10.3390/s26031056

Table 5. Comparison of variables between groups with and without diabetes mellitus (NO: $n = 79$, YES: $n = 65$).

Additional Parameters	NO (Mean ± SD)	YES (Mean ± SD)	*p* Value	Effect Size (d)
Age	60.06 (±10.45)	55.62 (±11.32)	0.008	0.408
Gender [F = 1, M = 0]	0.35 (±0.48)	0.47 (±0.50)	0.083	0.244
BMI	33.22 (±6.08)	30.71 (±5.56)	0.006	0.428
AHI	36.85 (±27.21)	28.56 (±24.55)	0.031	0.317
Heart Rate	66.58 (±16.52)	69.74 (±15.50)	0.123	0.196
t3_t1_mean	14.23 (±5.08)	15.24 (±5.52)	0.133	0.190
t4_t2_mean	12.76 (±4.23)	13.84 (±5.25)	0.090	0.228
delta_t_FP0_mean	50.20 (±10.64)	50.38 (±9.11)	0.457	0.018
delta_t_SpO_2_mean	33.32 (±5.35)	32.69 (±5.06)	0.237	0.120
mean_delta_SpO_2	6.63 (±2.74)	6.44 (±3.54)	0.359	0.061
mean_slope	0.24 (±0.13)	0.23 (±0.12)	0.357	0.079

Note: female = 1 (F), male = 0 (M). Effect size is reported as Cohen's *d* (absolute values), computed using the pooled standard deviation.

Table 6. Comparison of variables between groups with and without asthma/COPD (NO: $n = 79$, YES: $n = 65$).

Additional Parameters	NO (Mean ± SD)	YES (Mean ± SD)	*p* Value	Effect Size (d)
Age	57.28 (±10.68)	57.91 (±11.53)	0.367	0.057
Gender [F = 1, M = 0]	0.46 (±0.50)	0.38 (±0.49)	0.163	0.161
BMI	31.80 (±6.02)	31.88 (±5.85)	0.466	0.013
AHI	29.78 (±24.21)	34.38 (±27.41)	0.145	0.178
Heart Rate	68.21 (±12.20)	68.40 (±18.62)	0.472	0.012
t3_t1_mean	14.90 (±5.51)	14.70 (±5.21)	0.416	0.037
t4_t2_mean	13.27 (±5.18)	13.42 (±4.55)	0.427	0.030
delta_t_FP0_mean	49.98 (±9.60)	50.57 (±10.01)	0.361	0.060
delta_t_SpO_2_mean	32.65 (±5.17)	33.24 (±5.22)	0.249	0.113
mean_delta_SpO_2	6.19 (±3.19)	6.81 (±3.19)	0.126	0.194
mean_slope	0.23 (±0.12)	0.24 (±0.13)	0.234	0.080

Note: female = 1 (F), male = 0 (M). Effect size is reported as Cohen's *d* (absolute values), computed using the pooled standard deviation.

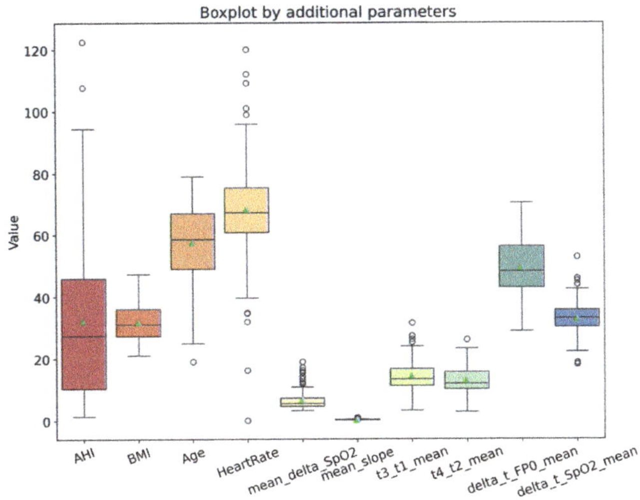

Figure 5. Box and whisker plots of selected clinical and signal-derived parameters used in the model. The central line indicates the median, the box the interquartile range (IQR), and whiskers extend to 1.5×IQR. Circles denote outliers, and triangles denote the mean.

https://doi.org/10.3390/s26031056

In addition to baseline comparisons, slope-based respiratory features were examined across AHI severity categories (Figures 6–8). The mean slope increases with higher AHI levels, particularly in the severe OSA group, indicating greater variability in respiratory signal dynamics with increasing apnea severity. When normalized by age and BMI, the same trend remains visible, suggesting that respiratory slope characteristics capture meaningful changes in breathing morphology across severity strata. Statistical testing across severity categories showed increasing separation between patients with and without comorbidities, reaching significance in the moderate OSA group ($p = 0.03$).

Overall, these observations support the subsequent modeling stage, in which both signal-derived features and clinical parameters are considered for comorbidity prediction. Even when univariate differences are modest, predictive information may arise from multivariate and nonlinear interactions that are not reflected in classical statistical comparisons.

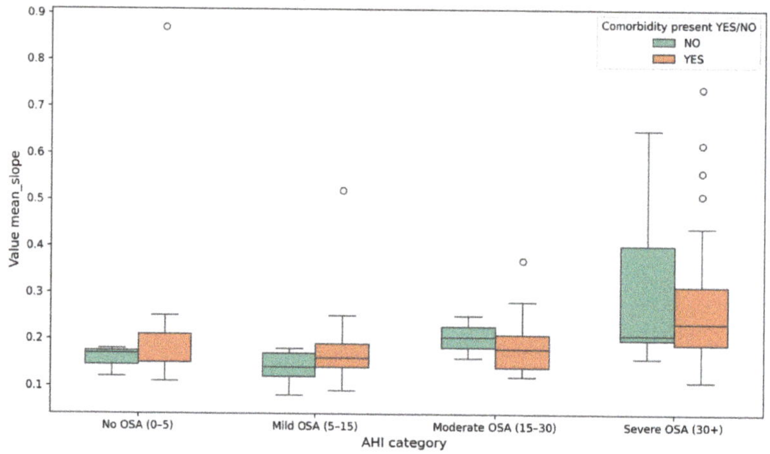

Figure 6. Distribution of the mean slope values across AHI categories for patients with and without comorbidities. Circles indicate outlier observations beyond the whiskers.

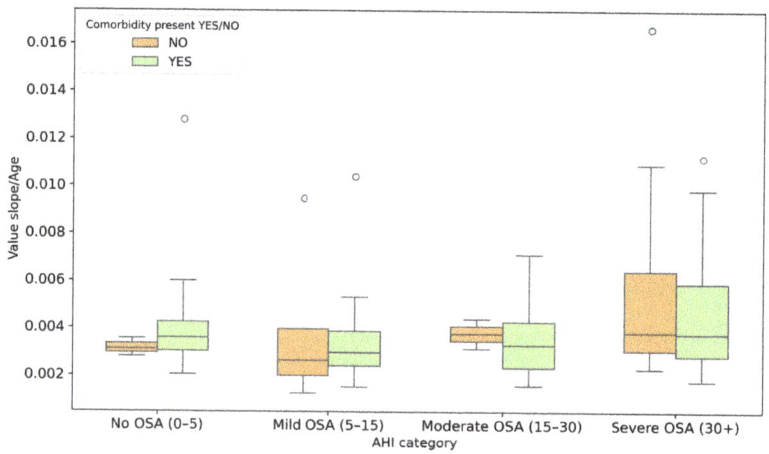

Figure 7. Distribution of slope-to-age ratio across AHI severity categories. Circles indicate outlier observations beyond the whiskers.

https://doi.org/10.3390/s26031056

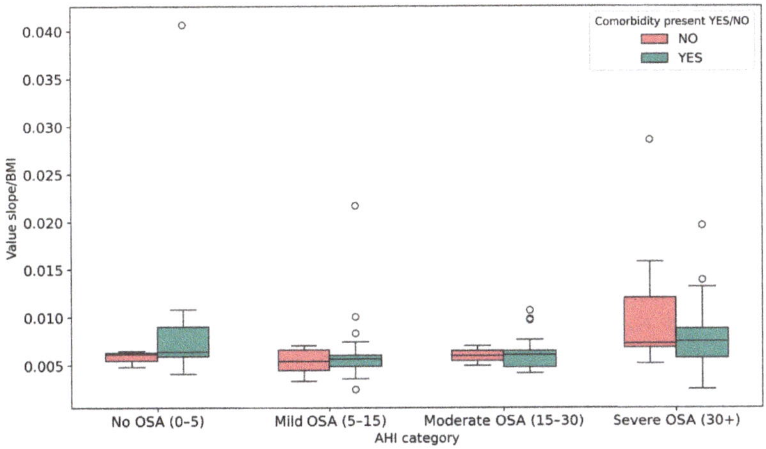

Figure 8. Distribution of slope-to-BMI ratio across AHI severity categories. Circles indicate outlier observations beyond the whiskers.

3.5. Limitations of Data

Although the dataset provides valuable clinical information, several limitations should be acknowledged. The label distribution is imbalanced: hypertension is considerably more prevalent than diabetes mellitus and asthma/COPD, while multi-label combinations are rare. This imbalance increases the difficulty of multi-label learning, may bias the model toward the most frequent conditions, and can reduce the stability of performance estimates for underrepresented comorbidities. In addition, the dataset does not include healthy control subjects, since all individuals were referred for PSG due to suspected or confirmed sleep-disordered breathing, which may limit generalizability to screening or population-based settings.

Although full PSG contains multiple physiological channels, this study focused on two core channels [69] (SpO_2 and FP0) for model development. Full PSG recordings include additional modalities (e.g., EEG, ECG, EMG, respiratory belts) that provide complementary information about sleep stages, autonomic regulation, and respiratory effort and could potentially improve classification performance. Therefore, restricting the input to two channels reduces the available multimodal context and may limit the model's ability to capture complex interactions between physiological systems. Finally, the dataset originates from a single clinical center and reflects local referral patterns, which may introduce selection bias and motivates further validation on independent cohorts.

4. Methods

4.1. Problem Definition

The goal of this study is to develop an MLC model capable of identifying three clinically relevant comorbidities commonly associated with OSA: hypertension, diabetes mellitus, and asthma/COPD. Each patient can simultaneously exhibit zero, one, two, or all three comorbidities. The predictive task therefore requires assigning a vector of three binary outputs, where each element indicates the presence or absence of a specific condition.

This setup differs from traditional single-label classification because labels are not mutually exclusive. The model must learn to capture shared patterns across conditions while also distinguishing features unique to each disease.

https://doi.org/10.3390/s26031056

4.2. 1D-CNN Architecture

Convolutional Neural Networks (CNNs) are a core DL architecture originally developed for image analysis, where they extract spatial patterns using trainable filters [70]. Their fundamental mechanism for learning local features through convolution extends naturally to one-dimensional data, making them highly suitable for biomedical time series signals. In the context of sleep medicine, 1D-CNNs are effective because physiological waveforms such as SpO_2 and airflow contain characteristic temporal structures associated with respiratory instability and oxygen desaturation events. These temporal signatures can be difficult to capture using traditional ML methods but can be efficiently learned through convolutional layers that scan the signal and detect recurring patterns [71].

In 1D form, each convolutional filter slides along the temporal axis of the signal and computes a dot product between the kernel and local segments of the waveform. This enables the model to detect short-term events such as rapid desaturation declines or airflow cessations, as well as more gradual patterns related to apnea severity or recovery dynamics. Additional components such as activation functions, padding, and stride control the nonlinearity and temporal resolution of the learned representations. The use of the ReLU activation function enhances gradient flow and prevents saturation effects, while padding ensures that the temporal length of the output remains aligned with the input signal [72].

The predictive task in this study is formulated as an MLC problem, where each patient may simultaneously exhibit several comorbidities rather than belonging to a single diagnostic category. This stands in contrast to traditional single-label classification, where each instance is associated with exactly one class. A simple visual illustration of this difference is shown in Figure 9, which compares mutually exclusive labels with multi-label assignments applicable to real-world biomedical data [73,74].

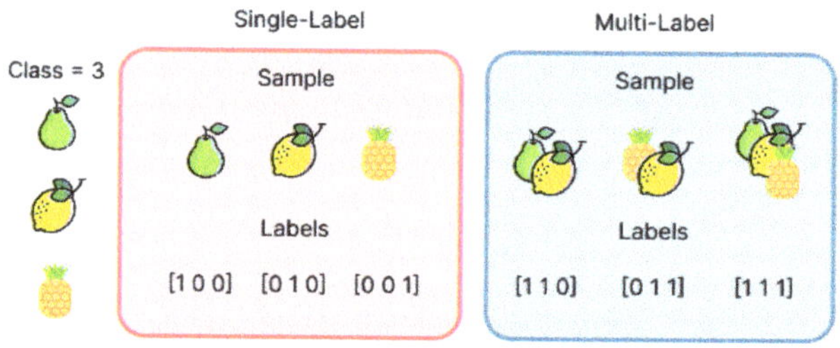

Figure 9. Example of single label vs. MLC.

Within this learning framework, convolutional layers play a key role in extracting temporal patterns from biomedical signals. A conceptual overview of how convolutional operations progressively transform the input signal through stacked feature extraction blocks is shown in Figure 10, which illustrates the hierarchical flow from raw time series data to deeper learned representations [71].

Building on these concepts, the proposed model uses a multi-branch 1D-CNN architecture designed to integrate PSG time series with clinical information. Two branches process the physiological signals independently: one for oxygen saturation (SpO_2), one for the derivated SpO_2 signal and one for nasal airflow ($FP0$). Each branch contains convolutional layers that learn relevant temporal motifs, followed by batch normalization to stabilize training and dropout to reduce overfitting. Global Average Pooling (GAP) condenses each feature map into a compact representation, emphasizing dominant temporal patterns rather than specific signal positions. In parallel, a third branch processes clinical and signal-derived parameters such as age, BMI, AHI, heart rate, and respiratory timing features. This structured input is passed through a fully connected pathway to generate a dense embedding compatible with the signal-based representations. The outputs of all three branches are then concatenated to form a unified feature vector that captures temporal dependencies in the SpO_2 waveform, airflow-related respiratory patterns, and broader patient-level characteristics. To support multi-label prediction, the final output layer uses three independent sigmoid units, enabling simultaneous estimation of hypertension, diabetes mellitus, and asthma/COPD. This design aligns the model with the multi-label nature of the task.

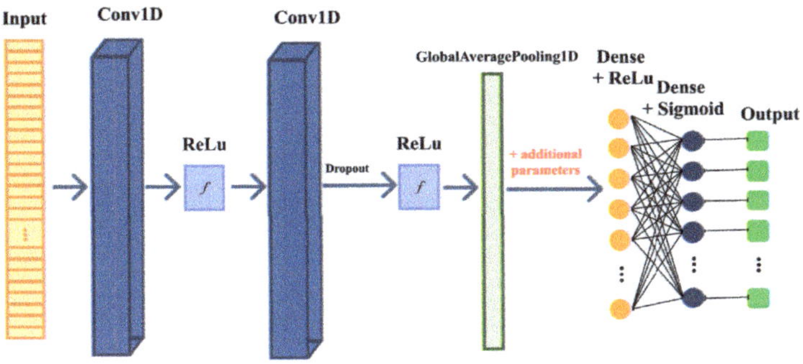

Figure 10. Conceptual overview of convolutional feature extraction in a CNN.

A detailed overview of the complete architecture, including convolutional hyperparameters, dense layers, dropout rates, and the focal loss configuration, is presented in Figure 11, which summarizes every component used in the final implementation.

Overall, the integration of convolutional feature extraction, clinical feature processing, and multi-label prediction enables the model to leverage diverse biomedical data and to learn both short-term physiological patterns and long-term patient characteristics. This architecture proved effective in identifying comorbidity-related signatures within PSG signals, supporting its use in automated risk assessment for OSA populations.

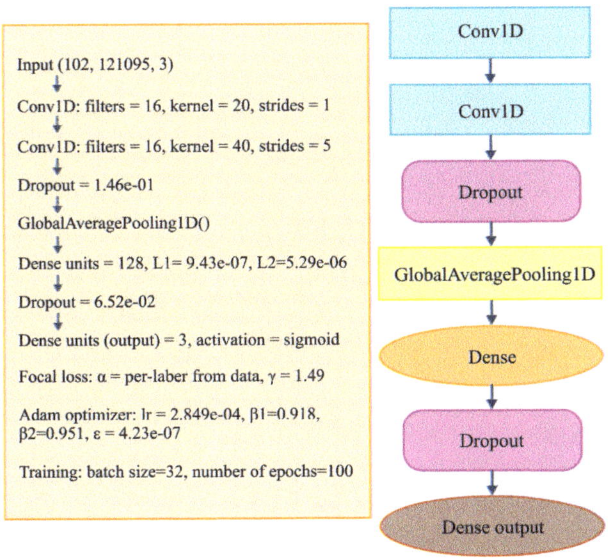

Figure 11. Multi-branch 1D-CNN architecture used for comorbidity prediction.

https://doi.org/10.3390/s26031056

4.3. Class Imbalance Handling

The dataset exhibits notable class imbalance, especially for diabetes mellitus and asthma/COPD, which occur less frequently than hypertension. Multi-label combinations further amplify this imbalance and can bias the model toward majority classes. To address this issue, the training process incorporates weighted binary cross entropy, where each label is assigned a class-specific weight inversely proportional to its frequency. This ensures that rare comorbidity classes contribute more strongly to the loss function, encouraging the model to learn from underrepresented cases. A detailed analysis of comorbidity distribution was performed to calculate appropriate weights and to identify the imbalance between single-label, dual-label, and triple-label cases.

4.4. Evaluation Metrics

The evaluation of MLC models requires metrics that capture the fact that each instance may contain multiple labels simultaneously. Unlike single-label classification, where each sample has exactly one true class, MLC allows partial correctness, meaning that a prediction may overlap with the true label set even when the match is not exact. For this reason, model performance was assessed using a combination of label-based, example-based, threshold-independent, and error-based metrics [75,76].

Label-based metrics evaluate each comorbidity independently by computing standard binary measures such as accuracy, precision, recall, and F1-score [77]. Here, TP, FP, TN, and FN denote the number of true positives, false positives, true negatives, and false negatives, respectively, and N denotes the total number of samples. These metrics rely on the following definitions:

$$Accuracy = \frac{TP + TN}{N} \tag{1}$$

$$Precision = \frac{TP}{TP + FP} \tag{2}$$

$$Recall = \frac{TP}{TP + FN} \tag{3}$$

$$F1 = \frac{2TP}{2TP + FP + FN} \tag{4}$$

To summarize results across all labels, macro and micro averaging were applied. Macro averaging assigns equal weight to each label, while micro averaging aggregates all true positives, false positives, true negatives, and false negatives across labels

$$B_{macro} = \frac{1}{q}\sum_{j=1}^{q} B(TP_j, FP_j, TN_j, FN_j) \tag{5}$$

$$B_{micro} = B\left(\sum_{j=1}^{q} TP_j, \sum_{j=1}^{q} FP_j, \sum_{j=1}^{q} TN_j, \sum_{j=1}^{q} FN_j\right) \tag{6}$$

Example-based metrics evaluate prediction correctness at the level of each patient. Subset accuracy is the strictest measure, requiring the entire predicted label set to match the true label set exactly,

$$SubsetAccuracy = \frac{1}{N}\sum_{i=1}^{N} I(Y_i = Z_i) \tag{7}$$

https://doi.org/10.3390/s26031056

Flat accuracy evaluates correctness at the level of individual labels,

$$FlatAccuracy = \frac{1}{Nq}\sum_{i=1}^{N}\sum_{j=1}^{q} I(y_{ij} = z_{ij}) \quad (8)$$

Partial accuracy quantifies the overlap between the predicted and true label sets,

$$PartialAccuracy = \frac{1}{N}\sum_{i=1}^{N}\frac{|Y_i \cap Z_i|}{|Y_i \cup Z_i|} \quad (9)$$

Threshold-independent metrics were also used. The area under the ROC curve (AUC-ROC) and the area under the precision–recall curve (AUC-PR) measure discriminative performance across different thresholds. AUC-PR is particularly informative for imbalanced datasets.

To quantify fine-grained prediction errors, Hamming loss was calculated,

$$HammingLoss = \frac{1}{Nq}\sum_{i=1}^{N}\sum_{j=1}^{q} I(y_{ij} \neq z_{ij}) \quad (10)$$

Finally, model errors were analyzed using a multi-label confusion matrix (MLCM). Unlike traditional confusion matrices, which assume a single true class, the multi-label version computes true positives, false positives, true negatives, and false negatives separately for each comorbidity. This enables detailed inspection of label-wise misclassifications and reveals dependencies between comorbidities [78–81].

The combined use of these complementary metrics provides a comprehensive evaluation framework for assessing the models' ability to detect multiple comorbidities simultaneously and supports a detailed interpretation of predictive performance.

5. Results

This section presents the quantitative evaluation of the proposed 1D-CNN architecture for MLC of comorbidities in patients with OSA. All experiments were conducted on a workstation equipped with an Intel® Core™ i5-1135G7 CPU (2.40 GHz) and 16 GB RAM. The complete training procedure for the final model required less than one hour, depending on the selected hyperparameters. At inference time, the model required only a few seconds per patient under the same hardware configuration.

The dataset was divided at the patient level into training (70%), validation (15%), and test (15%) subsets to prevent data leakage. Hyperparameter optimization was performed on the training and validation subsets, while the test subset was reserved exclusively for the final evaluation. The independent test set, fully unseen during model development, was used exclusively for the final evaluation. The model outputs three binary labels corresponding to hypertension, diabetes mellitus, and asthma/COPD.

Table 7 summarizes the raw MLCM, including class-wise precision and recall. The diagonal values represent correctly predicted labels, while non-diagonal entries represent misclassifications or clinically realistic co-occurrences.

https://doi.org/10.3390/s26031056

Table 7. Raw MLCM with class-wise recall and precision. Abbreviations: GT, ground truth; MLCM, multi-label confusion matrix; λ_1, hypertension; λ_2, diabetes mellitus; λ_3, asthma/COPD.

GT	λ_1	λ_2	λ_3	Recall
λ_1	4.0	0.0	4.0	0.50
λ_2	0.0	3.0	0.0	1.00
λ_3	0.5	2.5	7.0	0.70
Precision	0.89	0.55	0.64	

Label λ_2 demonstrates perfect recall (1.00), indicating that all true instances were successfully detected, despite its relatively small prevalence. Labels λ_1 and λ_3 exhibit moderate recall (0.50 and 0.70), reflecting typical overlaps between clinically related comorbidities. To investigate cross-label relationships, the precision and recall matrices were computed from the raw MLCM.

High diagonal values in both tables confirm that the 1D-CNN maintains stable precision and recall across all labels. Misclassifications primarily occur among physiologically or clinically related comorbidities, which is expected due to natural co-occurrence patterns.

To address the study objective of evaluating multi-label comorbidity identification performance, we report both label-wise metrics derived from the multi-label confusion matrix and global multi-label evaluation scores on the independent test set. The proposed 1D-CNN demonstrates stable and generalizable performance across all metrics. The high precision for λ_1 and λ_3 (0.89 and 0.64) indicates a low false positive rate (Table 8), while λ_2 achieves extremely high recall (1.00), confirming the model's ability to recognize all true cases of this comorbidity (Table 9). This behavior suggests that the network successfully differentiates subtle temporal features embedded in the SpO_2 and FP0 signals and effectively integrates structured clinical parameters.

Table 8. Precision matrix (column normalized) derived from the raw MLCM. Abbreviations: λ_1, hypertension; λ_2, diabetes mellitus; λ_3, asthma/COPD.

	λ_1	λ_2	λ_3
λ_1	0.89	0.00	0.36
λ_2	0.00	0.55	0.00
λ_3	0.11	0.45	0.64

Table 9. Recall matrix (row normalized) derived from the raw MLCM. Abbreviations: λ_1, hypertension; λ_2, diabetes mellitus; λ_3, asthma/COPD.

	λ_1	λ_2	λ_3
λ_1	0.50	0.00	0.50
λ_2	0.00	1.00	0.00
λ_3	0.05	0.25	0.70

Table 10 presents the full set of multi-label evaluation metrics. Subset accuracy (strictest measure) reached 0.286, indicating an exact match of all labels for 29% of samples. Flat and partial accuracy achieved markedly higher values (0.635), reflecting consistent partial correctness. F1-scores (macro, micro, and weighted) ranged between 0.53 and 0.55, demonstrating balanced performance across both frequent and rare labels. Macro AUC-ROC = 0.731 and AUC-PR = 0.750 indicate strong threshold-independent discriminative capability.

https://doi.org/10.3390/s26031056

Moderate recall for λ_1 and λ_3 primarily stems from the natural overlap between comorbidities (e.g., hypertension and metabolic disorders), not from instability of the model. Importantly, such confusions are clinically plausible, as several of the considered conditions frequently co-occur in OSA patients and share overlapping physiological patterns. Precision and recall matrices confirm this by showing the highest off-diagonal confusion occurring between clinically correlated labels.

Global metrics further support model robustness. While subset accuracy is intentionally strict and penalizes any partially incorrect prediction, flat/partial accuracy better reflects practical screening utility by quantifying how many comorbidity labels are correctly identified per patient. The model achieves approximately two-thirds correctness at the label level (flat/partial accuracy = 0.635) and balanced F1-scores despite class imbalance. High macro AUC-ROC and AUC-PR values reflect excellent ranking performance even when labels overlap.

Table 10. Summary of evaluation metrics. Abbreviations: AUC-ROC, area under the receiver operating characteristic curve; AUC-PR, area under the precision–recall curve; TP, true positives; FP, false positives; FN, false negatives; TN, true negatives.

Metric	Value	Definition	Interpretation
Subset accuracy	0.286	Exact match across all labels per sample.	Strictest metric, a sample counts as correct only if *all* labels are predicted correctly. Lower values are expected in multi-label tasks with partial hits.
Flat accuracy	0.635	Bit-level accuracy over all labels (flattened).	Indicates frequent partial correctness at the label (bit) level across samples.
Partial accuracy	0.635	Mean per sample label match ratio.	Aligns with flat accuracy, showing that, on average, about two-thirds of labels per sample are correct.
B_{macro} (F1-macro)	0.533	Unweighted mean F1 across labels.	Treats rare and frequent labels equally, lower due to class imbalance and harder labels.
B_{micro} (F1-micro)	0.549	Global F1 aggregating TP/FP/FN over all labels.	Reflects overall balance of precision/recall across the dataset.
$B_{weighted}$ (F1-weighted)	0.551	F1 weighted by label frequency.	Slight uplift vs. macro due to dominance of frequent labels.
AUC-ROC (macro)	0.731	Mean area under ROC curve across labels (one vs. rest).	Threshold independent discrimination, higher indicates better ranking of positives vs. negatives across labels.
AUC-PR (macro)	0.750	Mean area under precision–recall curve across labels.	More informative under class imbalance, higher indicates better detection of positives with fewer false alarms.
Hamming loss	0.365	Fraction of misclassified labels over all samples and labels.	Complement of flat accuracy (here $\approx 1 - 0.635$); lower is better.

Overall, these results demonstrate that the CNN reliably extracts meaningful temporal patterns from physiological waveforms. Comorbidities exhibit consistent and interpretable prediction behavior, not random confusion. The architecture generalizes well to unseen patients, confirming robustness for real-world deployment.

To address the objective of assessing robustness across demographic subgroups, we performed a stratified evaluation by age, gender, and BMI on the independent test set. Furthermore, stratified analysis by age, gender, and BMI indicates that the model performs consistently across all demographic subsets.

https://doi.org/10.3390/s26031056

Age groups (Figure 12): Most stable performance occurs in the 40–69 range groups with the largest representation and typical comorbidity prevalence. Slight deviations in the youngest and oldest ranges are attributable to small sample sizes. Gender (Figure 13): No significant differences. Minor fluctuations reflect natural prevalence differences rather than model bias. BMI categories (Figure 14): Highest stability occurs in overweight/obese class I ranges (BMI 25–34.9). Extremes (BMI > 40) show a moderate increase in errors due to physiological variability and fewer samples.

Overall, the observed fluctuations at the extremes of the distributions are primarily attributable to smaller subgroup sample sizes rather than systematic model bias.

These findings indicate that performance variability is driven by dataset distribution rather than any inherent bias, suggesting suitability for diverse clinical populations.

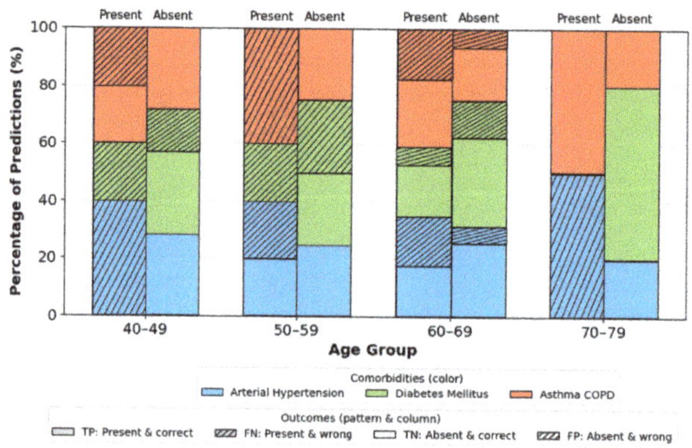

Figure 12. Correct and incorrect predictions per comorbidity by age group. Colors indicate comorbidity type (arterial hypertension, diabetes mellitus, asthma/COPD). For each age range, the left bar corresponds to comorbidity present and the right bar to absent; solid segments denote correct predictions (TP for present, TN for absent), and hatched segments denote incorrect predictions (FN for present, FP for absent).Abbreviations: TP, true positives; TN, true negatives; FP, false positives; FN, false negatives.

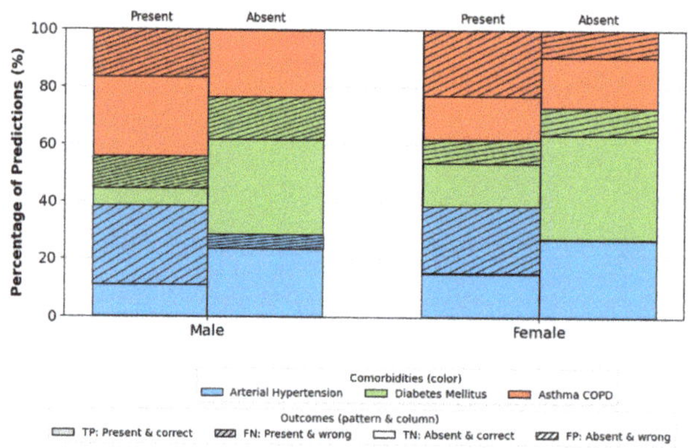

Figure 13. Correct and incorrect predictions per comorbidity by gender. Colors indicate comorbidity type (arterial hypertension, diabetes mellitus, asthma/COPD). For each gender, the left bar corresponds to comorbidity present and the right bar to absent; solid segments denote correct predictions (TP for present, TN for absent), and hatched segments denote incorrect predictions (FN for present, FP for absent). Abbreviations: TP, true positives; TN, true negatives; FP, false positives; FN, false negatives.

https://doi.org/10.3390/s26031056

The proposed 1D-CNN successfully captures short-term oxygen desaturation dynamics, airflow interruption patterns, and patient-level clinical characteristics. This multimodal integration enables reliable multi-label prediction of comorbidities directly from PSG-derived signals. Results confirm that SpO_2 and FP0 alone carry strong discriminative potential for identifying hypertension, diabetes mellitus, and asthma/COPD, supporting the development of cost-efficient screening tools. The strong threshold-independent performance (AUC-ROC, AUC-PR), balanced F1 scores, and clinically plausible confusion patterns highlight the models' potential for real-world deployment.

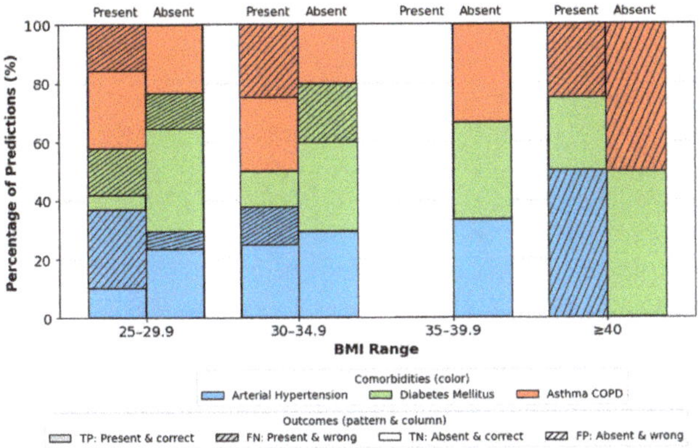

Figure 14. Correct and incorrect predictions per comorbidity by BMI range. Colors indicate comorbidity type (arterial hypertension, diabetes mellitus, asthma/COPD). For each BMI range, the left bar corresponds to comorbidity present and the right bar to absent; solid segments denote correct predictions (TP for present, TN for absent), and hatched segments denote incorrect predictions (FN for present, FP for absent). Abbreviations: TP, true positives; TN, true negatives; FP, false positives; FN, false negatives.

Analysis of the 1D-CNN Model and Comparison with Baseline Model Approach

Table 11 summarizes the MLC results of the proposed model and compares them with a baseline CNN model trained without additional clinical parameters. The baseline model used only the transformed time series signals as input, enabling a direct assessment of the contribution of the additional parameters to overall performance.

The proposed model achieves the best threshold-independent performance, with AUC-ROC (macro) = 0.731 and AUC-PR (macro) = 0.745. In contrast, the CNN baseline model, which uses only the transformed time series signals without additional clinical parameters, obtains substantially lower ranking performance (AUC-ROC = 0.459, AUC-PR = 0.599). This highlights the clear benefit of integrating additional clinical parameters alongside signal features in the proposed architecture, indicating that the proposed 1D-CNN ranks positive cases more reliably across labels and is better aligned with the underlying class imbalance. In threshold-dependent metrics, the CNN baseline also demonstrates inferior performance, with subset accuracy = 0.238 and Hamming loss = 0.413, while the proposed 1D-CNN achieves stronger performance, including Subset accuracy = 0.286 and Hamming loss = 0.365. Overall, the comparison confirms that predictive improvements stem not only from convolutional modeling but also from combining temporal features with clinically informative parameters.

 https://doi.org/10.3390/s26031056

Table 11. Comparison of multi-label classifiers on the test set.

Model	Subset Acc	Flat Acc	Partial Acc	F1-Macro	F1-Micro	F1-Weighted	AUC-ROC (Macro)	AUC-PR (Macro)	Hamming Loss
CNN (proposed)	0.286	0.635	0.635	0.533	0.549	0.551	0.731	0.750	0.365
CNN (baseline)	0.143	0.508	0.508	0.348	0.392	0.318	0.459	0.599	0.492

Note: Subset accuracy denotes exact match accuracy (all labels correct). Flat accuracy represents overall label-wise accuracy, while partial accuracy denotes average per-sample label accuracy. Macro/micro/weighted F1 are reported for MLC. AUC-ROC and AUC-PR are macro averaged across labels. Lower Hamming loss indicates fewer label-wise classification errors.

6. Discussion

The overall objective of this study was to develop and evaluate a multimodal DL framework for multi-label identification of major comorbidities in patients with OSA by integrating SpO_2, FP0 airflow, and structured clinical parameters. The findings of this study demonstrate that the proposed multi-branch 1D-CNN model can effectively extract clinically meaningful temporal patterns from SpO_2 and $FP0$ signals and integrate them with structured clinical variables to identify key comorbidities associated with OSA. The model achieved balanced multi-label performance across hypertension, diabetes mellitus, and asthma/COPD, despite notable class imbalance within the dataset. This indicates that weighted loss functions and multimodal feature fusion successfully mitigated the dominance of majority labels and encouraged the network to learn discriminative representations even for less frequent comorbidities.

Recent literature increasingly supports the use of DL models for automated analysis of physiological signals in OSA screening, particularly when leveraging multimodal signal fusion to improve robustness and generalizability [82–84]. The raw MLCM (Table 7) shows that hypertension and asthma/COPD achieved moderate recall (0.50 and 0.70), while diabetes mellitus reached perfect recall (1.00). This result is particularly noteworthy given the relatively low prevalence of diabetes within the dataset, suggesting that the model learned subtle temporal clinical signatures specific to the metabolic profile of diabetic patients. Precision remained high across all labels (0.89–0.64), indicating low false positive rates and confirming that the classifier avoids overpredicting comorbidities, which is crucial for clinical usability.

Analysis of the precision and recall matrices (Tables 8 and 9) further highlights that misclassifications predominantly occur between clinically related comorbidities, most notably hypertension and diabetes mellitus. This is consistent with well-known physiological and metabolic interactions in OSA patients, where sympathetic activation, intermittent hypoxia, and obesity contribute to overlapping risk profiles [85–87]. In addition, the bidirectional association between OSA and cardiometabolic dysfunction has been repeatedly highlighted in recent reviews and meta-analyses, supporting the clinical plausibility of these label overlaps [88]. These errors therefore likely reflect meaningful comorbidity co-occurrence rather than model instability.

Evaluation metrics (Table 10) reinforce these observations. Flat accuracy and partial accuracy of 0.635 show that approximately two-thirds of labels per patient were correctly predicted, while macro/micro/weighted F1-scores (0.533–0.551) indicate consistent performance across both frequent and rare labels. Threshold-independent metrics revealed strong discriminative capability (macro AUC-ROC = 0.731; AUC-PR = 0.750), confirming that the learned representations generalize well to unseen patient data. Combined, these results support the robustness of the proposed multimodal architecture. This aligns with recent methodological recommendations emphasizing threshold-independent evaluation

https://doi.org/10.3390/s26031056

(e.g., AUC-PR) for imbalanced clinical prediction tasks, where fixed threshold metrics may underestimate ranking performance [89,90].

Subgroup analyses, Figures 12–14, provide additional insights into demographic generalization. The model maintains stable performance across gender, with only minor variations reflecting natural prevalence differences rather than systematic bias. Age-based performance shows the highest stability in the 40–69 cohort, consistent with the highest sample density, while extremes of age exhibit greater variance due to limited representation. Similarly, accuracy remains highest within BMI ranges 25–35, aligning with typical OSA and comorbidity prevalence, whereas reduced stability in BMI ≥ 40 groups reflects physiological heterogeneity and smaller sample sizes. These findings suggest that performance variability is driven primarily by data distribution rather than architectural limitations.

Importantly, the study demonstrates that rich comorbidity-related physiological information is encoded within only two PSG-derived signals, SpO_2 and $FP0$. The ability of the 1D-CNN to detect comorbidities without relying on full PSG channels (EEG, EMG, ECG) underscores the potential for simplified and more accessible diagnostic workflows. This aligns with the growing need for scalable, low-cost screening tools in clinical and home-based environments [90]. A comparable trend is observed in the broader OSA literature, where multimodal but reduced sensor approaches (e.g., oxygen saturation combined with other accessible signals) can achieve competitive performance while improving practicality and scalability [82].

While the majority of prior work focuses on OSA detection and severity estimation, studies addressing comorbidity level prediction remain limited, which makes direct comparison challenging and highlights the clinical novelty of the presented multi-label framework [84]. Additionally, some studies report that simpler or traditional ML approaches can appear competitive under fixed threshold metrics, particularly when probability calibration or per-label threshold tuning is not applied. This may partly explain why differences between models are sometimes smaller for subset/flat accuracy than for AUC-based metrics, despite clear improvements in ranking performance.

Overall, the results show that 1D-CNN-based multimodal learning offers a promising direction for early identification of OSA-related comorbidities. The model captures both short-term respiratory dynamics and long-term clinical characteristics, achieving clinically interpretable and stable performance. These findings support the future integration of such models into decision support systems and telemedicine platforms.

7. Limitations and Future Work

Despite the encouraging results, several limitations should be acknowledged. First, the dataset size (144 patients) is modest and originates from a single clinical center, which restricts the models' exposure to broader population variability and may limit generalizability. Second, only two physiological channels (SpO_2 and FP0 nasal airflow) were used in this study. Although these signals are highly informative for capturing respiratory disturbances in OSA and contributed to strong predictive performance, the absence of additional PSG channels (e.g., EEG, ECG, EMG, and thoracoabdominal effort belts) reduces the physiological context available to the model. Future studies could incorporate a richer set of PSG modalities, supported by expert validation, to provide complementary information and potentially improve comorbidity classification. Future work should include external validation on datasets from other institutions and multi-center experiments to confirm generalizability across different clinical settings and patient populations.

Class imbalance remains another important challenge. Hypertension was substantially more prevalent than diabetes mellitus and asthma/COPD, while multi-label comorbidity

 https://doi.org/10.3390/s26031056

combinations were rare, reflecting the underlying clinical distribution rather than a sampling artifact. Although weighted loss functions improved learning stability, performance variability across labels persisted, indicating the need for additional strategies such as data augmentation, synthetic minority oversampling (e.g., GAN-based generation), and targeted rebalancing techniques in future work.

Finally, model interpretability was not explicitly addressed. Although convolutional architectures can provide more structured feature extraction than fully connected models, the present study did not incorporate explainable AI (XAI) methods such as Grad-CAM, SHAP, or LIME. Integrating XAI techniques in future research could improve clinical transparency and trust by highlighting the signal segments and clinical variables that most strongly influence comorbidity predictions.

8. Conclusions

This study demonstrates that a multimodal 1D-CNN can integrate SpO_2 and FP0 airflow signals with structured clinical variables to identify multiple OSA-related comorbidities within a unified multi-label framework. The findings show that the proposed fusion-based approach can reliably detect hypertension, diabetes mellitus, and asthma/COPD using a reduced set of PSG-derived inputs, supporting the feasibility of comorbidity screening without relying on full polysomnography.

The subgroup analyses indicate stable performance across age, BMI, and gender strata, suggesting that the learned representations capture clinically meaningful physiological patterns rather than systematic demographic bias. These results highlight the potential of simplified multimodal architectures to support scalable risk assessment in both clinical and home monitoring scenarios.

Despite limitations related to the modest single-center cohort and residual label imbalance, the proposed framework provides a methodological basis for further development toward clinical translation. Future work should focus on external multi-center validation, expansion of datasets, incorporation of additional PSG modalities, and the integration of explainable AI techniques to improve transparency and clinical trust. Overall, the study supports the use of deep-learning-based analysis of simplified PSG signals as a promising direction for automated decision support tools aimed at early identification of comorbidity profiles in OSA patients.

Author Contributions: Conceptualization, L.Š.; methodology, L.Š., I.P.D., R.P. and Z.Đ.; software, K.Z.; validation, K.Z., L.Š., T.P., I.P.D., R.P., Z.Đ. and P.Š.; formal analysis, K.Z., L.Š. and T.P.; investigation, K.Z.; resources, I.P.D., R.P. and Z.Đ.; data curation, I.P.D., R.P. and Z.Đ.; writing-original draft preparation, K.Z.; writing-review and editing, K.Z.; visualization, K.Z.; supervision, T.P., I.P.D., R.P., Z.Đ. and P.Š.; project administration, P.Š. All authors have read and agreed to the published version of the manuscript.

Funding: This work was funded by the Croatian Science Foundation under the project number [HRZZ-IP-2025-02-7836]. APC voucher.

Institutional Review Board Statement: The study was conducted in accordance with the Declaration of Helsinki and approved by the Ethics Committee of the School of Medicine, University of Split (Approval No. 003-08/23-03/0015; 17 October 2023).

Informed Consent Statement: Informed consent was obtained from all subjects for diagnostic procedures, data storage, and subsequent processing of their data.

https://doi.org/10.3390/s26031056

Data Availability Statement: The PSG recordings and associated clinical data were de-identified prior to analysis and handled in compliance with applicable data protection regulations. Due to patient privacy and ethical restrictions, the raw data are not publicly available.

Conflicts of Interest: The authors declare no conflicts of interest. The funders had no role in the design of the study; in the collection, analyses, or interpretation of data; in the writing of the manuscript; or in the decision to publish the results.

References

1. Benjafield, A.V.; Ayas, N.T.; Eastwood, P.R.; Heinzer, R.; Ip, M.S.M.; Morrell, M.J.; Nunez, C.M.; Patel, S.R.; Penzel, T.; Pépin, J.; et al. Estimation of the global prevalence and burden of obstructive sleep apnoea: A literature-based analysis. *Lancet Respir. Med.* **2019**, *7*, 687–698. [CrossRef]
2. Iannella, G.; Pace, A.; Bellizzi, M.G.; Magliulo, G.; Greco, A.; De Virgilio, A.; Croce, E.; Gioacchini, F.M.; Re, M.; Costantino, A.; et al. The Global Burden of Obstructive Sleep Apnea. *Diagnostics* **2025**, *15*, 1088. [CrossRef]
3. Abrishami, A.; Khajehdehi, A.; Chung, F. A systematic review of screening questionnaires for obstructive sleep apnea. *Can. J. Anesth.* **2010**, *57*, 423. [CrossRef] [PubMed]
4. Deviaene, M.; Varon, C.; Testelmans, D.; Buyse, B.; Van Huffel, S. Assessing cardiovascular comorbidities in sleep apnea patients using SpO_2. In *Proceedings of the 2017 Computing in Cardiology (CinC)*; IEEE: New York, NY, USA, 2017; pp. 1–4. [CrossRef]
5. Chadia, K.; Archontogeorgis, K.; Drakopanagiotakis, F.; Bonelis, K.; Anevlavis, S.; Steiropoulos, P. Clinical and Sleep Characteristics and the Effect of CPAP Treatment on Obese Patients with Obstructive Sleep Apnea and Asthma—A Retrospective Study. *Healthcare* **2025**, *13*, 2240. [CrossRef] [PubMed]
6. Gentile, S.; Monda, V.M.; Guarino, G.; Satta, E.; Chiarello, M.; Caccavale, G.; Mattera, E.; Marfella, R.; Strollo, F. Obstructive Sleep Apnea and Type 2 Diabetes: An Update. *J. Clin. Med.* **2025**, *14*, 5574. [CrossRef]
7. Tondo, P.; Hoxhallari, A.; Lacedonia, D.; Magaletti, P.; Sabato, R.; Foschino Barbaro, M.P.; Scioscia, G. The CORE syndrome: An overlap of severe asthma, obstructive sleep apnea, rhinosinusitis, and esophageal reflux. *Sleep Breath.* **2024**, *28*, 1761–1765. [CrossRef]
8. Kainulainen, S.; Töyräs, J.; Oksenberg, A.; Korkalainen, H.; Sefa, S.; Kulkas, A.; Leppänen, T. Severity of desaturations reflects OSA-related daytime sleepiness better than AHI. *J. Clin. Sleep Med.* **2019**, *15*, 1135–1142. [CrossRef]
9. Demko, B.G. The Evolution of Oral Appliance Therapy for Snoring and Sleep Apnea: Where Did We Come From, Where Are We, and Where Are We Going? *Sleep Med. Clin.* **2018**, *13*, 467–487. [CrossRef] [PubMed]
10. Marin, J.M.; Carrizo, S.J.; Vicente, E.; Agusti, A.G. Long-term cardiovascular outcomes in men with obstructive sleep apnoea-hypopnoea with or without treatment with continuous positive airway pressure: An observational study. *Lancet* **2005**, *365*, 1046–1053. [CrossRef]
11. Bahammam, A.; Gacuan, D.; George, S.; Acosta, K.L.; Pandi-Perumal, S.R.; Gupta, R. Polysomnography I: Procedure and Technology. In *Synopsis of Sleep Medicine*; Apple Academic Press Inc.: Palm Bay, FL, USA, 2016; pp. 443–456. [CrossRef]
12. Gottlieb, D.J.; Punjabi, N.M. Diagnosis and management of obstructive sleep apnea: A review. *JAMA* **2020**, *323*, 1389–1400. [CrossRef]
13. Slowik, J.M.; Sankari, A.; Collen, J.F. Obstructive Sleep Apnea. In *StatPearls*; StatPearls Publishing: Treasure Island, FL, USA, 2025. [PubMed]
14. Lipton, Z.; Kale, D.; Elkan, C.; Wetzel, R. Learning to Diagnose with LSTM Recurrent Neural Networks. *arXiv* **2015**, arXiv:1511.03677.
15. Pattipati, M.; Gudavalli, G.; Zin, M.; Dhulipalla, L.; Kolack, E.; Karki, M.; Devarakonda, P.K.; Yoe, L. Continuous Positive Airway Pressure vs Mandibular Advancement Devices in the Treatment of Obstructive Sleep Apnea: An Updated Systematic Review and Meta-Analysis. *Cureus* **2022**, *14*, e21759. [CrossRef] [PubMed] [PubMed Central]
16. Hussein, O.; Alkhader, A.; Gohar, A.; Bhat, A. Home Sleep Apnea Testing for Obstructive Sleep Apnea. *Mo. Med.* **2024**, *121*, 60–65. [PubMed] [PubMed Central]
17. Espinosa, M.A.; Ponce, P.; Molina, A.; Borja, V.; Torres, M.G.; Rojas, M. Advancements in Home-Based Devices for Detecting Obstructive Sleep Apnea: A Comprehensive Study. *Sensors* **2023**, *23*, 9512. [CrossRef]
18. Zovko, K.; Šerić, L.; Perković, T.; Belani, H.; Šolić, P. IoT and health monitoring wearable devices as enabling technologies for sustainable enhancement of life quality in smart environments. *J. Clean. Prod.* **2023**, *413*, 137506. [CrossRef]
19. Hüsken, M.; Stagge, P. Recurrent neural networks for time series classification. *Neurocomputing* **2003**, *50*, 223–235. [CrossRef]
20. M, I.A.C.; Ansari, M.Y.; Paul, S.; Halabi, O.; Alataresh, E.; Shah, J.; Hamze, A.; Aboumarzouk, O.; Al-Ansari, A.; Dakua, S.P. Development and Validation of a Class Imbalance-Resilient Cardiac Arrest Prediction Framework Incorporating Multiscale Aggregation, ICA and Explainability. *IEEE Trans. Biomed. Eng.* **2025**, *72*, 1674–1687. [CrossRef]
21. Liu, S.; Fu, B.; Wang, W.; Liu, M.; Sun, X. Dynamic Sepsis Prediction for Intensive Care Unit Patients Using XGBoost-Based Model With Novel Time-Dependent Features. *IEEE J. Biomed. Health Inform.* **2022**, *26*, 4258–4269. [CrossRef]

 https://doi.org/10.3390/s26031056

22. Kim, Y.; Koo, J.; Lee, S.; Song, H.; Lee, M. Explainable AI Warning Model Using Ensemble Approach for In-Hospital Cardia Arrest Prediction: A Retrospective Cohort Study. *J. Med. Internet Res.* **2023**, *25*, e48244. [CrossRef]
23. Kobir, M.; Machado, P.; Lotfi, A.; Haider, D.; Ihianle, I. Enhancing Multi-User Activity Recognition in an Indoor Environmer with Augmented Wi-Fi Channel State Information and Transformer Architectures. *Sensors* **2025**, *25*, 3955. [CrossRef]
24. Hossen, M.K.; Peng, Y.T.; Shao, A.; Chen, M. An ODE based neural network approach for PM2.5 forecasting. *Sci. Rep.* **202** *15*, 24830. [CrossRef]
25. Xie, J.; Wang, Z.; Yu, Z.; Ding, Y.; Guo, B. Prototype Learning for Medical Time Series Classification via Human–Machin Collaboration. *Sensors* **2024**, *24*, 2655. [CrossRef]
26. Sirrianni, J.; Sezgin, E.; Claman, D.; Linwood, S. Medical Text Prediction and Suggestion Using Generative Pretrained Transforme Models with Dental Medical Notes. *Methods Inf. Med.* **2022**, *61*, 195–200. [CrossRef] [PubMed]
27. Tian, M.; Chen, B.; Guo, A.; Jiang, S.; Zhang, A. Reliable generation of privacy-preserving synthetic electronic health record tim series via diffusion models. *J. Am. Med Inform. Assoc. JAMIA* **2024**, *31*, 2529–2539. [CrossRef] [PubMed]
28. Huo, Z.; Booth, J.; Monks, T.; Knight, P.; Watson, L.; Peters, M.; Pagel, C.; Ramnarayan, P.; Li, K. Dynamic mortality prediction i critically Ill children during interhospital transports to PICUs using explainable AI. *Npj Digit. Med.* **2025**, *8*, 108. [CrossRef]
29. Lin, P.K.; Chiu, Y.H.; Huang, C.J.; Wang, C.Y.; Pan, M.L.; Wang, D.W.; Liao, H.Y.; Chen, Y.S.; Kuan, C.H.; Lin, S.Y.; et al. PADA Physician-oriented artificial intelligence-facilitating diagnosis aid for retinal diseases. *J. Med Imaging* **2022**, *9*, 044501. [CrossRef [PubMed]
30. V J, S.; D, J.F. Deep Learning Algorithm for COVID-19 Classification Using Chest X-Ray Images. *Comput. Math. Methods Me* **2021**, *2021*, 9269173. [CrossRef]
31. Alp, S.; Akan-R.Farshi, T.; Bhuiyan, M.S.; Disbrow, E.; Conrad, S.; Vanchiere, J.; Kevil, C.; Bhuiyan, M.A.N. Joint transforme architecture in brain 3D MRI classification: Its application in Alzheimer's disease classification. *Sci. Rep.* **2024**, *14*, 8996. [CrossRef
32. Ahmad, S.; Ahmad, Z.; Kim, J.M. A Centrifugal Pump Fault Diagnosis Framework Based on Supervised Contrastive Learning *Sensors* **2022**, *22*, 6448. [CrossRef]
33. Rahaman Wahab Sait, A.; Alkhurayyif, Y. Lightweight hybrid transformers-based dyslexia detection using cross-modality data *Sci. Rep.* **2025**, *15*, 17054. [CrossRef]
34. Jovic, A.; Frid, N.; Brkic, K.; Cifrek, M. Interpretability and accuracy of machine learning algorithms for biomedical time series analysis—A scoping review. *Biomed. Signal Process. Control* **2025**, *110*, 108153. [CrossRef]
35. Saikumar, K.; Rajesh, V.; Srivastava, G.; Lin, J.C.W. Heart disease detection based on internet of things data using linear quadratic discriminant analysis and a deep graph convolutional neural network. *Front. Comput. Neurosci.* **2022**, *16*, 964686. [CrossRef]
36. Heydarian, M.; Doyle, T.E.; Samavi, R. MLCM: Multi-Label Confusion Matrix. *IEEE Access* **2022**, *10*, 19083–19095. [CrossRef]
37. Kimura, A.; Mitsukura, Y.; Oya, A.; Matsumoto, M.; Nakamura, M.; Kanaji, A.; Miyamoto, T. Objective characterization of hip pain levels during walking by combining quantitative electroencephalography with machine learning. *Sci. Rep.* **2021**, *11*, 3192 [CrossRef]
38. Patil, S.; Kukreja, D. Deep Reinforced Cognitive Analytics Algorithm (DRCAM): An Advanced Method to early detection of Cognitive skill impairment using Deep Learning and Reinforcement Learning. *MethodsX* **2025**, *14*, 103277. [CrossRef] [PubMed]
39. Khan, A.; Basit, M.S.; Farooq, O.; Khan, Y.U.; Shameem, M. Mitigating the class imbalance effect in Sleep Apnea Classification In *Proceedings of the 2023 International Conference on Recent Advances in Electrical, Electronics & Digital Healthcare Technologies (REEDCON)*; IEEE: New York, NY, USA, 2023; pp. 530–535. [CrossRef]
40. Sheta, A.; Turabieh, H.; Thaher, T.; Too, J.; Mafarja, M.; Hossain, M.S.; Surani, S.R. Diagnosis of Obstructive Sleep Apnea from ECG Signals Using Machine Learning and Deep Learning Classifiers. *Appl. Sci.* **2021**, *11*, 6622. [CrossRef]
41. Kumar, C.B.; Bhongade, A.; Gandhi, T.K.; Panigrahi, B.K. Recognition of Obstructive Sleep Apnea from a Single Lead Electrocardiogram Signal Using a ResNet Model. In *Proceedings of the 2023 14th International Conference on Computing Communication and Networking Technologies (ICCCNT)*; IEEE: New York, NY, USA, 2023; pp. 1–5. [CrossRef]
42. Kumar, C.B.; Mondal, A.K.; Bhatia, M.; Panigrahi, B.K.; Gandhi, T.K. Self-Supervised Representation Learning-Based OSA Detection Method Using Single-Channel ECG Signals. *IEEE Trans. Instrum. Meas.* **2023**, *72*, 15. [CrossRef]
43. Zhang, Y.; Shi, Y.; Su, Y.; Cao, Z.; Li, C.; Xie, Y.; Niu, X.; Yuan, Y.; Ma, L.; Zhu, S.; et al. Detection and severity assessment of obstructive sleep apnea according to deep learning of single-lead electrocardiogram signals. *J. Sleep Res.* **2025**, *34*, e14285. [CrossRef]
44. Khan, A.; Biswas, S.K.; Chunka, C. An Optimized Obstructive Sleep Apnea Detection Model Using Particle Swarm Optimization and Machine Learning. In *Proceedings of the 2025 10th IEEE International Conference on Integrated Circuits, Design, and Verification (ICDV)*; IEEE: New York, NY, USA, 2025; pp. 1–6. [CrossRef]
45. Khan, A.; Biswas, S.K.; Chunka, C.; Barman, S. Ensembled Obstructive Sleep Apnea Detection Using Extra Tree Ensemble Technique. In *Proceedings of the 2024 2nd International Conference on Advancement in Computation & Computer Technologies (InCACCT)*; IEEE: New York, NY, USA, 2024; pp. 342–347. [CrossRef]

https://doi.org/10.3390/s26031056

36. Satapathy, S.K.; Pattnaik, S.; Rath, R. Automated Sleep Staging Classification System Based On Convolutional Neural Network Using Polysomnography Signals. In *Proceedings of the 2022 IEEE Delhi Section Conference (DELCON)*; IEEE: New York, NY, USA, 2022; pp. 1–10. [CrossRef]
37. Jain, S.; Singhal, A.; Rai, J.K.; Sharma, P. Polysomnography based Sleep Stage Classification using Deep Learning for Sleep Apnea Pediatric Subjects. In *Proceedings of the 2025 4th OPJU International Technology Conference (OTCON) on Smart Computing for Innovation and Advancement in Industry 5.0*; IEEE: New York, NY, USA, 2025; pp. 1–7. [CrossRef]
38. M, S.; M, G.K.; Dillon P, D.; S, A.I.; S P, S.; N, M. SomnoDx: A Real-Time Deep Learning Framework for Multimodal Sleep Disorder Diagnosis. In *Proceedings of the 2025 3rd International Conference on Self Sustainable Artificial Intelligence Systems (ICSSAS)*; IEEE: New York, NY, USA, 2025; pp. 840–846. [CrossRef]
39. Jirakittayakorn, N.; Manupibul, U.; Wongsawat, Y.; Mitrirattanakul, S. RespNet: A Dual-Network Approach for Automated OSA Severity Classification Utilizing PSG Type III Signals. *IEEE Access* **2024**, *12*, 148538–148552. [CrossRef]
40. Hanif, U.; Leary, E.; Schneider, L.; Paulsen, R.; Morse, A.; Blackman, A.; Schweitzer, P.; Kushida, C.; Liu, S.; Jennum, P.; et al. Estimation of Apnea-Hypopnea Index Using Deep Learning On 3-D Craniofacial Scans. *IEEE J. Biomed. Health Inform.* **2021**, *25*, 4185–4194. [CrossRef]
41. He, Z.; Xiao, Y.; Wu, X.; Liang, Y.; Zhou, Y.; An, G. An Automatic Assessment Model of Adenoid Hypertrophy in MRI Images Based on Deep Convolutional Neural Networks. *IEEE Access* **2023**, *11*, 106516–106527. [CrossRef]
42. Qiu, X.; Wang, C.; Li, B.; Tong, H.; Tan, X.; Yang, L.; Tao, J.; Huang, J. An audio-semantic multimodal model for automatic obstructive sleep Apnea-Hypopnea Syndrome classification via multi-feature analysis of snoring sounds. *Front. Neurosci.* **2024**, *18*, 1336307. [CrossRef] [PubMed]
43. Singh, S.; Anisi, M.H.; Jindal, A.; Jarchi, D. Smart Multimodal In-Bed Pose Estimation Framework Incorporating Generative Adversarial Neural Network. *IEEE J. Biomed. Health Inform.* **2024**, *28*, 3379–3388. [CrossRef]
44. Kuan, Y.C.; Hong, C.T.; Chen, P.C.; Liu, W.T.; Chung, C.C. Logistic regression and artificial neural network-based simple predicting models for obstructive sleep apnea by age, sex, and body mass index. *Math. Biosci. Eng. MBE* **2022**, *19*, 11409–11421.
45. Javeed, A.; Berglund, J.S.; Dallora, A.L.; Saleem, M.A.; Anderberg, P. Predictive Power of XGBoost BiLSTM Model: A Machine Learning Approach for Accurate Sleep Apnea Detection Using Electronic Health Data. *Int. J. Comput. Intell. Syst.* **2023**, *2023*, 188. [CrossRef]
46. Kim, Y.J.; Jeon, J.S.; Cho, S.E.; Kim, K.G.; Kang, S.G. Prediction Models for Obstructive Sleep Apnea in Korean Adults Using Machine Learning Techniques. *Diagnostics* **2021**, *11*, 612. [CrossRef] [PubMed]
47. Troncoso-García, A.R.; Martínez-Ballesteros, M.; Martínez-Álvarez, F.; Lora, A.T. Explainable machine learning for sleep apnea prediction. *Procedia Comput. Sci.* **2022**, *207*, 2930–2939. [CrossRef]
48. Shi, Y.; Ma, L.; Chen, X.; Li, W.; Feng, Y.; Zhang, Y.; Cao, Z.; Yuan, Y.; Xie, Y.; Liu, H.; et al. Prediction model of obstructive sleep apnea-related hypertension: Machine learning-based development and interpretation study. *Front. Cardiovasc. Med.* **2022**, *9*, 1042996. [CrossRef]
49. Li, E.; Ai, F.; Liang, C. A machine learning model to predict the risk of depression in US adults with obstructive sleep apnea hypopnea syndrome: A cross-sectional study. *Front. Public Health* **2024**, *11*, 1348803. [CrossRef] [PubMed]
50. Xu, Y.; Duan, S.; Yin, W.; Yang, Y.; Zhang, X.; Wang, J. Machine learning-enhanced prediction model for atrial fibrillation development in patients with concurrent type 2 diabetes and obstructive sleep apnea syndrome: A comorbidity perspective. *Nutr. Metab.* **2025**, *22*, 158. [CrossRef]
51. Li, A.; Roveda, J.M.; Powers, L.S.; Quan, S.F. Obstructive sleep apnea predicts 10-year cardiovascular disease-related mortality in the Sleep Heart Health Study: A machine learning approach. *J. Clin. Sleep Med.* **2022**, *18*, 497–504. [CrossRef] [PubMed]
52. Korompili, G.; Amfilochiou, A.; Kokkalas, L.; Mitilineos, S.A.; Tatlas, N.A.; Kouvaras, M.; Kastanakis, E.; Maniou, C.; Potirakis, S.M. PSG-Audio, a scored polysomnography dataset with simultaneous audio recordings for sleep apnea studies. *Sci. Data* **2021**, *8*, 197. [CrossRef]
53. Philips Healthcare. Alice 6 LDe Diagnostic Sleep System. 2024. Available online: https://www.philips.com.bh/healthcare/product/HC1063311/alice-6-lde-diagnostic-sleep-system (accessed on 17 December 2025)
54. Wikimedia Commons. Sleep. Available online: https://commons.wikimedia.org/wiki/File:Sleep_studies.jpg (accessed on 30 October 2025)
55. VanderPlas, J. Python Data Science Handbook: Essential Tools for Working with Data. In *Python Data Science Handbook: Essential Tools for Working with Data*; O'Reilly Media: Sebastopol, CA, USA, 2016.
56. Crenna, F.; Rossi, G.B.; Berardengo, M. Filtering Biomechanical Signals in Movement Analysis. *Sensors* **2021**, *21*, 4580. [CrossRef] [PubMed]
57. Kawala-Sterniuk, A.; Podpora, M.; Pelc, M.; Blaszczyszyn, M.; Gorzelanczyk, E.J.; Martinek, R.; Ozana, S. Comparison of Smoothing Filters in Analysis of EEG Data for the Medical Diagnostics Purposes. *Sensors* **2020**, *20*, 807. [CrossRef]

68. Larner, A.J. Effect Size (Cohen's d) of Cognitive Screening Instruments Examined in Pragmatic Diagnostic Accuracy Studie *Dement. Geriatr. Cogn. Disord. Extra* **2014**, *4*, 236–241. [CrossRef] [PubMed]
69. Levendowski, D.J.; Hamilton, G.S.; St. Louis, E.K.; Penzel, T.; Dawson, D.; Westbrook, P.R. A comparison between auto-score apnea-hypopnea index and oxygen desaturation index in the characterization of positional obstructive sleep apnea. *Nat. Sc Sleep* **2019**, *11*, 69–78. [CrossRef]
70. Kelleher, J.D. *Deep Learning*; MIT Press: Cambridge, MA, USA, 2019; Chapter 1, pp. 1–38.
71. Kim, P. Matlab deep learning. *Mach. Learn. Neural Netw. Artif. Intell.* **2017**, *130*, 151.
72. Albawi, S.; Mohammed, T.A.; Al-Zawi, S. Understanding of a convolutional neural network. In *Proceedings of the 2017 Internationa Conference on Engineering and Technology (ICET)*; IEEE: New York, NY, USA, 2017; pp. 1–6. [CrossRef]
73. Gibaja, E.; Ventura, S. Multi-label learning: A review of the state of the art and ongoing research. *Wiley Interdiscip. Rev. Data Mi Knowl. Discov.* **2014**, *4*, 411–444. [CrossRef]
74. Koyejo, O.O.; Natarajan, N.; Ravikumar, P.K.; Dhillon, I.S. Consistent multilabel classification. *Adv. Neural Inf. Process. Syst.* **201** *28*, 3321–3329.
75. Du, J.; Chen, Q.; Peng, Y.; Xiang, Y.; Tao, C.; lu, Z. ML-Net: Multi-label classification of biomedical texts with deep neura networks. *J. Am. Med Inform. Assoc. JAMIA* **2019**, *26*, 1279–1285. [CrossRef]
76. Pereira, R.B.; Plastino, A.; Zadrozny, B.; Merschmann, L.H. Correlation analysis of performance measures for multi-labe classification. *Inf. Process. Manag.* **2018**, *54*, 359–369. [CrossRef]
77. Krstinić, D.; Braović, M.; Šerić, L.; Božić-Štulić, D. Multi-label classifier performance evaluation with confusion matrix. *Compu Sci. Inf. Technol.* **2020**, *1*, 1–14.
78. Koço, S.; Capponi, C. On multi-class classification through the minimization of the confusion matrix norm. In *Proceedings of th Asian Conference on Machine Learning*; PMLR: Cambridge, MA, USA, 2013; pp. 277–292.
79. Canbek, G.; Sagiroglu, S.; Temizel, T.T.; Baykal, N. Binary classification performance measures/metrics: A comprehensiv visualized roadmap to gain new insights. In *Proceedings of the 2017 International Conference on Computer Science and Engineerin (UBMK)*; IEEE: New York, NY, USA, 2017; pp. 821–826.
80. Labatut, V.; Cherifi, H. Evaluation of performance measures for classifiers comparison. *arXiv* **2011**, arXiv:1112.4133. [CrossRef]
81. Fawcett, T. An introduction to ROC analysis. *Pattern Recognit. Lett.* **2006**, *27*, 861–874. [CrossRef]
82. Zhang, W.; Li, X.; Chen, M.; Wang, R. Construction and validation of a machine learning-based risk prediction model for slee quality in patients with obstructive sleep apnea. *J. Sleep Res.* **2025**, *34*, e13789. [CrossRef]
83. Hemrajani, P.; Dhaka, V.S.; Rani, G.; Verma, S.; Kavita.; Wozniak, M.; Shafi, J.; Ijaz, M.F. Integrating physiological signals fo enhanced sleep apnea diagnosis with SleepNet. *Sci. Rep.* **2025**, *15*, 31715. [CrossRef] [PubMed]
84. Bazoukis, G.; Bollepalli, S.C.; Chung, C.T.; Li, X.; Tse, G.; Bartley, B.L.; Batool-Anwar, S.; Quan, S.F.; Armoundas, A.A. Applicatio of artificial intelligence in the diagnosis of sleep apnea. *J. Clin. Sleep Med.* **2023**, *19*, 1337–1363. [CrossRef]
85. Shiina, K. Obstructive sleep apnea-related hypertension: A review of the literature and clinical management strategy. *Hypertens Res.* **2024**, *47*, 3085–3098. [CrossRef]
86. Javaheri, S.; Javaheri, S.; Somers, V.K.; Gozal, D.; Mokhlesi, B.; Mehra, R.; McNicholas, W.T.; Zee, P.C.; Campos-Rodriguez, F. Martinez-Garcia, M.A.; et al. Interactions of Obstructive Sleep Apnea With the Pathophysiology of Cardiovascular Disease, Par 1: JACC State-of-the-Art Review. *J. Am. Coll. Cardiol.* **2024**, *84*, 1208–1223. [CrossRef]
87. Maniaci, A.; Lavalle, S.; Parisi, F.M.; Barbanti, M.; Cocuzza, S.; Iannella, G.; Magliulo, G.; Pace, A.; Lentini, M.; Masiello, E.; et al Impact of Obstructive Sleep Apnea and Sympathetic Nervous System on Cardiac Health: A Comprehensive Review. *J. Cardiovasc Dev. Dis.* **2024**, *11*, 204. [CrossRef]
88. Huang, H.; Chen, Z. Association between obstructive sleep apnea syndrome and type1/type2 diabetes mellitus: A systematic review and meta-analysis. *J. Diabetes Investig.* **2025**, *16*, 521–534. [CrossRef] [PubMed]
89. Hoang, N.H.; Liang, Z. AI-driven sleep apnea screening with overnight blood oxygen saturation: Current practices and future directions. *Front. Digit. Health* **2025**, *7*, 1510166. [CrossRef] [PubMed]
90. Kuo, N.Y.; Tsai, H.J.; Tsai, S.J.; Yang, A.C. Efficient Screening in Obstructive Sleep Apnea Using Machine Learning Models: Development and Validation Study. *J. Med. Internet Res.* **2024**, *26*, e51615. [CrossRef]

 https://doi.org/10.3390/s26031056

sensors

MDPI

Article

Radar Multiple Bin Selection for Breathing and Heart Rate Monitoring in Acute Stroke Patients in a Clinical Setting

Benedek Szmola [1,2,3,*], Lars Hornig [3], Jan Paul Vox [3], Thomas Liman [1,4], Andreas Radeloff [5,6], Birger Kollmeier [2,6], Karen Insa Wolf [3] and Karsten Witt [1,4,6]

1 Department of Neurology, School of Medicine and Health Science, Carl von Ossietzky Universität Oldenburg, 26129 Oldenburg, Germany; thomas.liman@uni-oldenburg.de (T.L.); karsten.witt@uni-oldenburg.de (K.W.)
2 Medizinische Physik, Carl von Ossietzky Universität Oldenburg, 26129 Oldenburg, Germany; birger.kollmeier@uni-oldenburg.de
3 Fraunhofer Institute for Digital Media Technology IDMT, Oldenburg Branch for Hearing, Speech and Audio Technology HSA, Marie-Curie-Straße 2, 26129 Oldenburg, Germany; lars.hornig@idmt.fraunhofer.de (L.H.); jan.paul.vox@idmt.fraunhofer.de (J.P.V.); karen.insa.wolf@idmt.fraunhofer.de (K.I.W.)
4 Department of Neurology, Evangelical Hospital Oldenburg, Carl von Ossietzky Universität Oldenburg, 26122 Oldenburg, Germany
5 Division of Otolaryngology, Head and Neck Surgery, Carl von Ossietzky Universität Oldenburg, 26129 Oldenburg, Germany; andreas.radeloff@uni-oldenburg.de
6 Research Center of Neurosensory Sciences, Carl von Ossietzky Universität Oldenburg, 26129 Oldenburg, Germany
* Correspondence: benedek.ernoe.szmola@uni-oldenburg.de

Abstract

Simple to use and accurate monitoring of stroke patients' breathing and heart rate in sleep is needed to lower the risk of secondary strokes and prevent worse functional outcomes due to disturbed sleep. In this study, we computed breathing and heart rates from clinical radar sleep recordings of 49 acute ischemic stroke patients. Parallel polysomnography served as the reference for evaluation. We compared radar rates computed using previously developed multiple and single range bin selection methods. Multiple selection yielded lower mean absolute errors (breathing: 0.39 vs. 0.87 breaths per min; heart rate: 0.84 vs. 3.99 beats per min) and higher correlations with the reference (breathing: 0.95 vs. 0.85; heart rate: 0.96 vs. 0.56). However, single range bin selection produced rates for a larger proportion of recording time (breathing: 93.49% vs. 73.38%; heart rate: 81.85% vs. 19.93%). Our results indicate that multiple range bin selection provides more accurate estimates of breathing and heart rate, but it has lower temporal coverage. Easy to use radar systems could facilitate the clinical adoption of contactless breathing and heart rate monitoring in sleep, improving the care provided to stroke patients.

Keywords: FMCW radar; clinical monitoring; stroke; acute ischemic stroke; sleep monitoring; breathing rate; heart rate; multiple range bin selection; single range bin selection

1. Introduction

Sleep disturbances and stroke risks are interlinked [1]. Although this link is recognized [2,3], sleep disturbances are often undiagnosed [4], leading to a gap in the care received by stroke patients. New simple to use approaches could spread the clinical use of sleep monitoring. By detecting sleep disturbances early on, better outcomes could be achieved for stroke patients.

A recent analysis of the global burden of diseases has found that stroke is among the leading causes of death and disability [5]. Patients with sleep disturbances have a higher chance of suffering a stroke [6]. Furthermore, patients who have suffered a stroke and are affected by sleep disturbances have worse functional outcomes and a higher risk of a secondary stroke [7]. Studies have demonstrated this link for various types of sleep disturbances [8], among them insomnia [9,10] and sleep disordered breathing, including sleep apnea and hypopnea [11–13]. Therefore, for patients with an elevated risk of stroke and those who have already suffered a stroke, sleep monitoring should be considered [14].

The current gold standard for sleep monitoring is polysomnography (PSG) [15,16]. PSG applies a collection of mainly contact-based sensors to monitor a wide range of physiological signals during sleep in a dedicated sleep laboratory with staff supervision. Although PSG is a sensitive method, several drawbacks limit its application: accessibility [17], patient comfort [18], and the first night effect [19,20]. Thus, alternative sleep monitoring methods are needed.

Various alternative sleep monitoring solutions have been explored in the literature. There are approaches that still use contact-based sensors but in configurations that are less uncomfortable for the patient [21]. Multiple contactless approaches have also been tested [22], such as using a camera [23], ambient microphones [24], or radars [25].

Biomedical radars have received increasing attention in the field of sleep monitoring [26–29]. They provide a contactless monitoring method that is convenient for both the patient and the caregivers. Radars are advantageous in terms of privacy concerns, as the types of radar applied for sleep monitoring do not have the angular resolution to resolve the facial features of the person. Furthermore, radars emit their own signal and, therefore, do not require additional lighting, which simplifies the recording. Different types of radars have been implemented for sleep monitoring, but frequency modulated continuous wave radars (FMCW) [30] provide a good balance between cost, complexity, and the information provided. FMCW radars transmit electromagnetic waves with a frequency that changes over a period of time. The transmitted waves and the received reflections are used to separate the space in front of the FMCW radar into multiple sections and to detect objects in these sections. These sections are referred to as range bins.

In a previous publication [31], we introduced multiple range bin selection and tested its feasibility in a small group of healthy volunteers sleeping in an office setting. We developed multiple range bin selection to make breathing and heart rate computation more robust by using all valid signals reflected from the person's body. In contrast, with the more common single range bin selection method [25,29,32], only one range bin's signal is used. When the radar is set up at the foot end of the bed and pointed at the person at an oblique angle, the FMCW radar's range bins capture body motions from different segments of the body concurrently [33,34]. Therefore, motions from different body parts do not overlap, as is the case when the radar is perpendicular to the body. This separation facilitates the parallel monitoring of breathing and heartbeat motions, as the smaller heartbeat motion (0.287 to 0.568 mm [35]) can be monitored separately from the larger breathing motion (1 to 5 mm [36]). Our previous study was limited by the low number of participants and by including only healthy individuals. Because stroke can disrupt the autonomic nervous system (ANS), impairing cardiovascular functions [37,38], the performance of breathing and heart rate monitoring based on data from healthy individuals might not generalize to stroke patients.

This work aims to evaluate the use of multiple radar range bin selection in acute stroke patients sleeping in a clinical setting. The radar range bin selection was used to detect breathing and heart rates. We tested the radar technique against the gold standard of electrocardiography (ECG) and thoracic and abdominal respiratory inductance plethysmog-

https://doi.org/10.3390/s26010251

raphy (RIP) belts using a standard PSG. This study addresses the two main limitations of our previous study. Here we have a larger group (49 instead of 6), and instead of measuring healthy volunteers in a quiet office environment, we are measuring acute stroke patients in a clinical ward. In addition to multiple range bin selection, we also test our previously developed single bin selection approach [33] and compare the results.

2. Materials and Methods

2.1. FMCW Radar

We used the Texas Instruments (Dallas, TX, USA) IWR6843ISK-ODS FMCW radar (see [26,28,31] for FMCW radar principles in vital sign monitoring). This radar has a carrier frequency of 60 GHz, with monotonically increasing frequency modulation in a sawtooth pattern. See Table 1 for details on the radar configuration. The radar board is connected to a DCA100EVM real-time measurement board from Texas Instruments. These components are enclosed in a custom designed box (see the black box with a green sticker in Figure 1) and are connected via wires to the measurement tablet. On the tablet, we used the Lab Streaming Layer (LSL, version v1.16.2) [39] to record the data.

Table 1. Radar configuration.

Frequency band	60–63 GHz
Range resolution	0.05 m
Azimuth and elevation FoV	120°
ADC samples per chirp	64
Chirp count per frame	20
Frame rate	20 Hz
Number of transmit antennas used	1
Number of receive antennas used	1
Maximal range of detection	2.56 m

FoV: field of view; ADC: analog to digital converter.

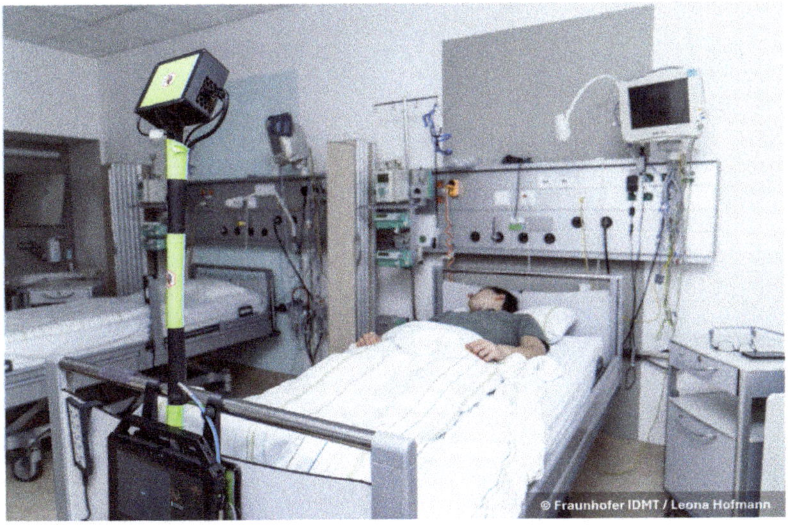

Figure 1. The measurement setup mounted on a clinical bed in the stroke unit. The setup itself is in the foreground. The measurement tablet is on the bottom, showing the graphical user interface. Above the tablet, the hooks holding the setup are visible. The radar box is held up by a pole which also leads the cables to the radar.

https://doi.org/10.3390/s26010251

For computing the breathing and heart rate, we used the displacement time series. The displacement is computed in each radar range bin from the phase values. We summarized the information of each frame by taking the median phase value of the 20 chirps in one frame for each range bin. In [31], we showed the advantage of applying this chirp median method. By taking one phase value for each frame, we obtained a time series with a sampling rate of 20 Hz for each range bin.

To detect motion from the radar recording, we calculated a motion parameter based on radar Doppler FFT [40]. This parameter summarizes velocity information from an epoch composed of multiple frames. The steps for computing the motion parameter in an epoch with multiple frames are as follows:

1. Compute the Doppler FFT for each frame in the epoch. To compute the Doppler FFT, an FFT operation is performed for each range bin along all chirps in one frame. This returns velocity information for each radar range bin.
2. Each Doppler FFT frame is reduced from a range–velocity representation to a velocity-only representation by summing along the range bins for each velocity bin.
3. Each velocity bin is cleaned of clutter by subtracting its median over all frames.
4. For each frame, a Hamming window is applied to the velocity bins to reduce the influence of low-velocity bins.
5. Finally, the velocity bins and frames are summed up to a single value.

This motion parameter highlights high velocities in the recording; therefore, it is appropriate to identify faster body movements during the recording.

2.2. Polysomnography Setup

We conducted sleep studies with parallel radar and PSG recordings. For PSG recordings, we used the SOMNOmedics HD eco device (Randersacker, Bavaria, Germany) with the following sensors: RIP abdominal and thorax belts, three-channel ECG, finger photoplethysmography (PPG) for pulse oximetry, three-channel electroencephalogram-electrooculogram combination (EEG-EOG) and a microphone attached to the neck. The listed sensors are connected to a small head unit, which is attached to the patient's abdomen with the abdominal RIP belt. Our PSG setup did not include video recording.

2.3. Patients

The study was conducted in the post-stroke unit of the Evangelisches Krankenhaus Oldenburg (Oldenburg, Germany). The study was registered in the German Clinical Trials Register (DRKS, identifier: DRKS00028189). Patients were recruited from acute stroke patients who came through the ward after being transferred from the stroke unit. We recruited 49 patients (14 women, 35 men) who suffered an acute ischemic stroke (AIS). The median age was 68 years (minimum 45 years, minimum 86 years); the median body mass index (BMI) was 28.1 (minimum 21.3, maximum 37). The study was reviewed and approved by the medical ethics committee of the Carl von Ossietzky Universität Oldenburg (votum number 2022-016; date of approval: 14 July 2023), and all patients gave their written informed consent. Sleep-associated breathing abnormalities were not included in the inclusion criteria. The exclusion criteria included dementia, aphasic syndromes, and delirium. The ability to give consent was determined during the informational discussion by a physician.

2.4. Measurement Setup

We have assembled a custom radar measurement setup. See Figure 1 for a depiction of the setup at the stroke unit. The main components are the radar box and the recording

 https://doi.org/10.3390/s26010251

tablet. The tablet is mounted on a backplate that holds two hooks to attach the setup to the bed frame. The beds were standard clinical beds, measuring 2.1 m in length. A pole mounted on the backplate holds the radar box. The radar is directed at the middle of the bed surface, while also ensuring that the entire bed is within its field of view. For handling the measurements, an intuitive graphical user interface (GUI) was created using the PyQt6 framework (version v6.5.1). The setup is powered through a power cable connected behind the patient's bed. For the connection to the electrical grid of the clinic, we used a connector with an inbuilt circuit breaker; thus, any malfunction of the measurement setup cannot affect the clinical systems. Furthermore, the setup can easily be removed and set aside in one motion in case the patient must be transported elsewhere in an emergency.

2.5. Measurement Synchronization

To ensure synchronicity of the PSG and radar measurements, we have developed a custom synchronization procedure. The manufacturer of the PSG system offers an optocoupler for transmitting external signals to the PSG head unit. We used this optocoupler for synchronization. With the measurement software, we send a synchronization signal consisting of 20 markers through the optocoupler to the PSG head unit and record this signal simultaneously on the measurement tablet. The synchronization signal is a sequence of 20 square-wave signals, with each signal level change serving as a marker for synchronization. Thus, we have precisely defined time points in both recordings, which can be used in postprocessing to align all measurements to one time axis. The delay between the signal on the tablet and the PSG caused by the optocoupler was determined by a calibration measurement. Figure 2 shows the recording tablet, the PSG head unit, and the optocoupler (the small box on top of the tablet) that connects them. The same synchronization process is performed at the beginning and end of the measurement. The recordings are aligned using the markers sent at the beginning, while the markers at the end serve as an indication of whether a significant temporal drift occurred between the tablet and the PSG clock during the night.

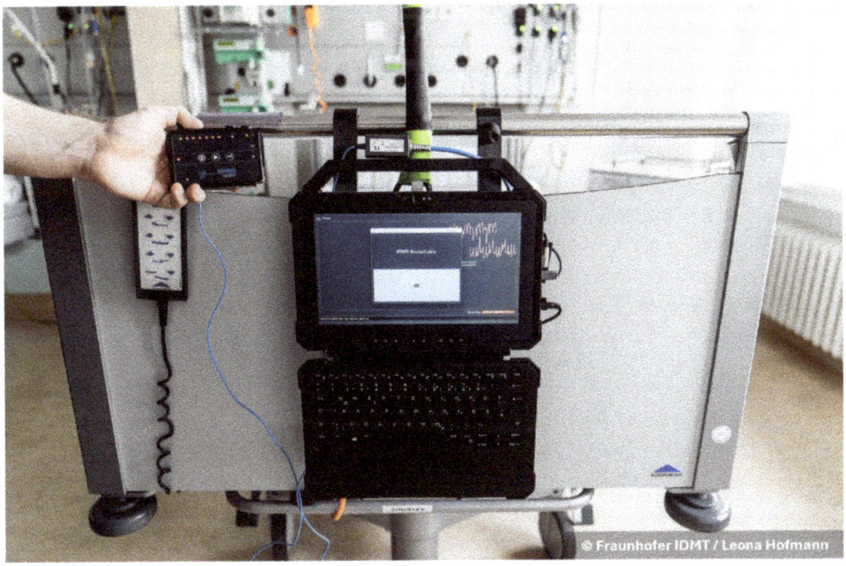

Figure 2. The graphical user interface of the measurement setup. The photo shows the process of synchronization, with the PSG head unit (held in the hand) connected to the measurement tablet (in the middle) over the manufacturer provided optocoupler (above the tablet).

 https://doi.org/10.3390/s26010251

2.6. Study Protocol

On the day of recording, the study personnel go to the patient between 6 and 7 p.m. First, the radar measurement setup is mounted on the bed. The tablet is started up, and the measurement personnel log into the study account. The measurement GUI starts automatically after a successful login. The GUI has only one button, which starts and stops the recording. Next, synchronization (see Section 2.5) between the radar and the PSG system is performed. The synchronization is also integrated into the GUI, guiding the personnel with a pop-up window (see Figure 2). After successful synchronization, the user account on the radar measurement tablet is locked for the night. The optocoupler is disconnected from the PSG system for the duration of the recording. The personnel then attach the PSG sensors to the patient. From then on, the patient can freely move around in the clinic and decide when to go to sleep. When sleeping, the patient is free to choose their sleeping posture. The next morning, the study personnel go to the patient at 7 a.m. First, they remove the PSG sensors. The measurement is then stopped, and the end synchronization is completed. The radar recording is automatically saved to the tablet.

2.7. Radar Range Bin Selection

For single bin selection, the breathing and heartbeat range bins are ranked using temporal phase coherence (TPC) [32]. From the range bins with the five highest TPC values, breathing and heart rates are computed. The final rate for the given epoch is computed from the range bin that has the highest quality breathing or heartbeat signals from the preselected group of five (see details in [33]).

The rationale for multiple over single range bin selection for computing breathing and heart rates is that the summarization of information from multiple spatial sources makes the computation more robust. The method for multiple bin selection is also considerably stricter in its choices, reducing the chance of false positives. Because single bin selection only performs a ranking using TPC, there is a higher chance that incorrect bins get through. This difference in range bin selection was explored in detail in [31].

The methodology for multiple bin selection is based on persistence homology [41,42], exploiting the fact that breathing and heartbeat signals have a specific shape in the radar phase signal. We chose this complex method for range bin selection because of the low specificity of more classical approaches, such as spectrum- or autocorrelation-based range bin selection. Although these classical approaches can often identify valid breathing and heartbeat signals, they are not reliable in rejecting unrelated signals that happen to share spectral characteristics. When developing persistence homology-based bin selection, we empirically derived thresholds for evaluating persistence diagrams computed from radar signals. In this article, we evaluate how well these settings generalize to a larger dataset from a different population in a different setting. For a detailed description of the algorithms, we refer the interested reader to the original publication [31].

2.8. Breathing and Heart Rate Computation

Breathing rates were computed using an autocorrelation-based method, while heart rates were computed based on peak detection. The reference rates were computed from the PSG sensors using the same approaches. We have described the details of these algorithms in [33]. The algorithms were implemented in the Python programming language (version 3.12.2) [43]. The computations were executed offline using a computing server with two Intel (Santa Clara, CA, USA) Xeon Gold 6240 CPUs and 768 GB of RAM.

https://doi.org/10.3390/s26010251

2.9. Adaptations in the Algorithms

Compared to the original implementation [31], we adapted two areas. First, we adjusted the expected breathing rate and heart rate intervals, meaning the minimal and maximal rates that the algorithm considers. This change was based on our observation that the reference sensors showed breathing and heart rates exceeding the boundaries we used previously. We changed the breathing rate boundaries from 10–22 breaths per minute (BPM) to 6–30 BPM, which covers the expected breathing rates in a more elderly population [44]. The heart rate boundaries were originally 40–120 beats per minute (BPM); here, we used 40–150 BPM. This new interval covers normal heart rate ranges [45] and also accounts for sudden increases in heart rate.

Second, we targeted the slow running time of the multiple bin selection algorithm that we have described in [31]. We implemented CPU parallelization at multiple stages of the algorithm using the *joblib* Python library (version 1.4.0). For timing the algorithms, we used the *perf_counter* function of the Python *time* module.

2.10. Description of the Dataset

The 49 sleep recordings comprise a total duration of 611 h and 26 s. The goal of this study was to compute breathing and heart rates during sleep. Due to the study protocol (see Section 2.6), the recordings include long intervals during which the patients were not asleep. To focus the analysis on intervals when patients were most likely to be asleep, we restricted the recordings to the time window between 10 p.m and 6 a.m. This reduced the total duration of the recordings to 394 h, 2 min, and 35 s.

Furthermore, we excluded intervals with high levels of motion using the motion parameter described in Section 2.1. Periods in which the level of movement exceeds the overnight average are indicative of wakefulness [46]. To identify such intervals, we computed the motion parameter in 60 s epochs with a 55 s overlap. Next, we applied a moving-average filter with a window length of 5 min and then calculated the average motion level over the entire recording, removing all segments exceeding this threshold. After excluding high-motion intervals, the total duration of the 49 recordings was further reduced to 244 h, 15 min, and 25 s.

Breathing and heart rates were computed after segmenting the recordings into epochs. Each patient's recording was split into 60 s epochs, with a 55 s overlap, providing fine temporal resolution of the breathing and heart rate variations throughout the night. Both single bin selection and multiple bin selection methods were applied using this epoching scheme. This represents a change from our previous publication [31], where single bin selection used a 40 s overlap, consistent with the original publication [33]. Using the same 55 s overlap for both methods facilitates a more interpretable comparison.

2.11. Evaluation Metrics

To evaluate the performance of the breathing and heart rate computations, we used the following metrics: mean absolute error (MAE)

$$\text{MAE} = \frac{1}{N}\sum_{n=1}^{N} |f_{PSG}(n) - f_{Radar}(n)|, \tag{1}$$

and mean absolute percent error (MAPE)

$$\text{MAPE} = 100 \cdot \frac{1}{N}\sum_{n=1}^{N} \frac{|f_{PSG}(n) - f_{Radar}(n)|}{f_{PSG}(n)}, \tag{2}$$

https://doi.org/10.3390/s26010251

where N is the total number of epochs, while $f_{Radar}(n)$ and $f_{PSG}(n)$ correspond to the breathing or heart rates of the radar and PSG of the nth epoch, respectively.

In addition to the error metrics, we also computed Spearman's correlation coefficient to express how closely the radar breathing and heart rates follow the reference rates. Spearman's rank correlation is defined as

$$\rho_s = \frac{cov(R(x), R(y))}{\sigma(R(x)) \cdot \sigma(R(y))}, \tag{3}$$

where $R(x)$ is the rank of the variable, $cov(R(x), R(y))$ is the covariance of the rank, and $\sigma(R(x))$ is the standard deviation of the rank.

We also report the ratio and count of epochs where the algorithms successfully computed the breathing and heart rates (hereafter referred to as recall). In addition, we calculated the duration for which no rate was computed. This is important to add to the previously mentioned metric because, given the overlap between epochs, it is not trivial to determine what the actual coverage of computed rates on the recordings is. The final metric is the ratio of epochs in which the radar breathing or heart rate error (difference to the PSG sensor) is lower than ± 1 BPM. This ratio is reported in relation to the epochs in which both reference and radar rates were successfully computed.

3. Results

We computed the breathing and heart rate results from the recordings of 49 patients, totaling 244 h, 15 min, and 25 s. In total, there were 175,425 epochs. We measured the running time of the algorithms with CPU parallelization, including epoching and computation. We excluded the time for loading the recording, as that varied depending on the server load. The average running time per patient for the breathing rate multiple bin selection algorithms was 1 h, 3 min, and 7 s. The heartbeat multiple bin selection took an average of 25 min and 43.9 s to compute. With single bin selection, the average running time per patient for the breathing rate calculation was 12 min and 59.2 s, while for the heart rate calculation, it was 28 min and 13 s.

3.1. Distribution of Selected Range Bins

Figure 3 shows the distribution of the selected range bins for breathing (top) and heartbeat (bottom) using single (left) and multiple (right) bin selection. These plots highlight the different spatial segments in which the algorithms identify the breathing and heartbeat signals.

The selected range bins vary between patients, but there is a distinct distribution for breathing and heartbeat. The breathing distribution starts farther away from the radar compared to that of the heartbeat. Furthermore, the peak of the breathing range bins' distribution is wider.

The single and multiple bin selection distributions have a similar shape, both for breathing and heartbeat. There are only slight differences, such as the breathing multiple selection distribution having a wider peak and the heartbeat multiple selection distribution having a more prominent peak than the single selection. The overall counts are higher for the multiple selection distributions, as it can select more than one range bin for each epoch.

https://doi.org/10.3390/s26010251

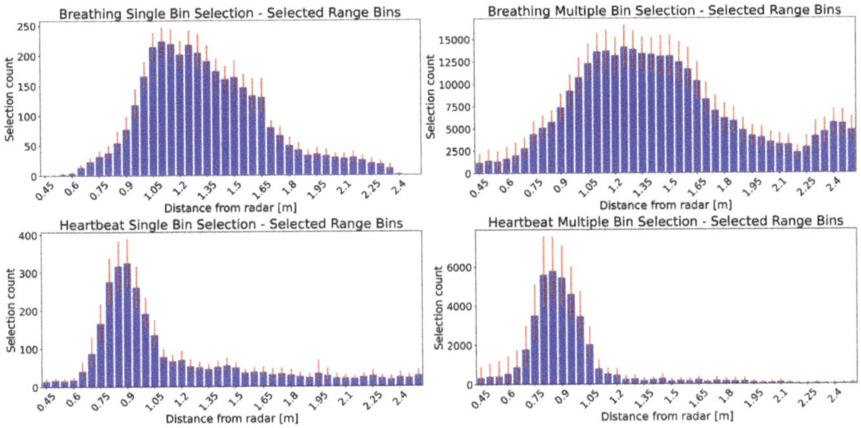

Figure 3. Distribution of selected range bins from the results of 49 patients. The horizontal axis corresponds to the range bins, starting on the left with those closer to the radar. The vertical axis shows how many times a range bin was selected. The blue bars show the mean selection count for each range bin over all 49 patients. The red error bars show the 95% confidence interval. Panels in the **upper** row show breathing selections, while those in the **lower** row show the heartbeat range bin selections. The distribution of range bins selected with single bin selection are in the **left** panels, while those selected with multiple bin selection are in the **right** panels.

3.2. Breathing Rate

Table 2 shows the comparison of the breathing rate computation results for single and multiple bin selection. With single bin selection, the recall for the radar breathing rate was 93.49%, while with multiple bin selection, it was 73.38%. In terms of errors, multiple bin selection outperformed single bin selection, with MAE and MAPE values 2.2 and 2.3 times lower, respectively. Furthermore, in the epochs in which rates were calculated for both reference and radar, 8.36% more of those epochs had lower than $\pm$ 1 BPM errors. Multiple bin selection had a higher correlation with the reference values than single bin selection (0.95 vs 0.85). Figure 4 presents the per-patient results using box plots, with each patient's result individually represented by gray circles. The values of the box plots are presented in tabular format in the supplementary materials (see Supplementary Tables S1–S4).

Table 2. Breathing rate results, computed from 49 overnight recordings. Comparison between single and multiple radar range bin selection.

	Single Range Bin Selection [33]	Multiple Range Bin Selection [31]
PSG recall [% (count)]	93.71 (164,393)	
Radar recall [% (count)]	93.49 (163,999)	73.38 (128,728)
Duration where no PSG rate was computed [hh:mm:ss]	00:28:25	
Duration where no radar rate was computed [hh:mm:ss]	02:19:30	35:35:35
Epochs with <±1 BPM error (for epochs with PSG and radar rate computed) [% (count)]	84.90 (132,680)	93.26 (116,508)
Mean absolute error [1/min]	0.87	0.39
Mean absolute percent error [%]	5.71	2.48
Spearman's correlation coefficient	0.85	0.95

BPM: breaths per minute.

https://doi.org/10.3390/s26010251

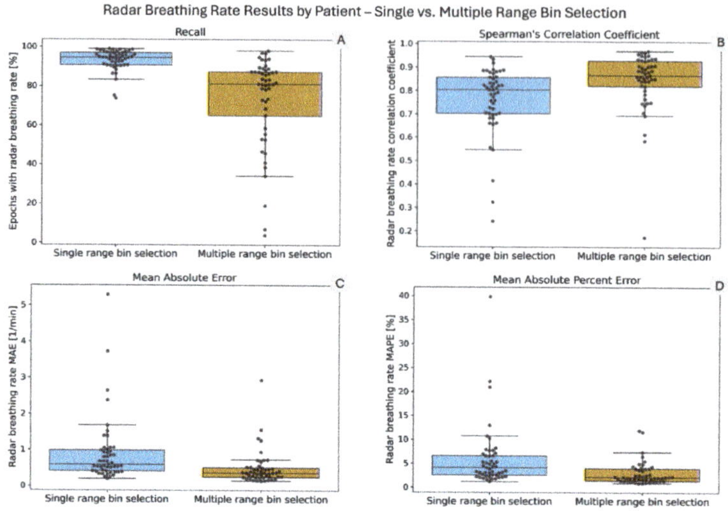

Figure 4. Box plots showing the distribution of per-patient radar breathing rate performance metrics. The overlaid points each correspond to one patient. In each panel, the blue box on the left shows the single range bin selection results, while the orange box on the right shows the multiple range bin selection results. (**A**) shows the radar breathing rate recall. (**B**) presents Spearman's correlation coefficient. (**C**) shows the mean absolute error (MAE), and (**D**) shows the mean absolute percent error (MAPE) of the computed radar breathing rates.

Figure 5 shows Bland–Altman plots of the breathing rate results from single (left panel) and multiple (right panel) bin selection. The mean breathing rate error with single bin selection is −0.20 BPM, while with multiple bin selection it is 0.04 BPM. The 95% confidence interval of the errors is approximately twice as wide with single bin selection ([−4.87, 4.47] vs. [−2.31, 2.39]). For single bin selection, 3.31% of the points are below the lower limit of the confidence interval, and 1.67% are above the upper limit. For multiple bin selection, these values are 1.49% and 1.54%. The distributions of the plots show no appreciable differences. Both are symmetric and do not show any obvious trends.

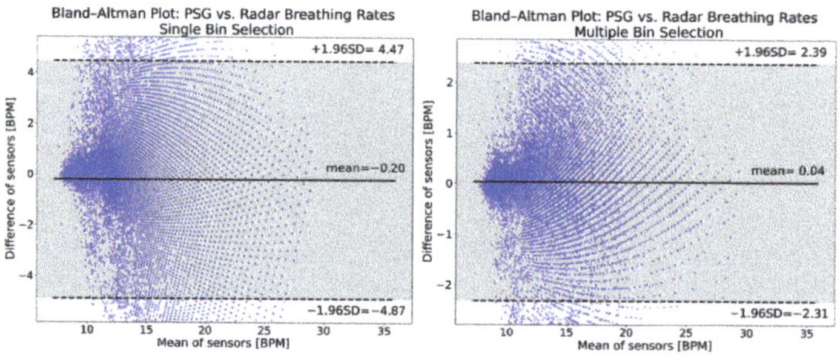

Figure 5. Breathing rate Bland–Altman plots for single (**left panel**) and multiple bin selection (**right panel**). The plots were made from the data of all 49 patients, after cutting the recordings and removing high motion intervals. The horizontal axis shows the mean of the reference and radar breathing rates. On the vertical axis, the difference between the computed breathing rates is shown. Both are expressed in breaths per minute (BPM). The solid horizontal line in the middle is the mean of differences, while the two dashed lines show the upper and lower limits of the 95% confidence interval. All of the values indicated are in BPM. The 95% confidence interval is also indicated with the gray shading.

https://doi.org/10.3390/s26010251

The overnight breathing rates for the same example patient are shown in Figures 6 and 7, calculated using single and multiple bin selection, respectively. In both figures, the upper panel shows the breathing rates computed from the reference and radar. The middle panel shows the error of the radar breathing rates. The lower panel shows the range profile; that is, the range bins that were selected for the computation of the breathing rate. The gray shading in all panels shows the segments that were disregarded because of high levels of motion.

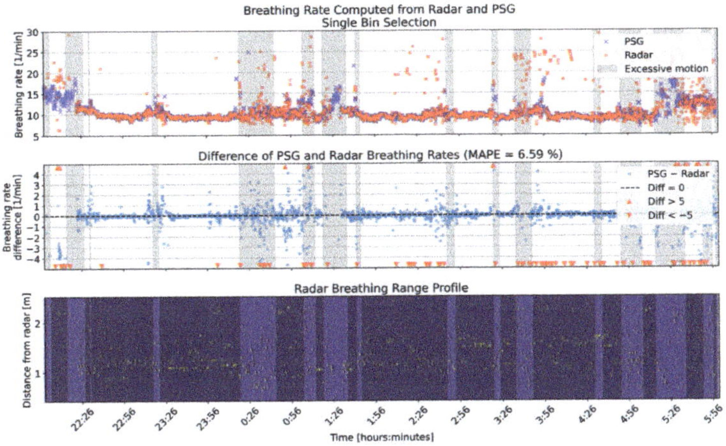

Figure 6. One example full night comparison of breathing rates computed from the PSG sensor and radar single bin selection. The **upper** panel shows the breathing rates in breaths per minute (BPM) for the two sensors. In the **middle** panel, the differences between the rates are shown in BPM. The **lower** panel shows the range profile, that is, the range bins that were selected for breathing rate computation (marked with yellow). Gray shading in each panel shows the segments that had high levels of motion based on the radar motion parameter.

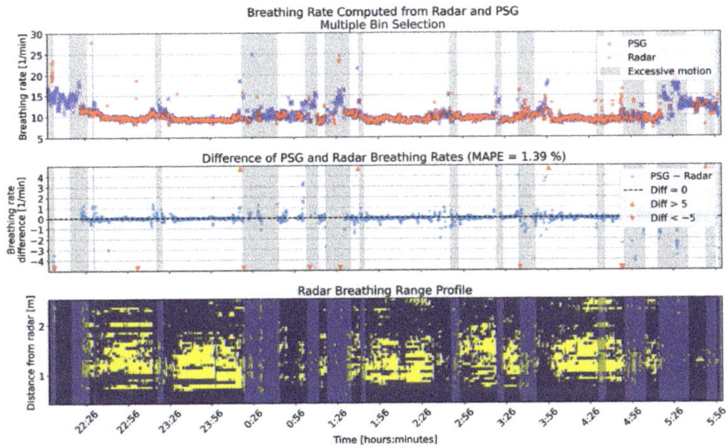

Figure 7. One example full night comparison of breathing rates computed from the PSG sensor and radar multiple bin selection. The **upper** panel shows the breathing rates in breaths per minute (BPM) for the two sensors. In the **middle** panel, the differences between the rates are shown in BPM. The **lower** panel shows the range profile, that is, the range bins that were selected for breathing rate computation (marked with yellow). Gray shading in each panel shows the segments that had high levels of motion based on the radar motion parameter.

https://doi.org/10.3390/s26010251

3.3. Heart Rate

Table 3 shows the result metrics for the heart rate calculation. The heart rate results show the same pattern as the breathing rates, although with larger differences. The recall is 4.1 times higher with single bin selection. However, the MAE and MAPE values are 4.8 and 5.3 times lower with multiple bin selection, respectively. Among the epochs in which both reference and radar heart rates were calculated, the ratio of errors lower than ±1 BPM is 1.6 times higher with multiple selection. Finally, heart rates computed with multiple bin selection have a 1.7 times higher correlation coefficient with the reference rates. Figure 8 presents the per-patient results with box plots, with gray circles representing individual patients. The values of the box plots are presented in tabular format in the supplementary materials (see Supplementary Tables S5–S8).

Table 3. Heart rate results, computed from 49 overnight recordings. Comparison between single and multiple radar range bin selection.

	Single Range Bin Selection [33]	**Multiple Range Bin Selection [31]**
PSG recall [% (count)]	90.77 (159,238)	
Radar recall [% (count)]	81.85 (143,582)	19.93 (34,963)
Duration where no PSG rate was computed [hh:mm:ss]	13:56:05	
Duration where no radar rate was computed [hh:mm:ss]	02:51:50	154:39:40
Epochs with <±1 BPM error (relative to epochs with PSG and radar rate computed) [% (count)]	50.94 (67,291)	80.09 (26,641)
Mean absolute error [1/min]	3.99	0.84
Mean absolute percent error [%]	7.67	1.44
Spearman's correlation coefficient	0.56	0.96

BPM: beats per minute.

The Bland–Altman plots for the heart rates computed with single and multiple bin selection are shown in Figure 9. Multiple bin selection (right panel) has a mean of −0.43 BPM, while single bin selection (left panel) has a mean of −3.05 BPM. The single bin selection 95% confidence interval is more than three times as wide ([−17.83, 11.73] vs. [−4.64, 3.78]). For single bin selection, 7.26% of the points are below the lower limit of the confidence interval, and 0.24% are above the upper limit. For multiple bin selection, these values are 1.68% and 0.40%. Both approaches have an overall negative bias and show a similar trend: with an increasing heart rate, the radar goes from underestimating to overestimating the reference rate. However, the distribution of the plots is noticeably different, especially with single bin selection having more values underestimating the reference rate.

Figures 10 and 11 show an example night of computed heart rates for the same patient, using single and multiple bin selection, respectively. The results shown are from the same patient as the breathing rate results in Figures 6 and 7. The layout of the panels is the same as in those figures. Gray shading shows periods with high levels of motion based on the radar motion parameter. The negative bias pointed out in Figure 9 is visible with more negative difference values present in the middle panel of the two overnight figures.

https://doi.org/10.3390/s26010251

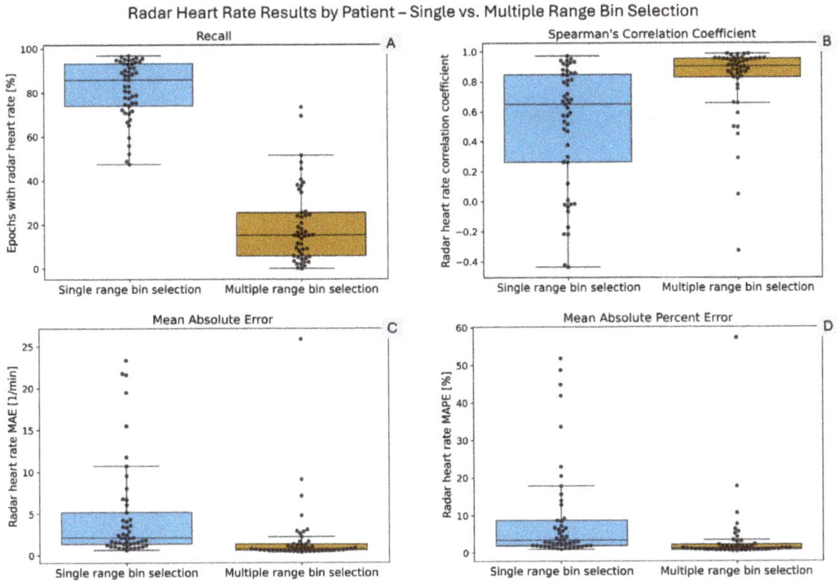

Figure 8. Box plots showing the distribution of per-patient radar heart rate performance metrics. The overlaid points each correspond to one patient. In each panel, the blue box on the left shows the single range bin selection results, while the orange box on the right shows the multiple range bin selection results. (**A**) shows the radar heart rate recall. (**B**) presents Spearman's correlation coefficient. (**C**) shows the mean absolute error (MAE), and (**D**) shows the mean absolute percent error (MAPE) of the computed radar heart rates.

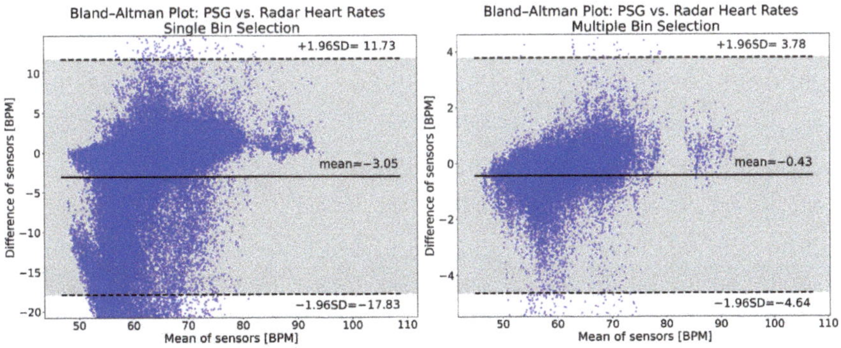

Figure 9. Bland–Altman plots of heart rates computed from the reference PSG and the radar. The **left** panel shows the single bin selection results, while the **right** panel shows the multiple bin selection results. The plots show data from 49 patients, after cutting the recordings and removing high motion intervals. The mean of the reference and radar heart rates is shown on the horizontal axis. The difference between the reference and the radar heart rates is represented by the vertical axis. Both are expressed in beats per minute (BPM). The solid horizontal line in the middle is the mean of differences, while the two dashed lines show the upper and lower limits of the 95% confidence interval. All of the values indicated are in BPM. The 95% confidence interval is indicated also with the gray shading.

https://doi.org/10.3390/s26010251

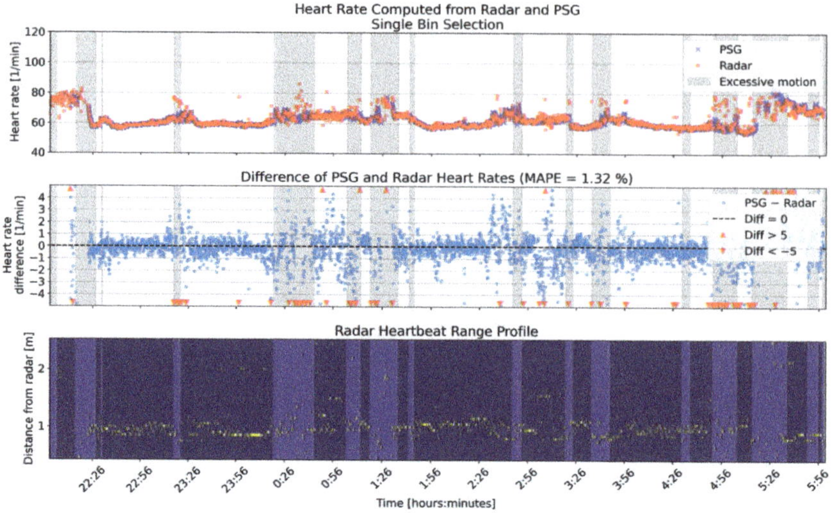

Figure 10. Overnight heart rates computed with single bin selection from one example patient, compared to the reference. The **upper** panel shows the heart rates in beats per minute (BPM) for the two sensors. In the **middle** panel, the differences between the rates are shown in BPM. The **lower** panel shows the range profile, that is, the range bins that were selected for heart rate computation (marked with yellow). Gray shading in each panel shows the segments that had high levels of motion based on the radar motion parameter.

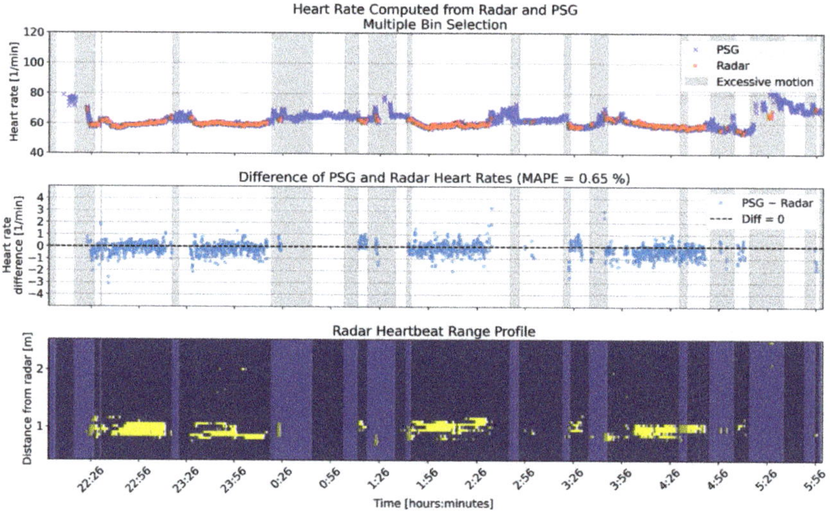

Figure 11. Overnight heart rates computed with multiple bin selection from one example patient, compared to the reference. The **upper** panel shows the heart rates in beats per minute (BPM) for the two sensors. In the **middle** panel, the differences between the rates are shown in BPM. The **lower** panel shows the range profile, that is, the range bins that were selected for heart rate computation (marked with yellow). Gray shading in each panel shows the segments that had high levels of motion based on the radar motion parameter.

https://doi.org/10.3390/s26010251

4. Discussion

In this article, we have evaluated two approaches for radar-based breathing and heart rate calculation in a clinical dataset of acute stroke patients. We have used a single- and multiple range bin selection approach from our previous work, with only minor modifications. Previously, we evaluated these methods only in a small sample of six healthy volunteers who slept in an office environment. This current study included 49 acute stroke patients sleeping in a clinical environment, which provides a better perspective on the robustness of the methods.

4.1. Performance of Algorithms

Multiple bin selection led to lower error values for both breathing and heart rate. The MAE and MAPE for the breathing were 0.39 BPM and 2.48%, while for the heart rate they were 0.84 BPM and 1.44%, respectively. These values are slightly worse than those in the healthy volunteer dataset (breathing rate MAE 0.29 BPM, MAPE 2.24%; heart rate MAE 0.66 BPM, MAPE 1.02%).

The results in the clinical dataset show similar patterns as in healthy volunteers, but with more exaggerated differences between the single- and multiple bin selection approaches. Single bin selection has a higher recall for both the breathing and heart rates, especially the heart rates, where there is a 4.1 times difference. For the breathing rate, this difference is comparatively small, with a factor of 1.3 difference. On the other hand, both the computed breathing and heart rates have substantially lower errors using multiple bin selection. For the breathing rates, the MAE is 2.2 times lower, while for the heart rates, it is 4.8 times lower.

There is a large variation in the results between individual patients, as shown by the box plots in Figures 4 and 8. In particular, the recall values with multiple selection span a wide range, even disregarding extreme outliers. For breathing rates computed with multiple selection, the difference between the 10th and 90th percentiles was 53.35 percentage points (see Supplementary Table S1). For heart rates computed with multiple selection, the same difference was 38.55 percentage points (see Supplementary Table S5). Single bin selection performed more consistently in recall; however, the error and correlation values did show large variations. The Spearman correlation coefficient for heart rates with single bin selection had 10th and 90th percentiles of −0.09 and 0.93, respectively (see Supplementary Table S8).

4.2. Comparison with the Literature

To place our results in context, we searched the literature for related publications. Stroke disrupts the ANS [37,38], which can affect cardiovascular function, making monitoring more challenging. Therefore, our initial aim was to compare our findings with studies involving stroke patients. However, we did not find any studies on radar-based sleep monitoring specifically in stroke populations. Therefore, we expanded our search to recent studies that used radar-based overnight monitoring of breathing or heart rate, regardless of the study population. We identified five relevant works [47–51]. Table 4 summarizes these studies, including the radar type, study population, protocol, and reported breathing and heart rate results. For consistency, we extracted only the metrics that were also reported in our study.

Compared with studies reporting breathing rate results [47,48,50,51], our multiple bin selection approach achieved a lower MAE and MAPE, as well as a higher correlation. However, the limits of agreement (the limits of the 95% confidence interval) in our Bland–Altman analysis were wider than those reported in three of these studies [48,50,51].

 https://doi.org/10.3390/s26010251

Only two of the five studies reported heart rate results [49,51], and both provided only a subset of the metrics we reported. In [49], the authors validated their method using data from 62 healthy individuals. Their reported heart rate accuracy was lower than that achieved with our multiple bin selection but higher than that achieved with our single bin selection. However, the recall was higher than in both of our approaches. The study in [51] included elderly participants, both healthy individuals and patients with neurodegenerative diseases. However, the authors reported only correlation and Bland–Altman limits of agreement. Based on these metrics, our multiple bin selection performed better, whereas our single bin selection performed worse.

Table 4. Comparison of studies presenting radar-based breathing and heart rate monitoring during sleep. For the sake of comparison only the result metrics that were also included in our work are presented. The bottom two rows show our results with single and multiple range bin selection.

Study	Radar Type	Subjects	Study Protocol	Breathing Rate Results	Heart Rate Results
Do et al. 2022 [47]	FMCW 60 GHz (Albus Home™)	N = 32, 8 of them children; both healthy individuals and patients with chronic respiratory condition	Overnight measurements at home, 10 subjects had 2 h evaluated, others only 15 min	MAE = 0.6 BPM	-
Bujan et al. 2023 [48]	Doppler 24 GHz (Sleepiz One+)	N = 139; patients with suspected sleep apnea	Overnight measurements in sleep laboratory	MAE = 0.48 BPM LoA = [−0.88, 1.61]	-
Xu et al. 2023 [49]	FMCW 60 GHz (Google Nest Hub)	N = 122, 62 used for evaluation; healthy individuals	Overnight recordings	-	MAE = 1.69 BPM MAPE = 2.67% Recall = 88.53%
Ravindran et al. 2024 [50]	IR-UWB (Somnofy; VitalThings)	N = 17; elderly individuals, those with stable comorbidities were included	Overnight recordings in sleep laboratory	MAPE = 4.64% LoA = [−2.48, 1.47]	-
Yin et al. 2025 [51]	UWB (XeThru X4; Novelda)	N = 47; elderly participants, both healthy individuals and patients with neurodegenerative diseases	Overnight sleep recording in a research facility	r = 0.88 LoA = [−1.2, 1.2]	r = 0.65 LoA = [−6.7, 4.9]
Our results SRBS	FMCW 60 GHz (Texas Instruments)	N = 49; acute ischemic stroke patients	Overnight sleep recording in post-stroke unit	MAE = 0.87 BPM MAPE = 5.71% LoA = [−4.87, 4.47] r = 0.85 Recall = 93.49%	MAE = 3.99 BPM MAPE = 7.67% LoA = [−17.83, 11.73] r = 0.56 Recall = 81.85%
Our results MRBS	FMCW 60 GHz (Texas Instruments)	N = 49; acute ischemic stroke patients	Overnight sleep recording in post-stroke unit	MAE = 0.39 BPM MAPE = 2.48% LoA = [−2.31, 2.39] r = 0.95 Recall = 73.38%	MAE = 0.84 BPM MAPE = 1.44% LoA = [−4.64, 3.78] r = 0.96 Recall = 19.93%

LoA: Bland–Altman plot limits of agreement, the 95% confidence interval; IR-UWB, UWB: impulse-radio ultra-wideband; r: correlation coefficient; SRBS and MRBS: Single and multiple range bin selection.

4.3. Discussion of Key Findings

The contrast between the recall and error values highlights the fundamentally different characteristics of the two range bin selection methods. Single bin selection is more permissive in computing breathing and heart rates and, therefore, yields a higher proportion of epochs with estimated rates, albeit at the cost of larger errors. Multiple bin selection, in contrast, applies stricter criteria when selecting range bins. As a result, the recall is lower, particularly for the estimation of the heart rate (see [31] for an analysis of range bins rejected by the multiple bin selection method). However, when a rate is calculated, it is highly accurate, as reflected by the low MAE and MAPE values of the radar heart rates.

 https://doi.org/10.3390/s26010251

For 75% of patients, the heart rate MAE is below 1.34 BPM and the MAPE below 2.28% (see Figure 8, panels C and D and Supplementary Tables S6 and S7).

The heart rate computation with single bin selection has a higher recall and 2.5 times more epochs with errors lower than ±1 BPM. However, as panels B, C, and D in Figure 8 and the Bland–Altman plot in Figure 9 demonstrate, there are too many recordings in which the estimate is too unreliable. This demonstrates the inability of range bin selection solely based on ranking to discard signals where no accurate heart rate can be computed. A possible improvement would be to integrate the ranking produced by the TPC [32,33] into the decision step based on persistence homology [31]. This would combine the high recall of TPC with the specificity of persistence homology.

There are two factors independent of the algorithms that contribute to low heart rate recall with multiple bin selection (19.93%). Heartbeats are, in the best case, half the size of breathing motions but can be approximately 17 times smaller (0.287–0.568 mm [35] vs. 1–5 mm [36]). This makes accurate detection difficult even in an optimal setting, such as our study with healthy volunteers in a quiet office room [31,33]. In addition, the ANS of stroke patients is disrupted [37,38]. This can impact cardiovascular functioning in an inhomogeneous way, depending on the exact injury of the patient. The low recall rates, together with these two factors, point to the need for specifically designed heart rate computation algorithms for stroke patients. A general approach that can be fine tuned for individuals would address the inhomogeneity in stroke injuries.

In calculating breathing rates, multiple bin selection had a more comparable recall to single bin selection (73.38% vs. 93.49%); however, as panel A in Figure 4 shows, there was a large variation among patients. Given the more reliable accuracy of multiple selection (see panels B, C, and D of Figure 4) and the additional information provided by the range profile (see Figure 7), it presents a better option for monitoring breathing rates than single bin selection.

The distribution of selected range bins in this clinical dataset shows patterns similar to those observed in the healthy volunteer dataset. The breathing range bins are located farther from the radar than the heartbeat range bins and also span a wider spatial region. This indicates that the tendency of multiple range bin selection to associate breathing with range bins closer to the upper body and heartbeat with bins closer to the lower body is not dataset dependent. The clear spatial separation between the breathing and heartbeat range bins supports the use of lateral radar placement, specifically at the foot end of the bed. By achieving intrinsic separation of the signals, this configuration avoids the need for complex signal separation algorithms that are otherwise required when breathing and heartbeat signals overlap within the same range bin.

The implementation of CPU parallelization reduced the runtime by approximately a factor of five compared to the original implementation [31]. The observed runtime differences between single and multiple range bin selection reflect the differing computational complexity of the underlying algorithms. For multiple bin selection, we used two persistence homology methods: Vietoris–Rips filtration and sublevel set filtration [41]. Vietoris–Rips filtration is computationally intensive, while sublevel set filtration has a complexity comparable to the TPC method [32] used for single bin selection [33]. During breathing rate estimation, multiple range bin selection applies both filtration methods, while for heart rate estimation, only sublevel set filtration is used. This explains why multiple bin selection for breathing rate estimation is approximately five times slower than single bin selection, whereas for heart rate estimation, the runtimes are comparable.

https://doi.org/10.3390/s26010251

4.4. Potential of the Method

Accurate breathing and heart rates, especially when using multiple bin selection, show promise in the use of radar-based sleep monitoring for at-risk patients in clinical wards. The contactless nature of the radar avoids the burden of contact-based sensors on patients and caregivers while still providing useful insights into the patients' states. Although the pipelines introduced here only provide breathing and heart rates and not further evaluations, such as the detection of abnormal respiratory patterns or the classification of sleep stages, this information is already valuable for assessing patients' sleep. Breathing and heart rates outside the expected boundaries can indicate underlying disease. In addition, the overnight evolution of the rates can also provide caregivers with insights into whether there were many sleep interruptions or if the patient could sleep peacefully.

Having a good range bin selection method should also enable the detection of abnormal respiratory patterns, such as sleep apnea and hypopnea [52]. Sleep apnea or hypopnea occurs when a patient's airflow stops or is reduced. Therefore, if we have a good method for detecting breathing, that should be a good starting point to look for cessations in breathing. In particular, central events, where airflow stops or is reduced due to a lack of breathing effort, should be detectable with this approach.

4.5. Limitations

The sample of 49 patients provides a better basis for evaluating the efficacy of our methods than the six healthy volunteers whose data we tested before [31,33]. However, given the specific condition of the patients in this study—acute ischemic stroke patients—it is possible that the results do not reflect the method's performance in the general population, although we assume that the general population would have calmer sleep than this patient population, which should lead to better performance, not worse. Furthermore, the sexes in this study were not balanced (14 female, 35 male); therefore, the results might be less representative for monitoring the sleep of women.

We have cut each recording to focus on a typical sleeping window. In addition, we used a radar derived motion parameter to remove periods with high levels of motion. Although these are sensible steps to clean the dataset before computing breathing and heart rates, a more sophisticated set of algorithms might do a better job of keeping only sleep epochs for each individual. A bed presence detector with a more complex motion parameter should be implemented together with a dedicated sleep staging algorithm for optimal sleep monitoring.

The manual setting of parameters for the range bin selection algorithms is another limitation. A machine learning based approach to classifying range bins based on persistence homology features might provide a more optimal solution. The large hurdle for such an approach is the lack of clear labels for the range bins that the machine learning model could learn.

By setting the lower boundary of the expected breathing rate range to 6 BPM (see Section 2.9), there is a chance of treating apneas as normal breathing cycles. While the algorithms presented in this article are not meant for detecting apneas, it is still important to address this possibility. The breathing rate computation algorithm itself has a check that controls how consistent the breathing cycles are in an epoch (see [33] for details). Therefore, in epochs with apnea events, no breathing rate should be returned. However, if an apnea detection algorithm were to be combined with this breathing rate algorithm, it is an important case to investigate by comparing epochs where breathing is detected against expert apnea annotations.

The last limitation we would like to point out is that the method was not tested on more accessible computing platforms. To efficiently process the 2.5 TB of raw data in our study, we

https://doi.org/10.3390/s26010251

used a powerful computing server, and with CPU parallelization, we were able to achieve manageable running times. The algorithms we used are compatible with widely available modern computers for the intended offline evaluation. Although large file sizes might require users to process recordings in shorter segments instead of the whole night at once.

4.6. Outlook

We will investigate whether a combination of the single- and multiple range bin selection algorithms can improve the heart rate calculation recall in this dataset. Then, our next focus will be on developing a set of algorithms to investigate the potential of radar-based contactless screening of sleep apnea and hypopnea in acute stroke patients in a clinical setting. We will evaluate whether the range bin selection tested here can be successfully integrated into the detection of respiratory events. A simple-to-apply method in neurology clinics would be very beneficial for screening sleep apnea and hypopnea to aid in the better recovery of stroke patients.

5. Conclusions

We have demonstrated the performance of multiple range bin selection for radar-based breathing and heart rate computation in sleeping acute stroke patients. In terms of accuracy, multiple selection outperforms the more commonly used single selection. However, single selection has higher temporal coverage, especially for heart rates. Therefore, single bin selection could be a useful supplement, especially for heart rate computation. These results are a valuable contribution to developments that incorporate radar-based sleep monitoring in clinical wards in the future.

Supplementary Materials: The following supporting information can be downloaded at https://www.mdpi.com/article/10.3390/s26010251/s1, Table S1: Breathing Rate: Recall (%). Distribution of per-patient values.; Table S2: Breathing Rate: Mean Absolute Error (BPM). Distribution of per-patient values.; Table S3: Breathing Rate: Mean Absolute Percentage Error (%). Distribution of per-patient values.; Table S4: Breathing Rate: Spearman's Correlation Coefficient. Distribution of per-patient values.; Table S5: Heart Rate: Recall (%). Distribution of per-patient values.; Table S6: Heart Rate: Mean Absolute Error (BPM). Distribution of per-patient values.; Table S7: Heart Rate: Mean Absolute Percentage Error (%). Distribution of per-patient values.; Table S8: Heart Rate: Spearman's Correlation Coefficient. Distribution of per-patient values.

Author Contributions: Conceptualization, B.S., B.K., K.I.W. and K.W.; methodology, B.S., L.H., J.P.V., T.L., A.R., B.K., K.I.W. and K.W.; software, B.S., L.H. and J.P.V.; validation, B.S., L.H., B.K., K.I.W. and K.W.; formal analysis, B.S.; investigation, B.S.; resources, B.S., L.H., J.P.V., T.L. and K.W.; data curation, B.S. and L.H.; writing—original draft preparation, B.S.; writing—review and editing, B.S., L.H., J.P.V., T.L., A.R., B.K., K.I.W. and K.W.; visualization, B.S.; supervision, B.K., K.I.W. and K.W.; project administration, T.L., A.R., B.K., K.I.W. and K.W.; funding acquisition, T.L., A.R., B.K., K.I.W. and K.W. All authors have read and agreed to the published version of the manuscript.

Funding: This study was supported by an intramural grant (mHealth) from the Carl von Ossietzky Universität Oldenburg and by the Deutsche Forschungsgemeinschaft (DFG, German Research Foundation)–GRK2969–512960146.

Institutional Review Board Statement: The clinical study was conducted in accordance with the Declaration of Helsinki and approved by the medical ethics committee of the Carl von Ossietzky Universität Oldenburg (votum number 2022-016; date of approval: 14 July 2023).

Informed Consent Statement: The details of the study were explained to the patients, both verbally and in writing. Written informed consent was obtained from all patients involved in the study.

 https://doi.org/10.3390/s26010251

Data Availability Statement: The raw data supporting the conclusions of this article will be made available by the authors upon request, in accordance with the consent of the test subjects as per the data protection agreement. To avoid misunderstandings, we would like to point out that the radar system used here is a demonstrator exclusively for research and development purposes (research use only). It is not CE-certified as a medical device, and no performance evaluation has been carried out in accordance with the Medical Device Regulations. Data and analyses are not used in diagnostic or therapeutic decisions. The overnight plots of breathing and heart rate results for both single and multiple range bin selection for each patient are available upon request. The source codes used for computing the results presented in this article can be found in this repository: https://doi.org/10.5281/zenodo.17559602.

Acknowledgments: The authors thank every patient for agreeing to participate in our study. We thank the student assistants who were our measurement personnel. Finally, we thank Finn-Christian Dittkuhn from Fraunhofer IDMT-HSA for helping with the construction of the radar measurement setup.

Conflicts of Interest: The authors declare no conflicts of interest. The funders had no role in the design of the study; in the collection, analyses, or interpretation of data; in the writing of the manuscript; or in the decision to publish the results.

Abbreviations

The following abbreviations are used in this manuscript:

PSG	Polysomnography
FMCW	Frequency modulated continuous wave
ANS	Autonomic nervous system
FFT	Fast Fourier transform
ECG	Electrocardiography
RIP	Respiratory inductance plethysmography
LSL	Lab streaming layer
FoV	Field of view
ADC	Analog to digital converter
PPG	Photoplethysmography
EEG	Electroencephalogram
EOG	Electrooculogram
AIS	Acute ischemic stroke
BMI	Body mass index
GUI	Graphical user interface
TPC	Temporal phase coherence
BPM	Breaths per minute
BPM	Beats per minute
MAE	Mean absolute error
MAPE	Mean absolute percent error
LoA	Limits of agreement
IR-UWB	Impulse-radio ultra-wideband

References

1. Khot, S.P.; Morgenstern, L.B. Sleep and Stroke. *Stroke* **2019**, *50*, 1612–1617. [CrossRef]
2. Hermann, D.M.; Bassetti, C.L. Role of sleep-disordered breathing and sleep-wake disturbances for stroke and stroke recovery. *Neurology* **2016**, *87*, 1407–1416. [CrossRef]
3. Seiler, A.; Camilo, M.; Korostovtseva, L.; Haynes, A.G.; Brill, A.K.; Horvath, T.; Egger, M.; Bassetti, C.L. Prevalence of sleep-disordered breathing after stroke and TIA: A meta-analysis. *Neurology* **2019**, *92*, e648–e654. [CrossRef]

Brown, D.L.; Jiang, X.; Li, C.; Case, E.; Sozener, C.B.; Chervin, R.D.; Lisabeth, L.D. Sleep apnea screening is uncommon after stroke. *Sleep Med.* **2019**, *59*, 90–93. [CrossRef] [PubMed]

Feigin, V.L.; Abate, M.D.; Abate, Y.H.; Abd ElHafeez, S.; Abd-Allah, F.; Abdelalim, A.; Abdelkader, A.; Abdelmasseh, M.; Abd-Elsalam, S.; Abdi, P.; et al. Global, regional, and national burden of stroke and its risk factors, 1990–2021: A systematic analysis for the Global Burden of Disease Study 2021. *Lancet Neurol.* **2024**, *23*, 973–1003. [CrossRef]

Clocchiatti-Tuozzo, S.; Rivier, C.A.; Renedo, D.; Huo, S.; Hawkes, M.A.; de Havenon, A.; Schwamm, L.H.; Sheth, K.N.; Gill, T.M.; Falcone, G.J. Life's Essential 8 and Poor Brain Health Outcomes in Middle-Aged Adults. *Neurology* **2024**, *103*, e209990. [CrossRef] [PubMed]

Mayer-Suess, L.; Ibrahim, A.; Moelgg, K.; Cesari, M.; Knoflach, M.; Högl, B.; Stefani, A.; Kiechl, S.; Heidbreder, A. Sleep disorders as both risk factors for, and a consequence of, stroke: A narrative review. *Int. J. Stroke* **2024**, *19*, 490–498. [CrossRef]

Wallace, D.M.; Ramos, A.R.; Rundek, T. Sleep disorders and stroke. *Int. J. Stroke* **2012**, *7*, 231–242. [CrossRef] [PubMed]

Wu, M.P.; Lin, H.J.; Weng, S.F.; Ho, C.H.; Wang, J.J.; Hsu, Y.W. Insomnia subtypes and the subsequent risks of stroke: Report from a nationally representative cohort. *Stroke* **2014**, *45*, 1349–1354. [CrossRef]

10. Huang, R.J.; Lai, C.H.; Lee, S.D.; Pai, F.Y.; Chang, S.W.; Chung, A.H.; Chang, Y.F.; Ting, H. Objective sleep measures in inpatients with subacute stroke associated with levels and improvements in activities of daily living. *Arch. Phys. Med. Rehabil.* **2018**, *99*, 699–706. [CrossRef]
11. Baillieul, S.; Dekkers, M.; Brill, A.K.; Schmidt, M.H.; Detante, O.; Pépin, J.L.; Tamisier, R.; Bassetti, C.L.A. Sleep apnoea and ischaemic stroke: Current knowledge and future directions. *Lancet Neurol.* **2022**, *21*, 78–88. [CrossRef]
12. Yaggi, H.K.; Concato, J.; Kernan, W.N.; Lichtman, J.H.; Brass, L.M.; Mohsenin, V. Obstructive sleep apnea as a risk factor for stroke and death. *N. Engl. J. Med.* **2005**, *353*, 2034–2041. [CrossRef]
13. Johnson, K.G.; Johnson, D.C. Frequency of sleep apnea in stroke and TIA patients: A meta-analysis. *J. Clin. Sleep Med.* **2010**, *6*, 131–137. [CrossRef]
14. Kernan, W.N.; Ovbiagele, B.; Black, H.R.; Bravata, D.M.; Chimowitz, M.I.; Ezekowitz, M.D.; Fang, M.C.; Fisher, M.; Furie, K.L.; Heck, D.V.; et al. Guidelines for the prevention of stroke in patients with stroke and transient ischemic attack: A guideline for healthcare professionals from the American Heart Association/American Stroke Association. *Stroke* **2014**, *45*, 2160–2236. [CrossRef]
15. Rundo, J.V.; Downey, R. III Polysomnography. In *Handbook of Clinical Neurology*; Elsevier: Amsterdam, The Netherlands, 2019; Volume 160, pp. 381–392. [CrossRef]
16. Markun, L.C.; Sampat, A. Clinician-focused overview and developments in polysomnography. *Curr. Sleep Med. Rep.* **2020**, *6*, 309–321. [CrossRef] [PubMed]
17. Flemons, W.W.; Douglas, N.J.; Kuna, S.T.; Rodenstein, D.O.; Wheatley, J. Access to diagnosis and treatment of patients with suspected sleep apnea. *Am. J. Respir. Crit Care Med.* **2004**, *169*, 668–672. [CrossRef]
18. Aalaei, S.; Amini, M.; Taghipour, A.; Afsharisaleh, L.; Rezaeitalab, F.; Asadpour, H.; Eslami, S. Adherence to prescribed overnight sleep study in patients suspected of sleep apnea: Problem size and influential factors. *Sleep Breath* **2021**, *25*, 1359–1368. [CrossRef] [PubMed]
19. Le Bon, O.; Staner, L.; Hoffmann, G.; Dramaix, M.; San Sebastian, I.; Murphy, J.R.; Kentos, M.; Pelc, I.; Linkowski, P. The first-night effect may last more than one night. *J. Psychiatr. Res.* **2001**, *35*, 165–172. [CrossRef] [PubMed]
20. Ding, L.; Chen, B.; Dai, Y.; Li, Y. A meta-analysis of the first-night effect in healthy individuals for the full age spectrum. *Sleep Med.* **2022**, *89*, 159–165. [CrossRef]
21. Yoon, H.; Choi, S.H. Technologies for sleep monitoring at home: Wearables and nearables. *Biomed. Eng. Lett.* **2023**, *13*, 313–327. [CrossRef]
22. Boiko, A.; Martínez Madrid, N.; Seepold, R. Contactless technologies, sensors, and systems for cardiac and respiratory measurement during sleep: A systematic review. *Sensors* **2023**, *23*, 5038. [CrossRef]
23. van Meulen, F.B.; Grassi, A.; Van den Heuvel, L.; Overeem, S.; van Gilst, M.M.; van Dijk, J.P.; Maass, H.; Van Gastel, M.J.; Fonseca, P. Contactless camera-based sleep staging: The healthbed study. *Bioeng* **2023**, *10*, 109. [CrossRef]
24. Dafna, E.; Tarasiuk, A.; Zigel, Y. Sleep staging using nocturnal sound analysis. *Sci. Rep.* **2018**, *8*, 13474. [CrossRef]
25. Turppa, E.; Kortelainen, J.M.; Antropov, O.; Kiuru, T. Vital sign monitoring using FMCW radar in various sleeping scenarios. *Sensors* **2020**, *20*, 6505. [CrossRef]
26. Boric-Lubecke, O.; Lubecke, V.M.; Droitcour, A.D.; Park, B.K.; Singh, A. *Doppler Radar Physiological Sensing*; John Wiley & Sons: Hoboken, NJ, USA, 2015. [CrossRef]
27. Liebetruth, M.; Kehe, K.; Steinritz, D.; Sammito, S. Systematic Literature Review Regarding Heart Rate and Respiratory Rate Measurement by Means of Radar Technology. *Sensors* **2024**, *24*, 1003. [CrossRef]
28. Paterniani, G.; Sgreccia, D.; Davoli, A.; Guerzoni, G.; Di Viesti, P.; Valenti, A.C.; Vitolo, M.; Vitetta, G.M.; Boriani, G. Radar-Based Monitoring of Vital Signs: A Tutorial Overview. *Proc. IEEE* **2023**, *111*, 277–317. [CrossRef]

https://doi.org/10.3390/s26010251

29. Choi, S.H.; Yoon, H. Convolutional Neural Networks for the Real-Time Monitoring of Vital Signs Based on Impulse Radi Ultrawide-Band Radar during Sleep. *Sensors* **2023**, *23*, 3116. [CrossRef]
30. Wang, Y.; Wang, W.; Zhou, M.; Ren, A.; Tian, Z. Remote monitoring of human vital signs based on 77-GHz mm-wave FMCW radar. *Sensors* **2020**, *20*, 2999. [CrossRef]
31. Szmola, B.; Hornig, L.; Wolf, K.I.; Radeloff, A.; Witt, K.; Kollmeier, B. Feasibility of Radar Vital Sign Monitoring Using Multipl Range Bin Selection. *Sensors* **2025**, *25*, 2596. [CrossRef] [PubMed]
32. Choi, H.I.; Song, W.J.; Song, H.; Shin, H.C. Improved Heartbeat Detection by Exploiting Temporal Phase Coherency in FMCW Radar. *IEEE Access* **2021**, *9*, 163654–163664. [CrossRef]
33. Hornig, L.; Szmola, B.; Pätzold, W.; Vox, J.P.; Wolf, K.I. Evaluation of Lateral Radar Positioning for Vital Sign Monitoring: A Empirical Study. *Sensors* **2024**, *24*, 3548. [CrossRef]
34. Hornig, L.; Appell, J. System und Verfahren zur Kontaktlosen Vitalparametererfassung Durch Erstellung eines Körpermodell Basierend auf der Körperunterteilung Entlang des Radar-Sichtfeldes. Patent DE102022208945B4, 31 July 2025.
35. Ramachandran, G.; Singh, M. Three-dimensional reconstruction of cardiac displacement patterns on the chest wall during the QRS and T-segments of the ECG by laser speckle inteferometry. *Med. Biol. Eng. Comput.* **1989**, *27*, 525–530. [CrossRef]
36. De Groote, A.; Wantier, M.; Chéron, G.; Estenne, M.; Paiva, M. Chest wall motion during tidal breathing. *J. Appl. Physiol.* **199** *83*, 1531–1537. [CrossRef]
37. Korpelainen, J.T.; Sotaniemi, K.A.; Myllylä, V.V. Autonomic nervous system disorders in stroke. *Clin. Auton. Res.* **1999**, *9*, 325–33 [CrossRef] [PubMed]
38. Mo, J.; Huang, L.; Peng, J.; Ocak, U.; Zhang, J.; Zhang, J.H. Autonomic disturbances in acute cerebrovascular disease. *Neurosc Bull* **2019**, *35*, 133–144. [CrossRef] [PubMed]
39. Kothe, C.; Shirazi, S.Y.; Stenner, T.; Medine, D.; Boulay, C.; Grivich, M.I.; Artoni, F.; Mullen, T.; Delorme, A.; Makeig, S. The la streaming layer for synchronized multimodal recording. *Imaging. Neurosci.* **2025**, *3*, 136. [CrossRef]
40. Rao, S. Introduction to mmWave sensing: FMCW radars. In *Texas Instruments (TI) mmWave Training Series*; Texas Instruments Inc Dallas, TX, USA, 2017; pp. 1–11.
41. Ravishanker, N.; Chen, R. An introduction to persistent homology for time series. *WIRES Comput. Stat.* **2021**, *13*, e1548. [CrossRef
42. Chung, Y.M.; Hu, C.S.; Lo, Y.L.; Wu, H.T. A persistent homology approach to heart rate variability analysis with an application t sleep-wake classification. *Front. Physiol.* **2021**, *12*, 637684. [CrossRef] [PubMed]
43. Van Rossum, G.; Drake, F.L. *Python 3 Reference Manual*; CreateSpace: Scotts Valley, CA, USA, 2009.
44. Rodríguez-Molinero, A.; Narvaiza, L.; Ruiz, J.; Gálvez-Barrón, C. Normal respiratory rate and peripheral blood oxygen saturatio in the elderly population. *J. Am. Geriatr. Soc.* **2013**, *61*, 2238–2240. [CrossRef]
45. Mason, J.W.; Ramseth, D.J.; Chanter, D.O.; Moon, T.E.; Goodman, D.B.; Mendzelevski, B. Electrocardiographic reference range derived from 79,743 ambulatory subjects. *J. Electrocardiol.* **2007**, *40*, 228–234. [CrossRef]
46. Yoo, Y.K.; Jung, C.W.; Shin, H.C. Unsupervised Detection of Multiple Sleep Stages Using a Single FMCW Radar. *Appl. Sci.* **2023** *13*, 4468. [CrossRef]
47. Do, W.; Russell, R.; Wheeler, C.; Lockwood, M.; De Vos, M.; Pavord, I.; Bafadhel, M. Performance of Contactless Respiratory Rat Monitoring by Albus HomeTM, an Automated System for Nocturnal Monitoring at Home: A Validation Study. *Sensors* **2022**, *22* 7142. [CrossRef]
48. Bujan, B.; Fischer, T.; Dietz-Terjung, S.; Bauerfeind, A.; Jedrysiak, P.; Große Sundrup, M.; Hamann, J.; Schöbel, C. Clinica validation of a contactless respiration rate monitor. *Sci. Rep.* **2023**, *13*, 3480. [CrossRef]
49. Xu, L.; Lien, J.; Li, H.; Gillian, N.; Nongpiur, R.; Li, J.; Zhang, Q.; Cui, J.; Jorgensen, D.; Bernstein, A.; et al. Soli-enabled noncontac heart rate detection for sleep and meditation tracking. *Sci. Rep.* **2023**, *13*, 18008. [CrossRef]
50. G Ravindran, K.K.; della Monica, C.; Atzori, G.; Lambert, D.; Hassanin, H.; Revell, V.; Dijk, D.J. Reliable Contactless Monitoring of Heart Rate, Breathing Rate, and Breathing Disturbance During Sleep in Aging: Digital Health Technology Evaluation Study *JMIR mHealth uHealth* **2024**, *12*, e53643. [CrossRef] [PubMed]
51. Yin, M.; Hadjipanayi, C.; Ravindran, K.K.G.; Bannon, A.; Rapeaux, A.; Monica, C.d.; Lande, T.S.; Dijk, D.J.; Constandinou, T Unobtrusive Sleep Health Assessment Using Impulse Radar: A Pilot Study in Older People. *IEEE Trans. Biomed Eng.* **2025** *72*, 2663–2674. [CrossRef] [PubMed]
52. Strollo, P.J., Jr.; Rogers, R.M. Obstructive sleep apnea. *N. Engl. J. Med.* **1996**, *334*, 99–104. [CrossRef] [PubMed]

https://doi.org/10.3390/s26010251

sensors

MDPI

rticle

ʼhe Effect of Deep Sedation with High Flow Nasal Oxygen ʼherapy on the Transcutaneous CO_2 and Mitochondrial ʼxygenation: A Single-Center Observational Study

nnika M. van Smaalen [1,*], Calvin J. de Wijs [1], Sanne E. Hoeks [2], Egbert G. Mik [1] and Floor A. Harms [1]

[1] Laboratory of Experimental Anesthesiology, Department of Anesthesiology, Erasmus MC University Medical Center Rotterdam, 3015 GD Rotterdam, The Netherlands
[2] Department of Anesthesia, Erasmus MC University Medical Center Rotterdam, 3015 GD Rotterdam, The Netherlands
* Correspondence: a.vansmaalen@erasmusmc.nl

Abstract: Deep Sedation (DS) allows for shorter recovery times, reduced complication rates and increased cost-effectiveness compared to general anesthesia. In prolonged DS, High Flow Nasal Oxygen Therapy (HFNOT) ensures adequate oxygenation. Concerns remain regarding potential masking of inadequate ventilation and induction of hyperoxia. In this single-center observational study, we continuously monitored $tcPCO_2$ and $mitoPO_2$ in 30 patients using the SenTec Monitoring System and Cellular Oxygen METabolism (COMET®, Photonics Healthcare, Utrecht, The Netherlands) device to observe the effect of prolonged DS with HFNOT on periprocedural ventilation and oxygenation. Measurements were taken at baseline and 30, 60, 90 and 120 min after starting DS. $tcPCO_2$ significantly increased after 30 (55.5 (34.5–61.9) mmHg, $p < 0.001$), 60 (54.8 (52.5–62.2) mmHg, $p < 0.001$), 90 (56.5 (53.1–69.3), $p < 0.001$) and 120 (55.8 (50.7–56.6) mmHg, $p = 0.02$) minutes of DS compared to baseline (37.3 (34.5–45.5) mmHg), surpassing the normal range (35–45 mmHg). $mitoPO_2$ increased non-significantly from baseline (69.6 (43.9–76.7) mmHg) compared to 30 (80.5 (65.7–98.9) mmHg, $p = 0.19$), 60 (78.6 (70.3–85.8) mmHg, $p = 0.19$), 90 (74.4 (52.7–86.3) mmHg, $p = 0.38$) and 120 (85.6 (82.5–98.0) mmHg, $p = 0.38$) minutes. We observed increased $tcPCO_2$ and a non-significant rise in $mitoPO_2$ over time, without adverse effects. These findings highlight the potential of continuous sensor-based monitoring to improve real-time detection of ventilation and oxygenation.

Keywords: deep sedation; transcutaneous CO_2; mitochondrial oxygenation; non-invasive monitoring; wearable sensors

1. Introduction

Procedural sedation induces a state of reduced consciousness, providing pain control and minimizing recollection [1]. The American Society of Anesthesiologists categorizes sedation into four levels based depth [2]. In moderate sedation, patients respond to verbal or tactile stimuli, whilst in deep sedation, responsiveness is limited to repeated or painful stimuli (Ramsay Score of 5–6). Deep Sedation (DS) involves greater ventilation suppression than moderate sedation [3]. Unlike general anesthesia, DS does not require intubation, with manual techniques like a jaw thrust or Mayo tube usually sufficing [2]. Sedation strategies depend on procedure duration and patient preferences. Dutch guidelines recommend propofol over midazolam for longer procedures requiring moderate to deep sedation [4]. DS offers several advantages over general anesthesia in minimally invasive procedures, including reduced recovery times, improved hemodynamic stability and minimized risk of nasopharyngeal damage [5]. Moreover, DS may have a lower carbon footprint and a reduced climate change score when compared to general anesthesia [6]. In the Netherlands, nurse anesthetists can become sedation practitioners after completing a one-year program, enabling them to independently perform DS under the supervision of an anesthesiologist, thereby improving cost-efficiency [4].

High Flow Nasal Oxygen Therapy (HFNOT) delivers heated and humidified air via a nasal canula at flow up to 70 L/min, with inspiratory oxygen fraction (FiO_2) up to 1.0, therefore minimizing hypoxic events during DS [7,8]. While it enhances patient comfort and improves alveolar ventilation [9], high FiO_2 could potentially induce hyperoxic vasoconstriction, reducing microvascular perfusion despite supranormal arterial oxygen levels. Hyperoxia has also been associated with increased oxidative stress and impairment of endothelial function [10,11]. However, its effects at the tissue level remain largely unknown, as current monitoring systems measure oxygenation in different physiological compartments, such as arterial or venous blood, rather than directly at the microcirculatory or cellular level.

A recently developed parameter to assess tissue oxygenation is the mitochondrial oxygen tension ($mitoPO_2$), measured non-invasively and in real-time using the Cellular Oxygen METabolism (COMET®) device. Mitochondria are the end user of oxygen, and $mitoPO_2$ therefore represents the balance between oxygen delivery and consumption at cellular level, offering direct insight into oxygen availability for ATP synthesis [12,13]. Conventional systemic parameters such as SpO_2 and PaO_2 remain essential, but they provide limited information about microcirculatory perfusion or cellular oxygen utilization. SpO_2 rapidly reaches a plateau at high FiO_2 levels, making it insensitive to further increases or decreases in tissue oxygenation. As high FiO_2 is administered continuously during DS, evaluating mitochondrial oxygenation could potentially help detect whether hyperoxygenation adversely affects tissue oxygen delivery or microcirculatory dynamics. Moreover, PaO_2 does not account for local changes in perfusion, metabolic demand, or oxygen extraction, whereas $mitoPO_2$ can detect such discrepancies because it reflects cellular oxygenation, and can reveal tissue hypoxia or impaired oxygen utilization even when blood oxygen levels appear normal [14,15]. Increases in $mitoPO_2$ can result from increased oxygen delivery (e.g., increased perfusion or partial pressure of arterial oxygen (PaO_2)) or reduced consumption (e.g., due to low metabolic demand or mitochondrial dysfunction). Because of this dual dependency, $mitoPO_2$ interpretation is context-dependent and ideally supported by simultaneous measurements of mitochondrial oxygen consumption ($mitoVO_2$) [16].

While HFNOT optimizes oxygenation during DS, high FiO_2 may mask hypoventilation, increasing the risks of hypercapnia. Capnography has been shown to reduce the incidence of hypoxic events during DS by enabling early detection of hypoventilation [17]. End-tidal CO_2 ($etCO_2$) monitoring, which relies on exhaled air, is less accurate in DS due to dilution by ambient air. Transcutaneous CO_2 ($tcPCO_2$) monitoring via the SenTec Monitoring System overcomes this by measuring CO_2 directly through the skin and therefore offering potential novel insights into the CO_2 dynamics during DS. Moreover, this method has been validated as a reliable reflection of $PaCO_2$ during DS by several studies [18–21].

The primary objective of this study was to assess the effect of DS with HFNOT on ventilation and tissue oxygenation, as measured by $tcPCO_2$ and $mitoPO_2$. The secondary objectives encompassed the effect of time on $tcPCO_2$ and $mitoPO_2$, length of hospital stay, and adverse events, as well as the effect of DS with HFNOT on the $mitoVO_2$. Lastly, this study explores the feasibility and potential clinical value of combining these technologies during prolonged DS.

2. Materials and Methods

In this single-center observational trial at the Erasmus Medical Center (Erasmus MC) Rotterdam, The Netherlands, we continuously and intraoperatively monitored $tcPCO_2$ and $mitoPO_2$ in patients undergoing DS with HFNOT (Fisher & Paykel Healthcare, Auckland, New Zealand). To be eligible for participation, patients had to be at least 18 years of age, scheduled for a procedure of at least 90 min requiring DS with HFNOT and have sufficient proficiency of the Dutch language. The exclusion criteria included a diagnosis of porphyria, known intolerance to components of the ALA-plaster, mitochondrial disease, pregnancy or lactation, skin lesions at the measurement location that could impede measurements and inability to provide informed consent.

A measurement was considered successful if the duration of DS with HFNOT and the monitoring period for $tcPCO_2$ and $mitoPO_2$ each exceeded 30 min. The stipulated minimum duration of 30 min was chosen to align with the statistical analysis plan, aiming to facilitate a comparison between baseline and those taken 30 min thereafter. Additionally, intraoperative monitoring data had to be available. Unsuccessful measurements were excluded from the analysis.

In December 2022, approval was granted by the Medical Ethics Committee of the Erasmus MC, Rotterdam, The Netherlands (MEC-2022–0421), and the trial was registered in the Clinical Trial Registry (NCT06124027). All participating patients provided written informed consent prior to any research-related activities. Patients in whom measurements were unfeasible due to logistical constraints or who withdrew their informed consent, were subsequently replaced. This manuscript adheres to the STROBE-guidelines [22].

2.1. *Perioperative Management*

Standard monitoring during DS included (SpO_2), electrocardiogram (ECG), and non-invasive blood pressure (NIBP). Additionally, measurements of $tcPCO_2$ and $mitoPO_2$ were incorporated for the purpose of this study. Preoperatively, HFNOT was initiated, with flow rates adjusted according to the patient's needs based on SpO_2 and clinical manifestations, which were continuously monitored by a sedation practitioner. SpO_2 levels were maintained above 93%. The FiO_2 delivered by the HFNOT devices was fixed at 100%, as the devices available did not allow for alteration of the FiO_2. Sedation induction was performed with propofol (0.4–1.0 mg/kg). Maintenance of anesthesia was achieved via a propofol infusion (4–6 mg/kg/h) and remifentanil infusion (2–4 μg/kg/h), aiming to maintain a Ramsay Score of 5–6. Blood pressure support was provided with noradrenaline as needed.

2.2. *$tcPCO_2$ Measurements*

$tcPCO_2$ was measured continuously at one-second intervals throughout the procedure using the SenTec Digital Monitoring System (SenTec AG, Therwil, Switzerland). By placing a heated sensor on the forehead, a hyperemic dermis is established resulting in the dilation of local capillaries. This hyperemia-driven vasodilation amplifies arterial blood flow, thereby enhancing the diffusion of CO_2 through the skin, as measured by the sensor [23]. As was previously described, several studies validated $tcPCO_2$ to be a reliable reflection of the $PaCO_2$, as opposed to the $etCO_2$ [18–21].

2.3. *$mitoPO_2$ Measurements*

$mitoPO_2$ was measured at one-minute intervals throughout the procedure using the non-invasive Cellular Oxygen METabolism (COMET®, Photonics Healthcare, Utrecht, The Netherlands) device, which utilizes the protoporphyrin IX Triplet State Lifetime technique (PpIX-TSLT). The PpIX-TLST employs oxygen-dependent quenching of PpIX, which acts as a mitochondrial located oxygen-sensitive dye after photo-excitation with a pulse of green light. The delayed fluorescence of protoporphyrin IX is inversely related to the available oxygen concentration in the mitochondria [24]. Detailed descriptions of background principles of the PpIX-TLST can be found elsewhere [12,13,25]. The PpIX-TLST has been validated and calibrated in healthy volunteers [26], and its feasibility has been demonstrated in the operating theatre [27,28], the intensive care unit [29,30] and patients with peripheral arterial disease undergoing endovascular therapy [31].

2.4. *mitoVO_2 Measurements*

The mitoVO_2 measurements are based on dynamic mitoPO_2 (1 Hz) measurements, during which local pressure is applied to the measurement probe for 60 s, inducing reproducible stop-flow conditions in the microcirculation. Halting the oxygen supply while mitochondria continue to consume oxygen, results in a time-dependent reduction in mitoPO_2. This enables the direct measurement of the oxygen disappearance rate, thereby providing quantifiable mitoVO_2 measurements. The calculation of mitoVO_2 is based on an adapted Michaelis-Menten fit procedure, which also accounts for the diffusion of oxygen back into the measurement volume [16]. This analysis results in the calculation of the maximal oxygen consumption (V_{max}) in mmHg s^{-1}. In order to consistently calculate the mitoVO_2, the Automated V_{max} Calculation COMET® Application (Erasmus MC, Rotterdam, The Netherlands) was utilized [32]. mitoVO_2 was measured approximately 5 min before the start and end of DS.

2.5. *Preparation and After Care*

The PpIX-TLST requires an upregulated concentration of PpIX [33]. Therefore, 8 mg of 5-aminolevulinic acid (ALA), a precursor of PpIX, was topically applied as a plaster (Alacare, Photonamic GmbH und Co. KG, Pinneberg, Germany) on both upper arms at least four hours before the measurement. Preparation of the plaster site involved shaving and gentle removal of the top layer of the stratum corneum with a fine abrasive pad. The mitoPO_2 measurements were performed at the plaster sites. After the measurement, the sites were covered with a light-shielding plaster (Aluderm® plaster, W.Söhngen GmbH, Taunusstein, Germany) to protect against sun exposure for at least 24 h. The day after the procedure, the patient was contacted to inquire whether they had experienced side effects caused by the plasters.

2.6. *Baseline Characteristics and Intra- and Postoperative Data*

Baseline characteristics, medical history, medication use, and intraoperative measurements were extracted from electronic patient records. Furthermore, electronic patient records were reviewed 30 days post-procedure to document the length of hospital stay (mean ± SD) and number of (serious) adverse events. Adverse events encompass any unfavorable occurrences experienced by a participating patient throughout the study, irrespective of the association with the measurements. A serious adverse event is any medical occurrence resulting in death, being life-threatening, requiring hospitalization or prolonging it, causing persistent or significant disability, or any other important medical event based on researcher judgment.

2.7. *Sample Size*

A clinically significant difference between baseline tcPCO_2 and 30 min after start of DS based on clinical expertise was established at 1.33 kPa (9.975 mmHg). The mean standard deviation, derived from a study examining the superiority of tcPCO_2 over end-tidal CO_2 measurements in non-intubated patients [20], was 11.6 mmHg (1.55 kPa). Using G*power [34] and a paired Wilcoxon signed-rank test, an effect size of 0.86 was calculated based on the clinically significant difference and the mean standard deviation. To achieve

95% power at a significance level of 0.01 with an effect size of 0.86, the required sample size was calculated to be 29. To account for potential measurements failures and participant attrition, the sample size was increased by 20%, resulting in a total of 35 patients.

2.8. Statistical Analysis

Statistical analyses were performed using R Statistical Software version 4.3.1 (R Foundation for Statistical Computing, Vienna, Austria) [35]. Distributions of standard hemodynamic and respiratory parameters, as well as the incidence of complications, were subjected to descriptive statistical analysis. The normality of continuous variables was assessed with the Shapiro–Wilk test. Normally distributed data were reported as mean ± standard deviation, while non-normally distributed data were reported as median (interquartile range). Categorical variables were summarized as frequencies and percentages. An alpha of 0.05 was considered significant for all analyses.

The paired Wilcoxon-signed rank test was used to compare $tcPCO_2$ and $mitoPO_2$ measurements at baseline with those 30, 60, 90 and 120 min after starting DS. The time points represent the average of measurements taken over 5 min intervals: 30 min (30–35 min), 60 min (60–65 min), 90 min (90–95 min), and 120 min (120–125 min) after starting DS. To account for multiple testing, the Benjamini–Hochberg correction method was used [36]. Baseline $mitoPO_2$ was defined as the mean of the first 30 measurements at a 1 s interval before the interval was set to one measurement per minute. Baseline $tcPCO_2$ was defined as the first 30 measurements after sensor calibration.

A linear mixed model with a random effects structure was fitted to investigate the effect of HFNOT with DS on the $tcPCO_2$ and $mitoPO_2$ over time. Depending on the level of non-linearity of the data, natural splines with three knots were added to improve the model fit. The ANOVA test was used to select the best-fitting model. Assumptions of the linear mixed model were tested, including an examination of the residuals.

3. Results

In total, 105 patients were screened for eligibility, and 54 patients were included. Of these, 25 were excluded before the measurements due to withdrawal of informed consent, insufficient preparation for $mitoPO_2$ measurements or logistical difficulties (Figure 1).

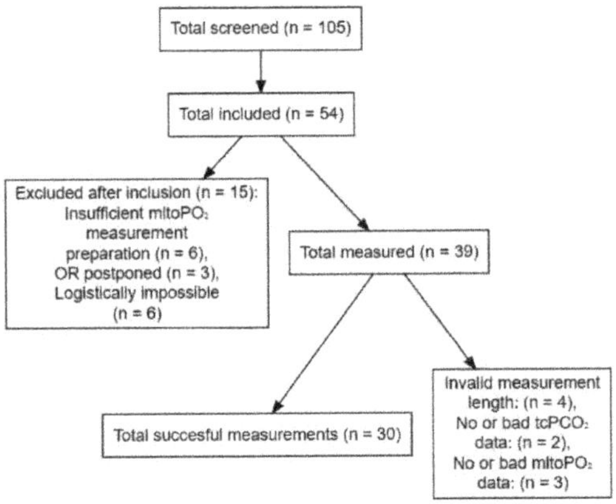

Figure 1. Flowchart of inclusion process. Abbreviations: $tcPCO_2$, transcutaneous CO_2; $mitoPO_2$, mitochondrial oxygenation; OR, operation room.

Between February and November 2023, measurements were conducted in 39 patients, of which 30 were successful. In four patients, measurements were considered unsuccessful according to the aforementioned criteria. Additionally, two patients had no or bad quality $tcPCO_2$ data, and three patients had no or bad quality $mitoPO_2$ data (Figure 1). All patients completed the follow-up.

3.1. Patient Characteristics

Baseline characteristics are shown in Table 1. The study sample included 30 patients, (21 males and 9 females), with a mean age of 60.0 ± 12.0. The median DS time was 89 (61–106) minutes, and the median HFNOT time was 80 (63–111) minutes. The median $tcPCO_2$ measurement time was 96 (63–116) minutes, and the median $mitoPO_2$ measurement time was 104 (71–116) minutes. The median SpO_2 was 98% (96–99). All patients underwent interventional radiologic or endoscopic procedures. Oncologic disease was the most prevalent comorbidity (76.7%). The median length of hospital stay was 1 (0–1.8) day. Two minor adverse events occurred: a skin abrasion from the preparation for $mitoPO_2$ measurements and a case of desaturation during transport, managed with oxygen therapy. Subsequent follow-up revealed no additional complications associated with these adverse events. No serious adverse events were reported during 30-day follow-up.

Table 1. Patient characteristics.

	Overall (n = 30)		**Overall (n = 30)**
Male	21 (70.0%)	Diabetes Mellitus	6 (20.0%)
Age (years)	60.0 ± 12.0	Neurodegenerative disease	1 (3.3%)
BMI (kg/m^2)	27.7 ± 4.8	Cerebrovascular disease	2 (6.7%)
Smoking history	14 (46.7%)	Hypercholesterolemia	1 (3.3%)
Former	12 (40.0%)	Respiratory disease	6 (20.0%)
Current	2 (6.7%)	Cardiovascular disease	15 (50.0%)
Alcohol use	24 (80.0%)	AF	3 (10.0%)
Former	7 (23.3%)	Arrhythmias	2 (6.7%)
Current	16 (53.3%)	DVT	2 (6.7%)
Missing	1 (3.3%)	MI	2 (6.7%)
Respiratory disease	6 (20.0%)	Heart valve disease	1 (3.3%)
OSAS	1 (3.3%)	PVD	1 (3.3%)
COPD	4 (13.3%)	Other	4 (13.3%)
Asthma	1 (3.3%)	Procedure type	
Oncologic disease	23 (76.7%)	Endoscopy	1 (3.3%)
Breast	2 (6.7%)	Colonoscopy	3 (10.0%)
Bladder	1 (3.3%)	Gastro intervention	2 (6.7%)
Colon/rectal	7 (23.3%)	Colon intervention	2 (6.7%)
Renal	4 (13.3%)	RFA kidney	3 (10.0%)
Liver	4 (13.3%)	RFA liver	9 (30.0%)
Lung	1 (3.3%)	TIPS	2 (6.7%)
Prostate	1 (3.3%)	Stenting	4 (13.3%)
Other	3 (10.0%)	Other	4 (13.3%)
Hypertension	16 (53.3%)	High Flow Nasal Oxygen Therapy duration (min)	80 (63–111)
Length of hospital stay (days)	1 (0–1.8)	$tcPCO_2$ measurement time (min)	96 (62–116)

Table 1. *Cont.*

	Overall (n = 30)		Overall (n = 30)
Adverse events	2 (6.7%)	mitoPO_2 measurement time (min)	104 (71–116)
Sedation duration (min)	89 (61–106)		
Oxygen saturation (%)	98 (96–99)		

Data reported as number (proportion), mean ± standard deviation if normally distributed or median (Q1–Q3) if not normally distributed. Abbreviations: Q1: first inter quartile range; Q3, third interquartile range; AF, atrium fibrillation; DVT, deep venous thrombosis; MI, myocardial infarction; PVD, peripheral vascular disease; OSAS, obstructive sleep apnoea syndrome; COPD, chronic obstructive pulmonary disease; RFA, radiofrequency ablation; TIPS, transhepatic intrajugular portosystemic shunt; min, minutes.

3.2. *Effect of DS with HFNOT on tcPCO_2*

Data was analyzed up to 120 min as only five patients underwent DS for a longer period. The median tcPCO_2 at 30 min was based on 29 patients due to a calibration error in one case. The sample size reduced over time due to procedure completion: 25 patients at 60 min, 16 at 90 min, and 7 at 120 min.

Baseline tcPCO_2 was 37.3 (34.5–45.5) mmHg, which significantly increased to 55.5 (34.5–61.9) mmHg after 30 min of DS ($p < 0.001$). This increase remained significant at 60 min (54.8 (52.5–62.2) mmHg, $p < 0.001$), 90 min (56.5 (53.1–69.3) mmHg, $p < 0.001$), and 120 min (55.8 (50.7–56.6) mmHg, $p = 0.016$) (Table 2, Figure 2A,B). The univariable model showed a significant effect of time on tcPCO_2 (Table 3 and Figure 2C).

Table 2. Median tcPCO_2 and mitoPO_2 at different timepoints with corresponding inter quartile range and sample size.

Timepoint	Sample Size	Median	Q1–Q3	*p*-Value
tcPCO_2 (mmHg)				
Baseline	30	37.3	34.5–45.5	
30 min	29	55.5 *	34.5–61.9	<0.001
60 min	25	54.8 *	52.5–62.2	<0.001
90 min	16	56.5 *	53.1–69.3	<0.001
120 min	7	55.8 *	50.7–56.6	0.02
mitoPO_2 (mmHg)				
Baseline	30	69.6	43.9–76.7	
30 min	30	80.5	65.7–98.9	0.19
60 min	24	78.6	70.3–85.8	0.19
90 min	14	74.4	52.7–86.3	0.38
120 min	6	85.6	82.5–98.0	0.38

* Denotes a significant effect between baseline and the corresponding timepoint. Abbreviations: Q1: first inter quartile range; Q3, third interquartile range; tcPCO_2, transcutaneous CO_2; mitoPO_2, mitochondrial oxygenation; min, minutes; mmHg, millimeters of mercury.

Table 3. Univariable mixed model of effect of time on tcPCO_2 and mitoPO_2.

	Estimate	Confidence Interval
tcPCO_2 (mmHg)		
Intercept	36.9	33.5–40.3
Spline (time 1)	11.9 *	11.8–12.1
Spline (time 2)	44.6 *	44.4–44.9
Spline (time 3)	12.3 *	12.1–12.4

Table 3. *Cont.*

	Estimate	Confidence Interval
mitoPO$_2$ (mmHg)		
Intercept	72.1	63.9–80.3
Spline (time 1)	−21.3 *	−25.3–−17.3
Spline (time 2)	30.0 *	25.1–34.9
Spline (time 3)	−2.0	−7.0–2.9

* Denotes a significant effect. Abbreviations: tcPCO$_2$, transcutaneous CO$_2$; mitoPO$_2$, mitochondrial oxygenation; mmHg, millimeters of mercury.

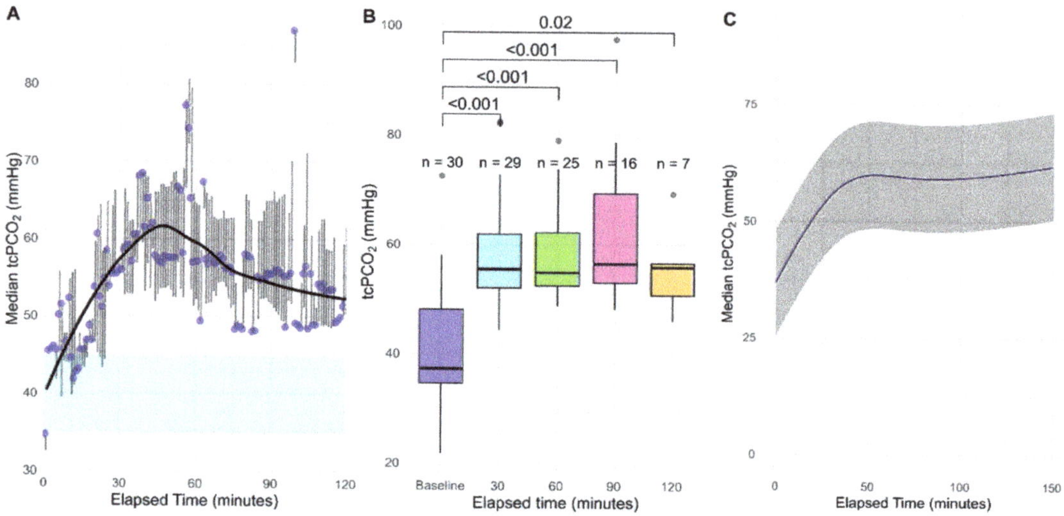

Figure 2. Median tcPCO$_2$ in mmHg grouped per minute denoted by the blue dots, with the error bars denoting the interquartile range, the black line denoting the Locally Estimated Scatterplot Smoothing (LOESS) regression line and the blue box denoting the normal range (**A**); baseline tcPCO$_2$ in mmHg compared to tcPCO$_2$ at 30, 60, 90 and 120 min after start of deep sedation using the paired Wilcoxon signed-rank (**B**); effect plot of univariable linear mixed model of tcPCO$_2$ in mmHg over time with the grey ribbon denoting the 95% confidence interval (**C**). Abbreviations: tcPCO$_2$, transcutaneous CO$_2$.

3.3. *Effect of DS with HFNOT on mitoPO$_2$*

Figure 3A shows mitoPO$_2$ data up to 120 min. Data from 30 patients was available at baseline and after 30 min of DS, which subsequently decreased over time due to procedure completion: 24 patients after 60 min, 14 after 90 min and 6 after 120 min. Median baseline mitoPO$_2$ was 69.6 (43.9–76.7) mmHg, increasing to 80.5 (65.7–98.9) mmHg after 30 min, though not significantly (p = 0.19). Similarly, non-significant increases were observed at 60 (78.6 (70.3–85.8) mmHg, p = 0.19), 90 (74.42 (52.7–86.3) mmHg, p = 0.38), and 120 min (85.6 (82.5–98.0) mmHg, p = 0.38) (Table 2, Figure 3B). Lastly, the univariable model showed a significant effect of time on mitoPO$_2$ in the first and second spline (Table 3 and Figure 3C).

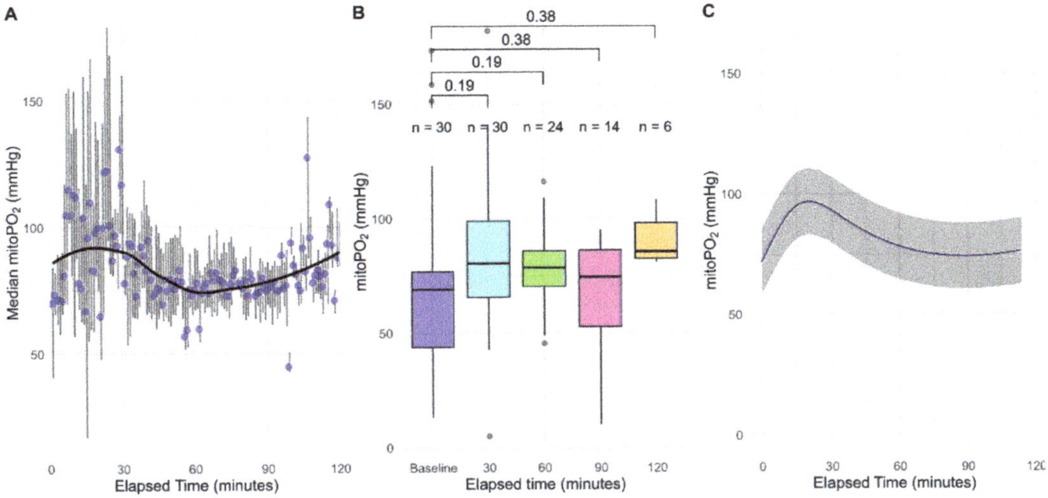

Figure 3. Median mitoPO_2 in mmHg grouped per minute denoted by the blue dots, with the error bars denoting the interquartile range and the black line denoting the Locally Estimated Scatterplot Smoothing (LOESS) regression line (**A**); baseline mitoPO_2 in mmHg compared to mitoPO_2 at 30, 60, 90 and 120 min after start of deep sedation using the paired Wilcoxon signed-rank test (**B**); effect plot of univariable linear mixed model of mitoPO_2 in mmHg over time with the grey ribbon denoting the 95% confidence interval (**C**). Abbreviations: mitoPO_2, mitochondrial oxygenation.

3.4. *Effect of DS with HFNOT on mitoVO$_2$*

The mitoVO_2 measurement before DS, after DS or both were infeasible in five patients due to logistical restraints. Additionally, in six patients, the analysis software had difficulty processing the data, leading to incomplete measurements. Therefore, the mitoVO_2 data consists of 19 patients. The median mitoVO_2 before the start of DS (4.12 (3.47–4.78) mmHg s^{-1}) did not significantly increase compared to the mitoVO_2 five minutes before the end of DS (4.32 (3.40–5.63) mmHg s^{-1}, $p = 0.37$), as is presented in Supplemental Table S1 and Supplemental Figure S2.

4. Discussion

In this study, we examined the effects of DS with HFNOT on tcPCO_2 and mitoPO_2. The analysis revealed a significant increase in the median tcPCO_2 at all four timepoints compared to baseline, most likely due to decreased respiratory drive after administration of DS induction medication [37–39]. This was further reiterated by the mixed model, indicating that tcPCO_2 increases over time during DS.

In DS, tcPCO_2 can be used as a viable non-invasive and continuously measured parameter to detect hypercapnia. Aarrestad et al. [18] validated tcPCO_2 measured with the SenTec Digital Monitoring System as a reliable reflection of $PaCO_2$, with no differences exceeding 1 kPa. In another study, prolonged tcPCO_2 monitoring was also well tolerated, and the correlation between tcPCO_2 and $PaCO_2$ remained highly significant [19]. Similarly, Lermuzeaux et al. [20] found a strong correlation between tcPCO_2 and PaC O_2, but a poor correlation between etCO_2 and $PaCO_2$ in non-intubated patients with acute respiratory failure. Lastly, De Oliveira et al. [21] demonstrated that tcPCO_2 monitoring was more sensitive in detecting hypercapnia than nasal capnography.

Notably, the median tcPCO_2 exceeded the normal range (35–45 mmHg) at all time points except baseline, indicating prevalent hypercapnia in this cohort. The persistent elevation in $tcPCO_2$ may have clinically relevant implications, as hypercapnia can increase intracranial pressure, contribute to respiratory acidosis, and place additional strain on the cardiovascular system [40]. Although hypoxemia was effectively prevented by HFNOT, the high FiO_2 may mask clinically important hypoventilation [17,41], meaning that hypercapnia could otherwise remain undetected without $tcPCO_2$ monitoring. These findings highlight the additional value of $tcPCO_2$ as an early-warning parameter during prolonged deep sedation, although further research is required to establish its precise clinical utility. However, no hypercapnia-related adverse events were observed in this cohort, nor was the study designed to detect these events. Future research is required to clarify the exact impact of hypercapnia in DS patients receiving HFNOT.

$mitoPO_2$ did not significantly increase from baseline at any time point. HFNOT is expected to increase cellular oxygenation due to the delivery of high concentrations of oxygen; however, this may also trigger hyperoxic vasoconstriction, potentially reducing tissue oxygenation [42–45]. At the same time, hypercapnia may develop, potentially masked by HFNOT, which could lead to hypercapnic vasodilation, increasing blood flow. This could possibly explain the observed effect, although adequately designed preclinical studies are required to clarify this physiological interaction.

In our study, the median $mitoPO_2$ was consistently higher than those reported in other studies using the COMET® device (healthy volunteer studies: 66 ± 16 mmHg [46] and 68 mmHg (61–77) [47]), studies in the operating theatre: 62 ± 23 mmHg [28], 60 ± 19 mmHg [27] and 39 (30 to 50) mmHg [48]). This may be due to the 100% FiO_2 provided by the HFNOT during DS, which is five times higher than the atmospheric oxygen concentration of 21% to which the healthy volunteers were subjected. Moreover, such high FiO_2 values are uncommon in the OR as they may increase the risk of long-term mortality [49]. Although $mitoPO_2$ values in our study were higher than in previous reports, there are currently no established thresholds for safe or toxic $mitoPO_2$ levels. Recent studies in cardiothoracic surgery patients have suggested that $mitoPO_2$ values below ~30 mmHg may be associated with an increased risk of postoperative complications, including CSA-AKI and elevated lactate levels [14,28,50]. In our cohort, $mitoPO_2$ remained well above this threshold. The absence of adverse events, combined with stable $mitoVO_2$, suggests that these supranormal values may not be clinically harmful in this setting. However, this study was not designed to detect these events.

Mitochondrial monitoring may have several potential clinical applications during prolonged DS. Continuous $mitoPO_2$ assessment could help detect microcirculatory impairment, hyperoxic vasoconstriction, or declining cellular oxygen availability before alterations appear in systemic parameters. Such early-warning capability may support individualized oxygen titration strategies or inform the need for ventilatory adjustments. Future controlled studies could evaluate whether $mitoPO_2$-guided sedation improves outcomes or reduces oxygen-related complications.

The mixed model found a significant initial increase in $mitoPO_2$, followed by a decrease and plateau near baseline values. Although pairwise comparisons at individual time points did not reach statistical significance, the spline-based mixed model did reveal a significant effect of time on $mitoPO_2$. This may indicate a time-dependent trend in mitochondrial oxygenation during DS with HFNOT, potentially reflecting physiological changes not captured in fixed-time comparisons. It is possible that the high FiO_2 provided by HFNOT increased $mitoPO_2$ initially, but vasoconstriction in response to hyperoxia may have caused the subsequent decline, causing a subsequent decrease in $mitoPO_2$. This was also noted in a recent study by Hilderink et al. [45] whom found that hyperoxia resulted in a decrease in $mitoPO_2$, likely due to a reduction in microcirculation.

No significant increase in $mitoVO_2$ was found, indicating that the oxygen consumption is likely not excessively affected by the high concentrations of oxygen administered. Moreover, this suggests that the observed increase in $mitoPO_2$ was more likely attributable to increased oxygen delivery rather than a reduction in mitochondrial oxygen consumption. This aligns with the expected physiological effect of HFNOT delivering high inspired oxygen concentrations.

Both the SenTec Monitoring System and the COMET® device offer the unique advantage of continuous and non-invasive parameter monitoring. Moreover, the SenTec Monitoring system allows for rapid and straightforward application, facilitating the seamless integration of this monitoring modality into perioperative logistics. Besides the plaster preparation, the COMET® Device is convenient in usage and is also easily integrated into perioperative logistics. Plaster preparation is an essential step in the monitoring process and requires extra effort from both the patient being monitored and the assessor. Aside from two minor skin abrasions, no complications regarding the plaster preparation process were reported. Beyond the physiological findings, this study highlights the technological and clinical innovation of integrating the SenTec and COMET® systems into the perioperative workflow. The SenTec Digital Monitoring System enabled continuous, high-resolution $tcPCO_2$ monitoring, providing real-time visualization of ventilation dynamics during DS. This underlines its potential as a reliable and non-invasive tool for early identification of hypoventilation during prolonged DS, while seamlessly fitting into existing procedural workflows. The COMET® system represents a novel advancement in clinical monitoring by quantifying $mitoPO_2$ in real time. Unlike conventional oxygenation parameters such as SpO_2 or PaO_2, which primarily reflect systemic oxygen delivery, $mitoPO_2$ provides direct insight into cellular oxygen utilization and microcirculatory dynamics. The ability to measure this parameter non-invasively and continuously introduces a new dimension to perioperative monitoring, bridging the gap between macro- and microcirculatory oxygen assessment.

From an implementation perspective, both systems were easily incorporated into routine sedation workflows with minimal setup time and without interference in procedural logistics. This demonstrates the feasibility of integrating advanced physiological monitoring technologies into daily clinical practice. These modalities have the potential to enhance diagnostic accuracy, optimize oxygen titration, and improve overall patient safety during prolonged DS. Future research should focus on validating these systems in larger, multicenter settings and exploring their potential to guide individualized sedation and oxygenation strategies.

Strengths & Limitations

This single center observational study allowed for the examination of ventilation and oxygenation during DS procedures with HFNOT in a real-world clinical setting, offering new insights into these parameters and their potential clinical application. A key strength is the continuous, non-invasive monitoring of both $tcPCO_2$ and $mitoPO_2$. These two parameters are not yet routinely assessed during procedural sedation and provide a more nuanced understanding of ventilation and tissue oxygenation dynamics.

However, this study design does not allow for the investigation of causal relationships because of the observational nature. Moreover, as the study was conducted in a single academic institution where DS is routinely performed using HFNOT with 100% FiO_2, the generalizability of our findings may be limited. Sedation protocols, including oxygen delivery strategies, can vary substantially between centers. The use of high FiO_2 during DS is common in many clinical settings to minimize the risk of hypoxemia [51]. Nevertheless, the physiological and clinical effects of lower or titrated FiO_2 levels during sedation have not been systematically studied. Future multicenter studies are therefore warranted to validate our findings and to explore the impact of different oxygenation strategies on patient outcomes.

Moreover, the observational nature of this study limited our ability to alter standard monitoring protocols during DS. While arterial blood gas (ABG) sampling at multiple intervals could have provided more direct insights into $PaCO_2$ and PaO_2 fluctuations, this approach was deemed too invasive and inconsistent with routine clinical practice. Frequent ABG sampling could also prolong the procedure and cause unnecessary discomfort to patients. Instead, two non-invasive monitoring modalities were added alongside standard monitoring. SpO_2 levels were maintained above 93% per protocol, ensuring the detection and management of hypoxia or hyperoxia as per standard guidelines.

Sedation practitioners were not blinded to the measured $tcPCO_2$ and $mitoPO_2$ measurements. To mitigate introduction of behavioral bias, sedation practitioners were advised to discard the observed values. Despite this, unconscious responses may have influenced care, potentially introducing bias.

The median duration of sedation was 89 min, with the longest nearing 4 h. Only a small number of patients underwent sedation for more than 120 min, resulting in limited data for these longer procedures (see Supplemental Figure S1). Consequently, formulating statements regarding extremely prolonged sedation procedures, exceeding 2 h, is challenging due to the infrequency of such events in this study.

The statistical power of this study was determined based on being able to find a significant difference in $tcPCO_2$. Consequently, this study may have been underpowered to detect significant differences in $mitoPO_2$. A well-powered study is necessary to draw robust conclusions regarding the effect of DS with HFNOT on $mitoPO_2$.

No adverse events were observed during the 30-day follow-up. However, the incidence of respiratory complications in DS is generally reported as low [52]. As this study was neither designed nor powered to address safety in terms of adverse event incidence, we cannot adequately assess this based on our data. Although no hyperoxia-related adverse events were observed in this study, the possibility of harm from prolonged exposure to high FiO_2 cannot be excluded. Therefore, further research is needed to assess the safety of sustained high FiO_2 levels in relation to hyperoxia and its consequences.

Both the SenTec and COMET® monitoring modalities do have limitations. In this study, $tcPCO_2$ measurements failed in two patients. One failure was due to a delayed membrane replacement by the technical service, while in another case, prolonged calibration resulted in insufficient data for analysis. Proper maintenance and user knowledge are crucial for effective use of the SenTec Monitoring System in clinical practice. Similarly, $mitoPO_2$ measurements failed in three patients, primarily due to improper adhesive application and malfunctioning of the device due to several instances of COMET® failures related to its sensitive light source. It is noteworthy that the manufacturer acknowledges this limitation and intends to address it in the development of a new version of the COMET® device.

5. Conclusions

This study found that $tcPCO_2$ levels increased from baseline during prolonged DS with HFNOT. Although $mitoPO_2$ showed a tendency to increase over time, this trend was not statistically significant compared to baseline. No significant adverse events attributable to elevated $tcPCO_2$ or $mitoPO_2$ levels were found. This study also demonstrates the feasibility of continuous, non-invasive monitoring of ventilation and mitochondrial oxygenation using the SenTec and COMET® systems in DS. Both technologies were smoothly integrated into perioperative care, without disrupting workflow.

Supplementary Materials: The following supporting information can be downloaded at https://www.mdpi.com/article/10.3390/s25247573/s1, Figure S1: Median $tcPCO_2$ over time, grouped per 5 min with the blue box denoting the normal range and the bars denoting the sample size (A), median mitoPO_2 over time grouped per 5 min and the bars denoting the sample size (B); Figure S2: Mean mitoVO_2 five minutes before the start and five min before the end of DS compared using the Wilcoxon signed-rank test; Table S1: Median mitoVO_2 five minutes before the start and five min before the end of DS compared using the Wilcoxon signed-rank test.

Author Contributions: Conceptualization, C.J.d.W. and F.A.H.; Methodology, C.J.d.W. and F.A.H.; Investigation, A.M.v.S.; Data Curation, A.M.v.S. and C.J.d.W.; Writing—Original Draft Preparation, A.M.v.S., C.J.d.W. and F.A.H.; Writing—Review and Editing, A.M.v.S., C.J.d.W., F.A.H., S.E.H. and E.G.M.; Visualization, A.M.v.S.; Supervision, F.A.H., S.E.H. and E.G.M.; Project Administration, A.M.v.S. All authors have read and agreed to the published version of the manuscript.

Funding: This research received no external funding.

Institutional Review Board Statement: The study was conducted in accordance with the Declaration of Helsinki and approved by the Medical Ethics Committee of the Erasmus MC, Rotterdam, the Netherlands (MEC-2022–0421, December 2022).

Informed Consent Statement: Informed consent was obtained from all subjects involved in the study.

Data Availability Statement: The raw data supporting the conclusions of this article will be made available on request from the corresponding author as publicly sharing the data was not included in the informed consent form signed by the participants.

Acknowledgments: Netherlands Institute for Health Sciences (NIHES) facilitated several epidemiological and statistical courses of which the obtained knowledge was implemented in the development of this research paper. Open access funding was provided by Erasmus University Rotterdam. We would like to extend our sincere gratitude to all the sedation practitioners who participated in this study. Your dedication and collaboration were instrumental in making this research possible.

Conflicts of Interest: E.G. Mik, inventor on patents for mitochondrial oxygen measurements owned by the Academic Medical Center Amsterdam and Erasmus Medical Center Rotterdam, is the founder and shareholder of Photonics Healthcare, which holds exclusive licenses and markets the COMET® system. E.G. Mik is also Head of the research group Experimental Anesthesiology at Erasmus MC. In this role he contributed as a supervisor and was involved in the conceptual development of the research. He had no role in data collection or analysis. Other authors report no relevant conflicts of interest.

Abbreviations

The following abbreviations are used in this manuscript:

ABG	Arterial blood gas
AF	Atrium fibrillation
ALA	5-aminolevulinic acid
COMET	Cellular Oxygen METabolism
COPD	Chronic obstructive pulmonary disease
DS	Deep Sedation
DVT	Deep venous thrombosis
ECG	Electrocardiogram
$etCO_2$	End-tidal CO_2
FiO_2	Inspiratory oxygen fraction
HFNOT	High Flow Nasal Oxygen Therapy
IQR	Interquartile range
LOESS	Locally Estimated Scatterplot Smoothing
MI	Myocardial infarction
min	Minutes

$mitoPO_2$	Mitochondrial oxygen tension
$mitoVO_2$	Mitochondrial oxygen consumption
mmHg	Millimeters of mercury
NIBP	Non-invasive blood pressure
OR	Operation room
OSAS	Obstructive sleep apnea syndrome
PaO_2	Partial pressure of arterial oxygen
PIF	Patient information
PpIX-TSLT	Protoporphyrin IX Triplet State Lifetime technique
PVD	Peripheral vascular disease
Q_1	First inter quartile range
Q_3	Third interquartile range
RFA	Radiofrequency ablation
SD	Standard deviation
SpO_2	Oxygen saturation
$tcPCO_2$	Transcutaneous CO_2
TIPS	Transhepatic intrajugular portosystemic shunt
V_{max}	Maximal oxygen consumption

References

1. Krauss, B.; Green, S.M. Procedural sedation and analgesia in children. *Lancet* **2006**, *367*, 766–780. [CrossRef]
2. Committee on Quality Management and Departmental Administration. Statement on Continuum of Depth of Sedation: Definitior of General Anesthesia and Levels of Sedation/Analgesia. Available online: https://www.asahq.org/standards-and-practice parameters/statement-on-continuum-of-depth-of-sedation-definition-of-general-anesthesia-and-levels-of-sedation-analgesia (accessed on 10 October 2025).
3. Ramsay, M.A.; Savege, T.M.; Simpson, B.R.; Goodwin, R. Controlled sedation with alphaxalone-alphadolone. *Br. Med. J.* **1974**, *2*, 656–659. [CrossRef]
4. Nederlandse Vereniging voor Anesthesiologie. Sedatie en Analgesie bij Volwassenen. Available online: https://richtlijnendatabase.nl/richtlijn/sedatie_en_analgesie_bij_volwassenen/startpagina_sedatie_en_analgesie_bij_volwassenen_2024.html (accessed on 18 March 2025).
5. Noordzij, P. *Klinische Anesthesiologie*; De Tijdstroom: Utrecht, The Netherlands, 2017; Volume 3.
6. Droog, W.; Grace, V.; Droog, L.; Hendriks, R.H.; van Oers, L.; Stolker, R.J.; Galvin, E.M. Substantiating 'green' healthcare decisions An explorative life cycle assessment study to identify differences in greenhouse gas emissions between general vs. regional anaesthesia for upper extremity surgery. *Eur. J. Anaesthesiol.* **2024**, *41*, 455–460. [CrossRef] [PubMed]
7. Al-Husinat, L.; Jouryyeh, B.; Rawashdeh, A.; Alenaizat, A.; Abushehab, M.; Amir, M.W.; Al Modanat, Z.; Battaglini, D.; Cinnella, G. High-Flow Oxygen Therapy in the Perioperative Setting and Procedural Sedation: A Review of Current Evidence. *J. Clin. Med.* **2023**, *12*, 6685. [CrossRef]
8. Thiruvenkatarajan, V.; Sekhar, V.; Wong, D.T.; Currie, J.; Van Wijk, R.; Ludbrook, G.L. Effect of high-flow nasal oxygen on hypoxaemia during procedural sedation: A systematic review and meta-analysis. *Anaesthesia* **2023**, *78*, 81–92. [CrossRef]
9. Möller, W.; Celik, G.; Feng, S.; Bartenstein, P.; Meyer, G.; Oliver, E.; Schmid, O.; Tatkov, S. Nasal high flow clears anatomical dead space in upper airway models. *J. Appl. Physiol.* **2015**, *118*, 1525–1532. [CrossRef] [PubMed]
10. Ottolenghi, S.; Sabbatini, G.; Brizzolari, A.; Samaja, M.; Chiumello, D. Hyperoxia and oxidative stress in anesthesia and critical care medicine. *Minerva Anestesiol.* **2020**, *86*, 64–75. [CrossRef] [PubMed]
11. Oldman, A.H.; Martin, D.S.; Feelisch, M.; Grocott, M.P.W.; Cumpstey, A.F. Effects of perioperative oxygen concentration on oxidative stress in adult surgical patients: A systematic review. *Br. J. Anaesth.* **2021**, *126*, 622–632. [CrossRef]
12. Ubbink, R.; Bettink, M.A.W.; Janse, R.; Harms, F.A.; Johannes, T.; Münker, F.M.; Mik, E.G. A monitor for Cellular Oxygen METabolism (COMET): Monitoring tissue oxygenation at the mitochondrial level. *J. Clin. Monit. Comput.* **2017**, *31*, 1143–1150. [CrossRef]
13. Mik, E.G.; Stap, J.; Sinaasappel, M.; Beek, J.F.; Aten, J.A.; van Leeuwen, T.G.; Ince, C. Mitochondrial PO2 measured by delayed fluorescence of endogenous protoporphyrin IX. *Nat. Methods* **2006**, *3*, 939–945. [CrossRef]
14. de Wijs, C.J.; Streng, L.; Stolker, R.J.; Ter Horst, M.; Hoorn, E.J.; Mahtab, E.A.F.; Mik, E.G.; Harms, F.A. Mitochondrial oxygenation monitoring and acute kidney injury risk in cardiac surgery: A prospective cohort study. *J. Clin. Anesth.* **2025**, *101*, 111715. [CrossRef]

15. Hilderink, B.N.; Crane, R.F.; Baysan, M.; Arbous, S.M.; van den Bogaard, B.; Mik, E.G.; Ince, C.; Pillay, J.; Juffermans, N.P. A simulation of skin mitochondrial Po_2 in circulatory shock. *J. Appl. Physiol.* **2023**, *134*, 1165–1176. [CrossRef]
16. Harms, F.A.; Mik, E.G. In Vivo Assessment of Mitochondrial Oxygen Consumption. In *Methods in Molecular Biology*; Springer: Berlin/Heidelberg, Germany, 2021; Volume 2277, pp. 175–185. [CrossRef]
17. Saunders, R.; Struys, M.; Pollock, R.F.; Mestek, M.; Lightdale, J.R. Patient safety during procedural sedation using capnography monitoring: A systematic review and meta-analysis. *BMJ Open* **2017**, *7*, e013402. [CrossRef] [PubMed]
18. Aarrestad, S.; Tollefsen, E.; Kleiven, A.L.; Qvarfort, M.; Janssens, J.P.; Skjønsberg, O.H. Validity of transcutaneous PCO_2 in monitoring chronic hypoventilation treated with non-invasive ventilation. *Respir. Med.* **2016**, *112*, 112–118. [CrossRef] [PubMed]
19. Janssens, J.P.; Perrin, E.; Bennani, I.; de Muralt, B.; Titelion, V.; Picaud, C. Is continuous transcutaneous monitoring of PCO_2 ($TcPCO_2$) over 8 h reliable in adults? *Respir. Med.* **2001**, *95*, 331–335. [CrossRef]
20. Lermuzeaux, M.; Meric, H.; Sauneuf, B.; Girard, S.; Normand, H.; Lofaso, F.; Terzi, N. Superiority of transcutaneous CO_2 over end-tidal CO_2 measurement for monitoring respiratory failure in nonintubated patients: A pilot study. *J. Crit. Care* **2016**, *31*, 150–156. [CrossRef] [PubMed]
21. De Oliveira, G.S., Jr.; Ahmad, S.; Fitzgerald, P.C.; McCarthy, R.J. Detection of hypoventilation during deep sedation in patients undergoing ambulatory gynaecological hysteroscopy: A comparison between transcutaneous and nasal end-tidal carbon dioxide measurements. *Br. J. Anaesth.* **2010**, *104*, 774–778. [CrossRef] [PubMed]
22. von Elm, E.; Altman, D.G.; Egger, M.; Pocock, S.J.; Gøtzsche, P.C.; Vandenbroucke, J.P. Strengthening the Reporting of Observational Studies in Epidemiology (STROBE) statement: Guidelines for reporting observational studies. *BMJ* **2007**, *335*, 806–808. [CrossRef] [PubMed]
23. Eberhard, P. The design, use, and results of transcutaneous carbon dioxide analysis: Current and future directions. *Anesth. Analg.* **2007**, *105*, S48–S52. [CrossRef] [PubMed]
24. Mik, E.G. Special article: Measuring mitochondrial oxygen tension: From basic principles to application in humans. *Anesth. Analg.* **2013**, *117*, 834–846. [CrossRef]
25. Mik, E.G.; Johannes, T.; Zuurbier, C.J.; Heinen, A.; Houben-Weerts, J.H.; Balestra, G.M.; Stap, J.; Beek, J.F.; Ince, C. In Vivo mitochondrial oxygen tension measured by a delayed fluorescence lifetime technique. *Biophys. J.* **2008**, *95*, 3977–3990. [CrossRef]
26. Harms, F.A.; Stolker, R.J.; Mik, E. Cutaneous Respirometry as Novel Technique to Monitor Mitochondrial Function: A Feasibility Study in Healthy Volunteers. *PLoS ONE* **2016**, *11*, e0159544. [CrossRef]
27. Harms, F.A.; Streng, L.; Wefers Bettink, M.A.; de Wijs, C.J.; Römers, L.H.; Janse, R.; Stolker, R.J.; Mik, E.G. Monitoring of mitochondrial oxygen tension in the operating theatre: An observational study with the novel COMET® monitor. *PLoS ONE* **2023**, *18*, e0278561. [CrossRef] [PubMed]
28. Harms, F.A.; Ubbink, R.; de Wijs, C.J.; Ligtenberg, M.P.; Ter Horst, M.; Mik, E.G. Mitochondrial Oxygenation During Cardiopulmonary Bypass: A Pilot Study. *Front. Med.* **2022**, *9*, 785734. [CrossRef]
29. Neu, C.; Baumbach, P.; Plooij, A.K.; Skitek, K.; Götze, J.; von Loeffelholz, C.; Schmidt-Winter, C.; Coldewey, S.M. Non-invasive Assessment of Mitochondrial Oxygen Metabolism in the Critically Ill Patient Using the Protoporphyrin IX-Triplet State Lifetime Technique-A Feasibility Study. *Front. Immunol.* **2020**, *11*, 757. [CrossRef] [PubMed]
30. Standke, A.; Neu, C.; Baumbach, P.; Plooij, A.K.; Skitek, K.; Götze, J.; Coldewey, S.M. Reversible impairment of non-invasively assessed mitochondrial oxygen metabolism in the long-term course of patients with sepsis: A prospective monocentric cohort study. *Intensive Care Med. Exp.* **2025**, *13*, 114. [CrossRef]
31. Zaid Al-Kaylani, A.H.A.; Schuurmann, R.C.L.; Slart, R.; Bokkers, R.P.H.; de Vries, J.P.M. Detecting Mitochondrial Oxygen Tension as a Measure of Local Tissue Oxygenation in Patients With Peripheral Arterial Disease Before and After Endovascular Therapy. *J. Endovasc. Ther.* **2025**, 15266028251344791. [CrossRef]
32. de Wijs, C.J.; Behr, J.R.; Streng, L.; van der Graaf, M.E.; Harms, F.A.; Mik, E.G. Automated mitochondrial oxygen consumption ($mitoVO_2$) analysis via a bi-directional long short-term memory neural network. *J. Clin. Monit. Comput.* **2025**, *39*, 947–956. [CrossRef]
33. Harms, F.A.; de Boon, W.M.; Balestra, G.M.; Bodmer, S.I.; Johannes, T.; Stolker, R.J.; Mik, E.G. Oxygen-dependent delayed fluorescence measured in skin after topical application of 5-aminolevulinic acid. *J. Biophotonics* **2011**, *4*, 731–739. [CrossRef]
34. Faul, F.; Erdfelder, E.; Buchner, A.; Lang, A.G. Statistical power analyses using G*Power 3.1: Tests for correlation and regression analyses. *Behav. Res. Methods* **2009**, *41*, 1149–1160. [CrossRef] [PubMed]
35. R Core Team. *R: A Language and Environment for Statistical Computing, Version 4.3.1*; R Foundation for Statistical Computing: Vienna, Austria, 2023.
36. Benjamini, Y.; Hochberg, Y. Controlling the False Discovery Rate: A Practical and Powerful Approach to Multiple Testing. *J. R. Stat. Soc. Ser. B (Methodol.)* **1995**, *57*, 289–300. [CrossRef]

37. Dahan, A.; Nieuwenhuijs, D.J.; Olofsen, E. Influence of propofol on the control of breathing. In *Advances in Experimental Medicir and Biology*; Springer: Berlin/Heidelberg, Germany, 2003; Volume 523, pp. 81–92. [CrossRef]
38. Bouillon, T.; Bruhn, J.; Radu-Radulescu, L.; Andresen, C.; Cohane, C.; Shafer, S.L. A model of the ventilatory depressant potenc of remifentanil in the non-steady state. *Anesthesiology* **2003**, *99*, 779–787. [CrossRef]
39. Olofsen, E.; Boom, M.; Nieuwenhuijs, D.; Sarton, E.; Teppema, L.; Aarts, L.; Dahan, A. Modeling the non-steady state respirator effects of remifentanil in awake and propofol-sedated healthy volunteers. *Anesthesiology* **2010**, *112*, 1382–1395. [CrossRef]
40. Almanza-Hurtado, A.; Polanco Guerra, C.; Martínez-Ávila, M.C.; Borré-Naranjo, D.; Rodríguez-Yanez, T.; Dueñas-Castell, C Hypercapnia from Physiology to Practice. *Int. J. Clin. Pract.* **2022**, *2022*, 2635616. [CrossRef] [PubMed]
41. Pattullo, G.G.; Culwick, M.D.; Endlich, Y.; MacPherson, R.D. Hypercarbia and high-flow nasal oxygen use during anaesthesia– Risking a failure to thrive? *Anaesth. Intensive Care* **2023**, *51*, 400–407. [CrossRef] [PubMed]
42. Smit, B.; Smulders, Y.M.; Eringa, E.C.; Oudemans-van Straaten, H.M.; Girbes, A.R.J.; Wever, K.E.; Hooijmans, C.R.; Spoelstra-d Man, A.M.E. Effects of hyperoxia on vascular tone in animal models: Systematic review and meta-analysis. *Crit. Care* **2018**, *2* 189. [CrossRef]
43. Farquhar, H.; Weatherall, M.; Wijesinghe, M.; Perrin, K.; Ranchord, A.; Simmonds, M.; Beasley, R. Systematic review of studies o the effect of hyperoxia on coronary blood flow. *Am. Heart J.* **2009**, *158*, 371–377. [CrossRef]
44. Rousseau, A.; Steinwall, I.; Woodson, R.D.; Sjöberg, F. Hyperoxia decreases cutaneous blood flow in high-perfusion area *Microvasc. Res.* **2007**, *74*, 15–22. [CrossRef] [PubMed]
45. Hilderink, B.N.; Crane, R.F.; van den Bogaard, B.; Pillay, J.; Juffermans, N.P. Hyperoxemia and hypoxemia impair cellula oxygenation: A study in healthy volunteers. *Intensive Care Med. Exp.* **2024**, *12*, 37. [CrossRef] [PubMed]
46. Baumbach, P.; Neu, C.; Derlien, S.; Bauer, M.; Nisser, M.; Buder, A.; Coldewey, S.M. A pilot study of exercise-induced changes i mitochondrial oxygen metabolism measured by a cellular oxygen metabolism monitor (PICOMET). *Biochim. Biophys. Acta Mo Basis Dis.* **2019**, *1865*, 749–758. [CrossRef] [PubMed]
47. Ubbink, R.; Wefers Bettink, M.A.; van Weteringen, W.; Mik, E.G. Mitochondrial oxygen monitoring with COMET: Verification o calibration in man and comparison with vascular occlusion tests in healthy volunteers. *J. Clin. Monit. Comput.* **2021**, *35*, 1357–136 [CrossRef] [PubMed]
48. Flick, M.; Vokuhl, C.; Bergholz, A.; Boutchkova, K.; Nicklas, J.Y.; Saugel, B. Personalized intraoperative arterial pressure management and mitochondrial oxygen tension in patients having major non-cardiac surgery: A pilot substudy of the IMPROVE trial. *J. Clin. Monit. Comput.* **2025**, *39*, 813–820. [CrossRef]
49. Meyhoff, C.S.; Jorgensen, L.N.; Wetterslev, J.; Christensen, K.B.; Rasmussen, L.S. Increased long-term mortality after a high perioperative inspiratory oxygen fraction during abdominal surgery: Follow-up of a randomized clinical trial. *Anesth. Analg* **2012**, *115*, 849–854. [CrossRef] [PubMed]
50. Hilderink, B.N.; Crane, R.F.; Arbous, S.M.; van den Bogaard, B.; Pillay, J.; Juffermans, N.P. Low postoperative mitochondria oxygen tension is an early marker of acute kidney injury after cardiac surgery: A prospective observational study. *J. Crit. Care* **2025**, *88*, 155088. [CrossRef] [PubMed]
51. Liu, H.Y.; Tam, K.W.; Loh, E.W.; Liu, W.C.; Kuo, H.C.; Li, C.C.; Cherng, Y.G.; Chen, J.T.; Tai, Y.H. High-flow nasal oxygenation reduces the risk of desaturation in adults receiving procedural sedation: A meta-analysis of randomized controlled trials. *Perioper Med.* **2021**, *10*, 41. [CrossRef] [PubMed]
52. Koers, L.; Eberl, S.; Cappon, A.; Bouwman, A.; Schlack, W.; Hermanides, J.; Preckel, B. Safety of moderate-to-deep sedation performed by sedation practitioners: A national prospective observational study. *Eur. J. Anaesthesiol.* **2018**, *35*, 659–666. [CrossRef] [PubMed]

sensors

MDPI

rticle

·easibility of Wearable Devices for Motivating Post-Stroke ?atients

:laudia Marek [1,*], Jan Górski [1], Piotr Karolczyk [1], Justyna Redlicka [1], Igor Zubrycki [2] and Elżbieta Miller [1,*]

[1] Department of Neurological Rehabilitation, Medical University of Lodz, Milionowa 14, 93-113 Lodz, Poland; jan.gorski1@student.umed.lodz.pl (J.G.); piotr.karolczyk@student.umed.lodz.pl (P.K.); justyna.redlicka@umed.lodz.pl (J.R.)

[2] Institute of Automatic Control, Lodz University of Technology, Stefanowskiego 18, 90-537 Lodz, Poland; igor.zubrycki@p.lodz.pl

* Correspondence: klaudia.marek@umed.lodz.pl (K.M.); elzbieta.dorota.miller@umed.lodz.pl (E.M.)

Abstract: The effectiveness of upper extremity rehabilitation in post-stroke patients significantly depends on patient motivation and adherence to therapeutic regimens. Rehabilitation-assistive technologies, including wearable sensors, have been adopted to facilitate intensive and repetitive exercises aimed at reducing hand dysfunction and enhancing quality of life. Building upon the previously introduced Przypominajka (reminder) system reported in this journal—a wearable sensory glove coupled with a mobile application providing exercise guidance and monitoring—we conducted a feasibility study to evaluate its effectiveness in supporting upper limb rehabilitation. Sixteen post-stroke patients with hemiparesis were equally randomized into experimental and control groups. Both groups performed upper limb exercises for 45 min daily for over two weeks. The experimental group utilized the sensor-equipped glove and tablet-based exercises, whereas the control group followed printed exercise instructions. Clinical improvements were measured using the Fugl–Meyer Assessment–Upper Extremity (FMA-UE), Functional Independence Measure (FIM), and MORE scales. The experimental group demonstrated a minimal clinically important difference (MCID) on the FMA-UE and reported greater overall improvement than the control group. This study confirms the feasibility and potential clinical benefit of supplementing post-stroke rehabilitation with sensor-augmented exercises provided by the previously described Przypominajka device.

Keywords: neurorehabilitation; rehabilitation robot; wearable technology

1. Introduction

Limb motor dysfunction is the most common post-stroke complication, affecting approximately 80% of patients who survive a stroke. Half of the symptoms persist throughout their lives, resulting in disability [1]. Neurological patients require continuous, ongoing rehabilitation and comprehensive care after a stroke. The use of technology supported by sensory and robotic devices can positively impact rehabilitation by providing intensive, specific, and repetitive training to patients and reducing the physical burden on physiotherapists [2]. Up to two-thirds of patients who discontinue rehabilitation after six months experience additional post-stroke deficits and complications [3,4]. Improving hand function after stroke requires a multidisciplinary and multifactorial approach [5]. Studies in primates demonstrate that, to permanently acquire simple but new motor skills, a significant number of exercise repetitions (from 300 to 1500) is required so that changes in motor programming and neuronal reorganization may occur [6]. In the case of brain damage, the flow of information to and from the entire musculoskeletal system is partially or completely impaired, in the case of information both received from and sent to the central nervous system (CNS); therefore, it is possible that it takes an even higher minimum number of repetitions, a longer duration and, above all, a greater frequency of training. For this reason, it is vital for the post-stroke patient to receive individually tailored training that is as intensive as possible [7].

Up to 65% of post-stroke patients experience limb hemiparesis of various levels of severity, as well as other neurological symptoms, depending on the location, size, and extent of the brain injury [8]. In the medical literature, hemiparesis is defined as weakness or the inability to move on one side of the body [8]. It is a severe disorder of motor function characterized by decreased muscle strength [9,10]. Low muscle strength results in a limited range of motion in the joints and impaired balance and coordination of the body, which directly affect the entire rehabilitation process, as the patient is unable to perform many simple activities of daily living and may also experience fatigue more quickly [11]. As a result of hemiparesis, the patient's posture deteriorates, stretch reflexes are reduced, and voluntary movements are partly or completely impaired [12]. The clinical picture of a patient with hemiparesis is heterogeneous, because, apart from motor disorders, they may also experience sensory disturbances affecting, i.e., touch, hearing, sight, taste, and smell, cognitive and emotional disorders, as well as medical problems related to multimorbidity, especially in the elderly [13]. About 40% of people develop increased muscle tone, or spasticity, one year after a stroke. This condition develops one, three months after a stroke or even later. While muscle strength may gradually improve in hemiparesis, increased muscle tone becomes worse over time. This phenomenon is part of upper motor neuron syndrome [14].

Results from meta-analyses and systematic reviews confirm that rehabilitation supported by technology and robotics can improve the recovery process for both therapists and patients [2,15]. We can observe the special value of using robotics in the case of hand problems. It allows us to perform precise and useful movements in different planes, activating many muscle groups [15]. Robotic therapy can help in the recovery of motor function in patients with subacute conditions. If there are no medical contraindications, rehabilitation should begin in the early stage of stroke, because at this point, due to the phenomenon of brain plasticity, the regenerative potential is high [16]. According to the results of a survey on the use of robotics in rehabilitation by Li et al., specialists emphasize the ease of use of devices, seamless adaptation, and, most importantly, increased therapy and exercise for stroke patients. The main barriers identified by professionals are high costs and human resources [17].

Smartwatches have been successfully applied in the rehabilitation of cardiac patients. These compact devices can monitor heart rhythm safety using electrocardiograms powered by artificial intelligence algorithms [18]. Many patients already utilize smartwatches with exercise apps to support their activity levels [19]. In a study by Fan et al. (2024), smartwatch ownership with health monitoring capabilities led to increased daily step counts and overall physical activity among patients [20].

Analysis of the literature published over the last 15 years reveals a much smaller number of studies on digital technology in neurological patients, including post-stroke patients [21]. In terms of functional abilities, digital technology has been used to record indicators of walking and hand use in post-stroke patients [22]. A critical review of the measurement properties is presented, and factors that hinder and facilitate the implementation of applications in clinical practice and research are identified. Mobile applications are important and dependable for step counting in chronic stroke patients [23].

The growing demand for technology and its rapid advancement, particularly in the development of artificial intelligence, has driven the emergence of mobile health (mHealth). Healthcare demonstrates significant potential for data collection, which can be used to predict health status, guide treatment choices, and support medical research. The use of sensors in healthcare shows great promise in gathering new insights about patients' conditions [24]. Mobile applications are increasingly being adopted across various branches of medicine, enabling health condition monitoring, fast communication, education, and treatment adherence, especially in the case of chronic diseases [25]. The use of mobile applications by patients is part of digital therapeutics (DTx), a specialized field of healthcare, as defined by the Digital Therapeutics Alliance. The term refers to "the use of information and communication technologies to support health and health-related areas" [26]. Mobile applications in neurology do not have to be about exercise and rehabilitation only. Adcock et al. used mHealth to target secondary prevention of stroke. Adults who have experienced a stroke often use mobile applications on a smartphone to support daily activity [27]. Despite widespread access to digital technologies, there is a paucity of information on the use of mHealth apps in post-stroke patients. The number of platforms available to patients is increasing each year. However, the pace is not as fast as in the case of other diseases [21].

The primary benefits of digital therapies include reducing the costs and time associated with patient visits to the hospital, optimizing communication and administrative tasks within healthcare facilities, and providing continuous monitoring of health indicators for week-to-week comparisons. By constant interaction through an application, patients gain a better understanding of their own limitations and strengths [28]. Mobile applications expand the scope of healthcare services and enhance health management through the use of statistical data, such as physiological measurements [29]. This technology can be employed under the supervision of a specialist, with family support, or independently by the patient [30].

Rehabilitation based on supplementing therapy with sensory devices has great potential for neurological patients with complications involving movement disorders [31]. Previously in this journal, we described the design and technical evaluation of the Przypominajka system—a sensor glove coupled with a tablet application to guide, monitor, and motivate self-training for patients with plegic or paretic hands [32]. That initial work confirmed the system's on-device machine learning capabilities and positive patient feedback in a particular case study. Building upon that foundation, the primary aim of the current study was to conduct a randomized controlled trial to evaluate the clinical feasibility and therapeutic effectiveness of the Przypominajka system in a cohort of post-stroke patients. Specifically, we sought to determine if this sensor-augmented rehabilitation approach leads to greater improvements in upper extremity function compared to a standard exercise program. The aim of the study was to validate the authors' device—a prototype wearable sensory device with a tablet application designed for hand exercises for post-stroke patients with hand disorders (paresis/spasticity). We hypothesized that exercises with use of the glove would contribute to changes in self-care, upper limb recovery and functional improvement, and motivation.

2. Materials and Methods

2.1. Study Design

This study, conducted from February to July 2024, conformed to the standards of the Declaration of Helsinki and received approval from the Bioethics Committee of the Medical University of Lodz (RNN/281/20/KE) for the project "Single-use and personalizable devices for hand rehabilitation" (LIDER/50/0203/L-11/19/NCBR/2020). The study is part of a grant awarded by the National Center for Research and Development of Poland. All the patients included in the study received verbal and written information about the study and gave written informed consent to participate in it. The participants were also informed about the option to withdraw from the study at any time, without consequences. Twenty post-stroke patients were recruited according to the inclusion and exclusion criteria of the study, using 1:1 randomization into an experimental group (EG) and a control group (CG).

In this study, we compared the effects of specially designed exercises with the use of a mobile application and a prototype sensory glove developed for neurological patients with the results achieved when performing the same exercises based on paper instructions and not supported with the device. The patients in the control group were first instructed on how to correctly perform the exercises and then practiced independently. In the experimental group, the study participants received training on how to use the device and how to turn on and operate the application and put on the glove, and then exercised under the supervision of a physiotherapist. Both groups exercised for two weeks, with assessments conducted at three points: before the study began, after the first week, and at the end of the second week.

All the patients enrolled in the study received routine conventional in-ward neurological rehabilitation, five days a week, excluding weekends. The participants were recruited from the Department of Neurological Rehabilitation, Dr. Karol Jonscher Municipal Medical Center, in Łódź, Poland. Only post-ischemic stroke patients with upper limb impairment were included in the study. The study was conducted by physiotherapists in charge of the patients, physicians, and engineers responsible for the equipment and technology. The study was approved by the head of the department.

2.2. Participants

The study included post-ischemic stroke patients with neurological complications (paresis, spasticity) affecting the upper limb. The inclusion criteria for patients in the study were as follows: patients diagnosed with a stroke and MMSE (Mini-Mental State Examination) score above 24—not indicative of significant cognitive impairment, preventing understanding of instructions and participation in research. The exclusion criteria for the study were as follows: inflammatory diseases with fever, severe general condition, systemic diseases, severe cardiovascular conditions (less than 30 days post myocardial infarction, unstable angina pectoris, circulatory insufficiency, severe arrhythmia), impaired ability to understand and perceive, significant general deterioration, impaired understanding of instructions, impaired perception or a significant general decline in cognitive function (with MMSE score as an indicator), uncompensated metabolic and endocrine diseases, and respiratory failure. We recruited 20 patients (ten women and ten men); however, in the course of the study, 4 patients (two women and two men) were excluded—one patient withdrew due to difficulties in understanding the exercises and low motivation, and three patients were transferred to the internal medicine ward due to the development of other stroke-related complications (Figure 1). Before the beginning of the upper extremity training program, the other 16 patients underwent medical assessments.

Sixteen patients (eight women and eight men) participated in the study. Approximately one month after stroke, three patients were in an acute condition, five patients were in the subacute phase for up to six months, and eight patients were in the chronic phase for more than six months. On average, it had been 15.5 months since the patients' strokes. Paresis occurred with equal frequency (50%) on the left and right sides, corresponding to a 1:1 ratio. The average age of the participants was 67.5 years.

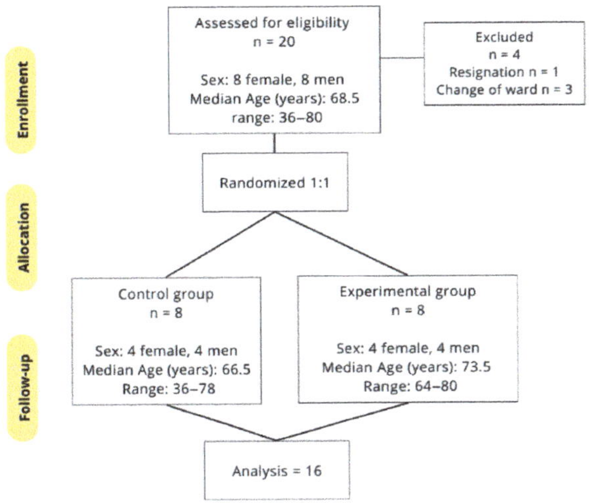

Figure 1. Scheme of the survey structure.

Among the 16 patients participating in the study, as many as 8 were found to have more than one comorbid condition (50%). The comorbid conditions present among participants occurred with the following frequencies: hypertension (62.5%), diabetes (25%), hypercholesterolemia (31.25%), nicotine addiction (50%), hypothyroidism (12.5%), ischemic heart disease (6.25%), sleep apnea (6.25%), and heart attack (6.25%).

2.3. *Assessment of Patients*

Prior to the study, patients were clinically assessed using specialized scales that provided experts with information on their functional state of motivation and the progression/regression of disorders present in the affected upper limb after stroke.

The recruited patients underwent tests using the following clinical scales:

- Fugl–Meyer Assessment–Upper Extremity (FMA-UE);
- Motivation scale (MORE);
- Functional Independence Measure (FIM).

2.3.1. Fugl–Meyer Assessment Upper Extremity (FMA-UE)

Functional assessment of the upper extremity after stroke was assessed using the Fugl–Meyer Upper Extremity Assessment (FMA-UE). This is a commonly used scale that also tests sensorimotor conditions and the associated dysfunction of the upper extremity resulting from stroke [Hassani]. The subscales included in the form allow for accurate and detailed assessment of the affected upper extremity (A—Upper Extremity, B—Wrist, C—Hand, D—Coordination/Speed, H—Sensation, I—Passive Joint Motion, and J—Joint Pain). The FMA-UE has been well known to clinicians for many years as a tool frequently used to measure outcomes. Studies have shown that, based on the FMA-UE scale, it is possible to predict the prognosis of functional status during the first days and weeks after a stroke. Thus, it is possible to plan the rehabilitation process and treatment and evaluate outcomes [33–35].

2.3.2. Motivation Scale (MORE)

The MORE scale is a recently published scale invented by Yoshida et al. Their goal was to develop a scale of motivation to rehabilitation for post-stroke patients according to standards based on the Consensus on the Selection of Health Measurement Instruments (COSMIN). The MORE scale addresses two factors that influence patient attitudes—personal factors and those related to social relations [36]. It consists of 17 items that address questions about rehabilitation, capacity, interpersonal relationships, and willingness.

2.3.3. Functional Independence Measure (FIM)

The FIM scale consists of 18 items. It is divided into smaller subscales related to self-care, sphincter control, mobility, locomotion, communication, and social awareness. The score obtained by the patient indicates their level of functional ability [37]. The maximum total score is 126, which corresponds to no problems at the level of functional independence and self-care.

2.4. *Przypominajka Device and Intervention*

The smartwatch-like device was named Przypominajka (Polish for Reminder), as its aim is to constantly remind patients to perform exercises throughout the day. The device consists of a sensory glove that connects to a tablet application via Bluetooth Low Energy. The application displays the exercises the patient should perform, specifically those focused on the wrist joint and forearm. During exercise sessions, the application collects data on how well the exercises are performed. The goal is to achieve five full stars for each exercise, which represents a high-intensity workout with a large number of repetitions. The application randomly selects exercises from a pre-selected set. Each exercise lasts five minutes and is followed by a five-minute break. Each single session includes five exercises. In total, the patient spends 25 min exercising and 20 min resting, as there is no break after the last exercise.

The study can be divided into five stages. The first stage involves medical assessment of the patients before the beginning of an exercise session. The second stage includes the first week of patient exercise using both graphic instructions and the device. The third stage involves assessment of the patients after the first week of exercise. The fourth stage includes assessment in the second week, and in the final fifth stage, the patients are assessed after completing two weeks of the training sessions (Figure 2).

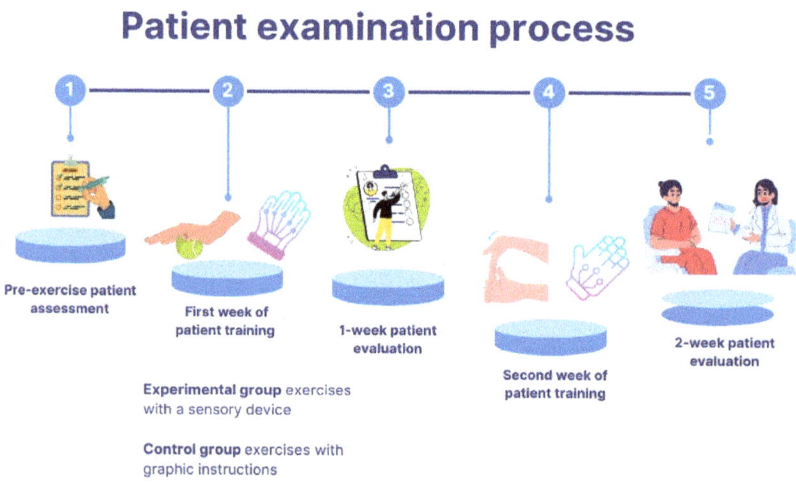

Figure 2. Scheme of the patient-training study.

Przypominajka is a sensory device in the form of a glove worn by a stroke patient on the middle finger, thumb, and wrist of the affected hand. Attached to the device is a tablet with an application that allows the patient to collect points (in the form of stars) that provide information on whether the patient has done enough repetitions and performed the exercises correctly. This is also feedback for the patient, to motivate them to practice further and to signal the correctness of completed tasks. Displayed exercises are randomly selected from among eight suggested movement tasks (Figure 3). When performing an exercise, the patient can receive from zero to five stars, depending on the accuracy of their movements. Five stars correspond to 80% accuracy. The device also allows a margin of error.

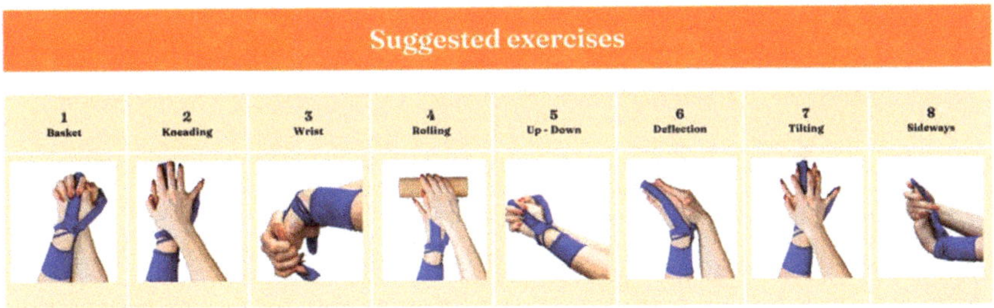

Figure 3. Suggested exercises available in the application.

The device is connected to the tablet via Bluetooth Low Energy (BLE). The multimedia application was created using MIT App Inventor 2 (AI2) (Cambridge, MA, USA). The program allows the start and end time of the exercises to be set. The application guides the patient step by step through each session (Figure 4). Once the time is set and the start button is clicked, the patient immediately proceeds to the exercise. The use of such a simple start screen greatly facilitates the use of the device for patients with cognitive function problems, which often occur as a post-stroke complication. After starting the exercise, the application allows the patient a short time to familiarize themself with the next task, which is described with simple commands and supported by a series of pictures illustrating the movement pattern. The tablet beeps at the end of the pause, and the patient clicks the start button to indicate that they are ready to resume the exercise. With this solution, the patient is not forced to control the break time, for fear of omitting the next task.

The device is based on a WEMOS LOLIN32 board (WEMOS Electronics, Shenzhen, China) with an ESP32 microcontroller (Espressif Systems, Shanghai, China), (Dual Core Tensilica LX6 240 MHz processor, 520 KB of SRAM, and 4 MB of external flash memory) and a custom-made circuit to collect data from the flexion sensors and from a six-axis IMU (acceleration, rotation) as the patient moves. The flexion sensors are located on the middle finger and thumb (Figure 5). The sensors on the device use a change in the flexion angle to change the resistance of the sensor (flex sensor, Spectra Symbol, Salt Lake City, UT, USA). A step change in the angle causes the change in sensor resistance to disappear. The flexion is measured by a voltage divider-type circuit with a fixed resistor, and the voltage is measured by the ADC circuit of the ESP 32 microcontroller. The sensors are not calibrated; instead, the raw ADC values are applied. The IMU (an MPU6080 integrated accelerometer and gyroscope) displays the angular velocity and acceleration via the I2C interface.

A machine learning-based approach is used to classify a two-second moving window of sensor data, which is sampled at a frequency of 21 Hz. The classification accuracy, which determines if an exercise was performed correctly or incorrectly, was evaluated in a previous study in a set of healthy participants. This evaluation yielded an overall accuracy of 91.3%, with a precision of 90%, a recall of 94%, and an $f1$ score of 91%.

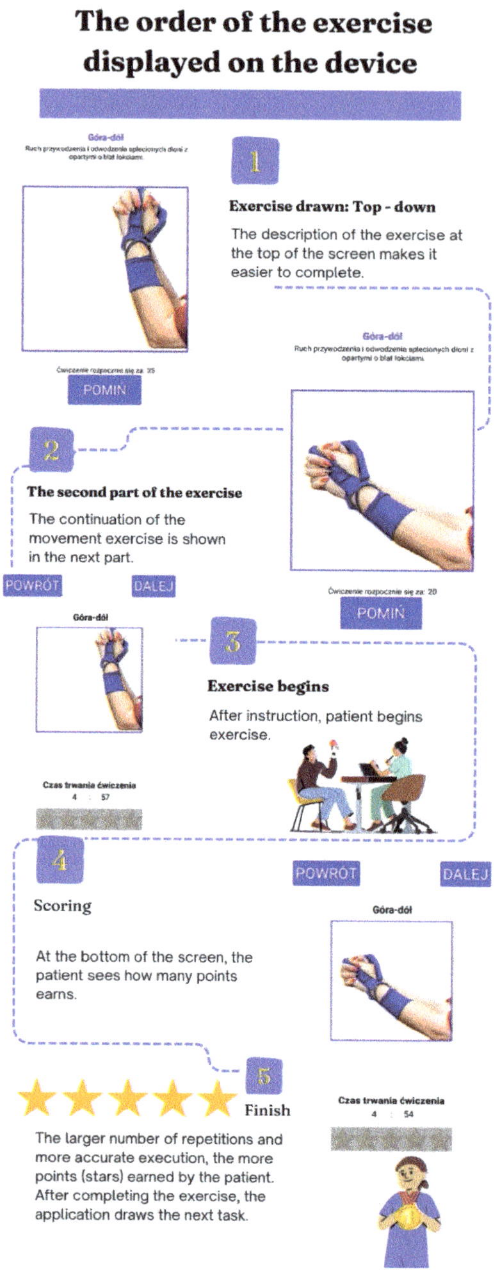

Figure 4. Scheme of application use during the exercise. Góra-dół—Up and down; Ruch przywodzenia i odwodzenia splecionych dłoni z opartymi o blat łokciami—Adduction and abduction movement of interlaced hands with elbows resting on the tabletop; Czas trwania ćwiczenia—Duration of exercise; Powrót—Back; Dalej—Next.

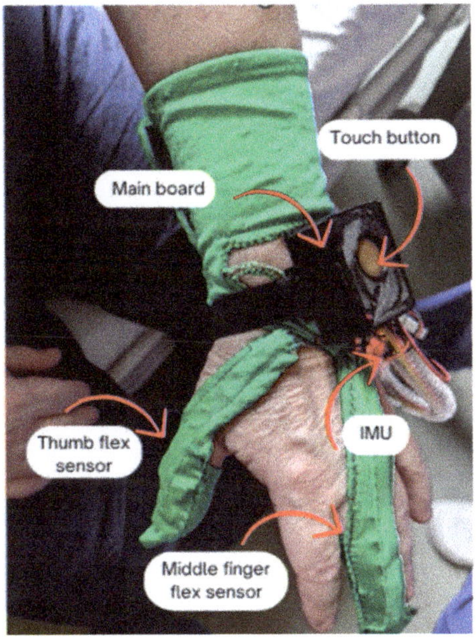

Figure 5. Construction of the device presented on the patient's hand.

The model, a convolutional neural network (CNN), uses a two-second input vector (containing 42 samples) composed of data from the flex sensors, accelerometer, and gyroscope. Due to the highly nonlinear transformations within the CNN, an ablation study was conducted to evaluate the importance of each sensor's data. This study revealed that the IMU (MPU6080 accelerometer + gyroscope, InvenSense (TDK) San Jose, CA, USA) data was the most critical feature set. Removing the IMU data caused the model's accuracy to drop significantly, from 91.3% to 80.3%. Conversely, the flex sensor data was found to be less important, as removing it only caused the categorization accuracy to decrease slightly, to 89.7%. More details can be found in a previous article in which we introduced the device and explained the machine-based approach [32].

3. Results

Statistical Analysis

Statistical analyses were performed in Python (Statsmodels 0.13.5) for each clinical scale (MORE, FIM, FMA-UE). Within-group changes (week 1 to week 3) were analyzed with paired *t*-tests; between-group differences in change scores were assessed with Student's *t*-test or Welch's *t*-test when Levene's test indicated unequal variances. Normality was evaluated using the Shapiro–Wilk test and visual inspection of Q–Q plots. Equal variance was tested with Levene's test. Effect sizes were calculated as Cohen's d for paired or independent samples, with 0.2, 0.5, and 0.8 interpreted as small, moderate, and large, respectively. Statistical significance was defined as $p < 0.05$. The results obtained are presented as boxplots (Figure 6).

Assumption checks indicated that MORE and FMA-UE change scores did not deviate from normality in either group, whereas FIM deviated from normality. Variances were equal for MORE and FIM and unequal for FMA-UE, for which Welch's *t*-test was applied for between-group comparison (Tables 1 and 2).

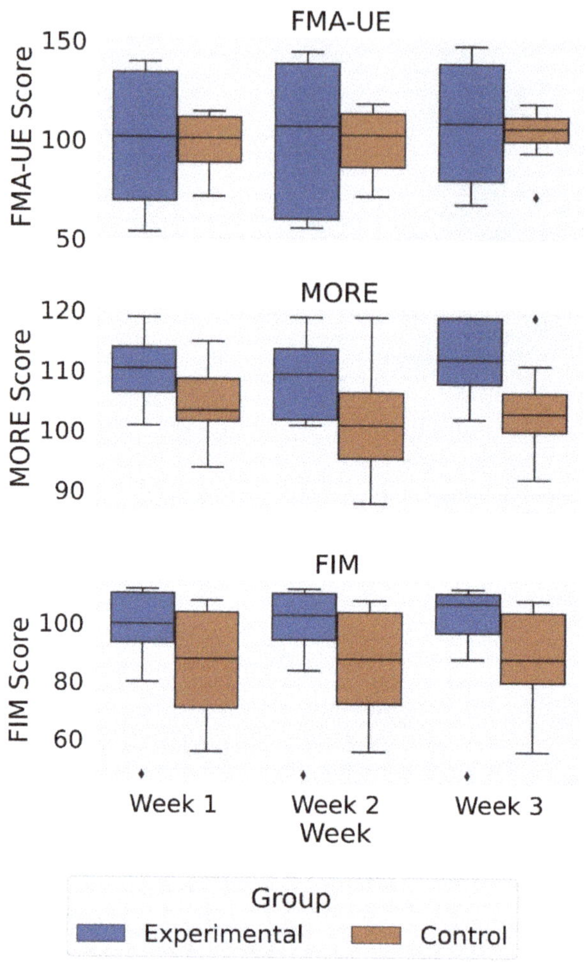

Figure 6. Box plot comparing outcomes for the experimental and control groups at weeks 1/2/3. Boxes denote the interquartile range with median lines; whiskers indicate 1.5 × IQR; individual points represent participants.

Table 1. Assumption checks and between-group comparisons.

Scale	Shapiro–Wilk p (Exp) (a)	Shapiro–Wilk p (Ctrl) (a)	Levene p (b)	Student's t-Test p (c)	Welch's t-Test p (d)	Cohen's d (e)
MORE	0.437	0.397	0.519	0.160	—	0.74
FIM	0.004	<0.001	0.436	0.515	—	0.34
FMA-UE	0.821	0.177	0.0058	0.657	0.660	0.23

(a) Shapiro–Wilk test for normality of change scores within each group; $p > 0.05$ indicates no evidence against normality. (b) Levene's test for equality of variances between groups; $p > 0.05$ indicates equal variances. (c) Between-group comparison of change scores assuming equal variances. (d) Between-group comparison of change scores, not assuming equal variances (reported when Levene's $p < 0.05$). (e) Cohen's d effect size for the between-group difference in change scores (small ≈ 0.2, moderate ≈ 0.5, large ≥ 0.8).

Table 2. Within-group paired *t*-tests.

Scale	Group	*n*	Mean Δ	SD Δ	*t* (*n* − 1)	*p*-Value	Cohen's d (f)
MORE	Experimental	8	2.25	4.10	−1.55	0.164	0.55
MORE	Control	8	−1.12	4.94	0.64	0.540	−0.23
FIM	Experimental	8	3.00	4.66	−1.82	0.111	0.64
FIM	Control	8	1.50	4.24	−1.00	0.351	0.35
FMA-UE	Experimental	8	9.38	9.90	−2.68	0.0316	0.95
FMA-UE	Control	8	5.38	22.88	−0.66	0.528	0.23

(f) Cohen's d for paired samples calculated as mean change divided by the standard deviation of change scores.

In the case of the MORE scale, the experimental group showed a mean increase of 2.25 points ($p = 0.164$; d = 0.55), while the control group decreased by 1.12 points ($p = 0.540$; d = −0.23). The between-group difference in change scores was not statistically significant (Student's *t*, $p = 0.160$; d = 0.74). The results for the FIM scale are as follows: the experimental group improved by 3.00 points ($p = 0.111$; d = 0.64), and the control group improved by 1.50 points ($p = 0.351$; d = 0.35). The between-group difference in change scores was not significant (Student's *t*, $p = 0.515$; d = 0.34). As a sensitivity check for non-normality, non-parametric tests (Wilcoxon within groups; Mann–Whitney between groups) yielded the same conclusions. Nevertheless, the FMA-EU scale is an exception: the experimental group showed statistically and clinically significant improvement (Δ = +9.38 points, $p = 0.0316$; d = 0.95), meeting or closely approaching commonly cited MCID ranges for upper extremity FMA (~9–10 points). The control group improved by 5.38 points ($p = 0.528$; d = 0.23). Levene's test indicated unequal variances; Welch's *t* test confirmed that the between-group difference in change scores was not significant ($t(9.53) = 0.454$, $p = 0.660$; d = 0.23).

4. Discussion

Our study answers the question of whether a relatively simple device, such as a glove with an attached tablet and an application that randomizes exercises, is useful in post-stroke hand rehabilitation. We find that the wearable Przypominajka device is helpful in the hand rehabilitation process. As an additional therapy, it has been shown to motivate patients and improve hand function and independence. The device allows for high-intensity multifactorial therapy that can improve the motor recovery process in the affected limb [38]. Passive and active movements of the upper limb, suggested as exercises in the application, can enhance motor recovery not only by activating somatosensory stimuli, but also through motor planning and soft tissue properties [16,39].

Smartphones and tablets have been increasingly used by many people, making the implementation of exercise applications relatively easy and inexpensive. Home-based mobile exercise applications for post-stroke patients show great efficacy, which was demonstrated by Chung et al. The results obtained by us confirm the findings of previous studies, namely that a mobile video-based exercise program is more effective than a standard paper-based exercise program. In our study, patients in the experimental group exercised with the application and a sensory glove, which had a significant impact on their sense of motivation in the rehabilitation process. They followed the application's exercise recommendations more carefully, which resulted in improvements in mobility [40]. An interesting solution was applied by Kim et al., who used scores to motivate patients to achieve better results. The team proposed a self-care rehabilitation system with automatic scoring of the movements made by the patient. Exercises are performed at home and recorded by an application installed on a smartphone. The automated system estimates the result of a completed task after analyzing the uploaded video. The completed task is scored from 0 to 3 points. After the exercise, the patient receives a report on progress or deterioration of the function and exercise recommendations [41]. Our application proposes a scoring system from 0 to 5 points, which allows for a greater variety of possible outcomes. The feedback is provided in real time, based on data fusion from an IMU and flex sensors. Also, by using a glove-based solution, the hand can be accurately tracked even when visual occlusions (due to specificity of exercises) happen.

This study used exercise applications for stroke patients, which may have a positive impact on the phenomenon of digital exclusion among elderly people with neurological conditions [42]. Patients relied on physiotherapists to operate the applications and switch exercises due to their lack of confidence in their ability to use such applications. This attitude, often observed among older adults, stems from digital exclusion, defined as inequality in access to and the ability to use information and communication technologies (ICTs), such as the Internet [43]. Digital disadvantage is most prevalent among elderly people, who make up the largest proportion of this group worldwide [44]. Despite the widespread use of smartphones, there is still a noticeable gap between particular age groups in terms of using ICT services [45]. In Poland, 82% of seniors aged 55–74 years show a low level of digital literacy. According to 2023 data, 75% of Polish seniors aged 60–74 years have never used the Internet [46]. Research has linked digital exclusion to poor physical and mental health in older adults [47,48]. The non-use of digital services is not only due to a lack of skills, but also to health-related barriers that limit older adults' ability to learn new technologies. These barriers include visual impairments, as well as motor impairments caused by musculoskeletal or neurological conditions, dementia, and difficulties with activities of daily living (ADLs) [49]. Factors contributing to digital exclusion include a lack of Internet skills, an inability to afford Internet access or digital devices, and a refusal to use the Internet, either by the individual or their family [43,50,51]. Older adults who are excluded from digital services are more likely to develop functional dependency, regardless of whether they live in high- or low-income countries [44].

The subacute phase begins approximately seven days after stroke. This phase is characterized by the onset of regenerative processes [52]. The subacute and chronic phases are associated with specific post-stroke repair processes, mainly neoangiogenesis and neurogenesis, respectively [53]. In the subacute phase, brain plasticity and neurorepair aim at restoring the lost core of brain tissue after stroke [54]. The chronic phase begins four weeks after stroke onset [53]. Scientific evidence in humans suggests that there is a spontaneous recovery of function within the first three months, which results from a complex pattern of brain reorganization [55]. In our study, we recruited patients in the subacute and chronic post-stroke phases and presented the rationale for prolonging rehabilitation. A greater improvement on the clinical scales was observed in the patients exercising with a sensory glove, while the control group, using graphic exercise instructions, showed a smaller increase on the FIM scales and in the FMA-UE total score.

Even in 2024, there is still a lack of information on the most effective neurological rehabilitation for post-stroke patients that could maximize the recovery process. We know that rehabilitation in the subacute phase can provide great functional benefits and reverse motor complications [56,57]. Rehabilitation and exercise should not be abandoned in the chronic phase, even though we know that the most significant recovery of motor function occurs within the first six months after stroke. The rate of recovery and return of function slows down significantly after six months; however, some improvement is still possible [58].

Rehabilitation using technology, including a smartwatch or robot, in conjunction with conventional rehabilitation can yield satisfactory outcomes in both the subacute and chronic phases [59,60]. This type of rehabilitation is easy to perform, can be delivered in non-hospital settings, and is widely available to a wide range of patients. It affects motor learning ability and improves hand function [61,62]. Many studies present robots, including exoskeletons that are large, heavy, and driven by rigid joints, that perform movement during training tasks [63]. This gives the option of performing precise movements; however, for many patients it is also a limitation, and there is often interference in the interaction [64]. Our device is made of a soft material, so its weight, even with cables attached, is low. It is handy, cheap, and easy to manufacture. It can be adjusted to fit the size of the patient's hand and can be used in different environments, such as in hospitals or at home. The COVID-19 pandemic [65] has shown us the importance of creating opportunities for full or continued rehabilitation at home. In this field, there is a need for strategies and technological support to ensure continuity of therapy for patients. A study by Chae et al. (2020) conducted during the pandemic showed that a home care system using a commercially available smartwatch can facilitate participation in home exercise and improve hand functional outcome in post-stroke patients [65]. The application for therapy that we propose is easy to use and intuitive, as subsequent steps are guided by arrows. Przypominajka is available for all devices based on the Android operating system. The application does not have unnecessary options or functions that could be confusing to the patient and cause problems with returning to the main panel and exercises.

The patients in the experimental group were given tablets with a mobile exercise application during the trial. All of the subjects had previous exposure to digital technology, as they had personal smartphones with mobile Internet and used them daily. One patient who withdrew from the study at his own request had no active contact with technology. He did not own a smartphone and felt confused when using a mobile application on a tablet. A similar form of glove was proposed by Nathan et al. to support grip function in self-care therapy for post-stroke patients. The glove was used to measure thumb and finger joint angles and grip. The device assisted the patient in performing a grasping movement. The study demonstrated the potential of measuring grip during functional tasks performed by patients. However, a significant number of researchers designing gloves use thick materials that cover the entire hand, making it difficult for the patient to perform a movement [66]. Wearable technology has proven to be a promising adjunctive therapy that can be delivered at home. Maintenance costs are low, and high availability allows for individualized rehabilitation [67].

Stroke patients often become angry and frustrated when it becomes clear that they have not achieved all their goals and have not regained their physical form. Rehabilitation should be designed in a way that motivates the patient and has a visible effect on their condition. If the patient is not motivated to exercise, even with the support of the best physiotherapists, they will not be able to achieve a satisfactory rehabilitation outcome [68]. Rehabilitation of stroke patients is long-term; it often takes time to obtain satisfactory results. Therefore, it is believed that rehabilitation of post-stroke patients is a lifelong process [69]. Currently, there is an ongoing discussion in the research community on how to increase motivation for rehabilitation in post-stroke patients [70]. In our study, we assessed motivation using the MORE scale. At the beginning of the therapy process, the patients in both groups showed low motivation to exercise, which increased in the experimental group during the second week of training compared to the control group; however, the level of motivation was still not very high. The results presented here confirm previous assumptions by other authors that motivating post-stroke patients to participate in rehabilitation can sometimes be difficult, so a social and psychological intervention model should be introduced in the future to provide social and psychological support to patients [68].

Our study has some limitations. It was carried out in 16 patients after a stroke, and the participants exercised for two weeks (14 days) only. More reliable results and conclusions can be drawn with a longer study period and a larger sample size. Due to the small sample size and short time period, it may not be possible to detect an existing effect, resulting in low statistical power. The potential for overestimating effects increases with a small number of patients, so large, randomized, open-label studies and blinded trials should be conducted after small pilot studies. The FMA-EU scale is an exception, as the experimental group improved by 9.38 points ($p = 0.0316$; d = 0.95, large). This exceeds commonly cited minimal detectable change (MDC) values for chronic stroke (~5.2 points) and meets or closely approaches minimal clinically important difference (MCID) estimates for subacute stroke (≈9–10 points), supporting both clinical and statistical significance [56,71]. The control group improved by 5.38 points ($p = 0.528$; d = 0.23), below MCID thresholds. Levene's test indicated unequal variances ($p = 0.0058$); Welch's t-test confirmed that the between-group difference was not significant ($t(9.53) = 0.454$, $p = 0.660$; d = 0.23). Regarding patient outcomes on the FIM scale, the experimental group improved by 3.0 points ($p = 0.111$; d = 0.64, moderate) and the control group by 1.5 points ($p = 0.351$; d = 0.35). Both changes are well below reported MCID values for stroke rehabilitation (≈22 points for total FIM; ≈17 points for the Motor subscore) [72], indicating that the observed gains are unlikely to be clinically meaningful over a two-week interval. Changes in FIM scores violated the normality assumption in both groups but had equal variances; non-parametric Wilcoxon and Mann–Whitney tests yielded the same conclusions as the parametric tests. In the case of the MORE scale, the experimental group increased by 2.25 points ($p = 0.164$; d = 0.55, moderate), while the control group decreased by 1.12 points ($p = 0.540$; d = −0.23). No between-group difference was statistically significant ($p = 0.160$; d = 0.74). To our knowledge, no MCID for the MORE scale has been published, so clinical significance must be inferred from effect size and direction of change rather than a threshold [73]. There are several reasons why p-values differ across scales. The FMA-UE measures impairment-level motor recovery and is typically more sensitive to short-duration, targeted upper-limb training, which explains the statistically and clinically significant within-group improvement in the experimental group. In contrast, the FIM reflects broader functional independence and requires larger or longer-term gains to surpass MCID thresholds, consistent with the small, non-significant changes observed here. Motivation (MORE) improved directionally with a moderate effect size, but large variability in score changes, particularly in the control group for FMA-UE, and the small sample size reduced the statistical power for between-group differences. These patterns are consistent with the differing constructs, responsiveness, and MCID benchmarks of the three scales.

Another limitation that arose during the study was the number of exercises presented by the application. According to the patients, it was low, and frequent repetition of the same exercises that had already appeared earlier in the session may have led to patient boredom. It was not uncommon for patients to ask for the exercise to be selected again. The patients also commented on the lack of stretching exercises, which are useful for spastic paresis. The digital exclusion of older patients seemed to be another limitation. Despite the large and bold font in the application, the patients were reluctant to use the tablet on their own. Before starting the exercises, they were given detailed instructions on how to use the application, and they read all the messages in the application on their own. Unfortunately, this was not enough to encourage older patients to use the application without assistance. They did not feel confident enough and sometimes had difficulty reading the words in the application. This is not surprising, as stroke patients often show cognitive impairment at various visuospatial levels, problems with orientation, attention focus, or memory. Delayed recovery of the above functions is an inherent part of the recovery process after stroke. It is related to cerebral ischemia and hypoxia during the development of a stroke lesion [74,75]. The prototype glove proved difficult for most patients to wear. A physiotherapist was always available during training; however, staff encouraged the patients to use the device themselves, with the aim of achieving independence. Unfortunately, in several cases, patients required assistance, cables got tangled, and the fitting process was prolonged. In one case, a cable broke, and the device had to be checked and repaired quickly. It should be noted that our device is a prototype with components printed on a 3D printer. These findings confirm and expand upon the ergonomic challenges identified in our initial case study. The difficulty patients experienced in putting on the glove and the prototype's durability issues highlight that, while the sensing and software concepts are viable, significant hardware refinement is necessary for independent use. Furthermore, a key technical limitation noted in our previous work was a drop in the classification accuracy of the machine learning model when applied to new users not included in the original training set. The positive clinical outcomes observed in this trial were achieved despite this known imperfection in the scoring algorithm's generalizability. This suggests that even a directionally correct, encouraging feedback system can be motivating and effective, but it also underscores the potential for even greater gains if the system incorporated methods for rapid personalization or on-device learning for new patients.

Our study has shown that additional training with a sensory glove and application leads to better scores on clinical scales. This means improvements in hand function, self-care, and functional independence and a greater motivation to exercise. The observed improvement was not significant in all cases, which clearly indicates that the challenge faced by physiotherapists and occupational therapists in relation to rehabilitation of the wrist in post-stroke patients is difficult. In terms of degrees of freedom, after the shoulder, the wrist is the second most complex upper limb joint. The complexity of its structure also makes it difficult to rehabilitate [76]. The use of adjunctive therapy with a wearable device in the form of a sensory glove with an application has added variety to routine rehabilitation and motivated patients to exercise. However, the therapy needs to be refined to be more useful in rehabilitation.

After completing the study, all patients received graphic instructions for the exercises they performed during the pilot program. It is planned to increase the number of participants in the future and conduct the study simultaneously in several international centers, which will allow for more reliable conclusions to be drawn regarding the future use of the device for stroke patients with hand paresis.

5. Conclusions

Additional upper limb exercises using an exercise application and a sensory glove that controls the precision and quantity of the exercises can have a positive impact on the post-stroke rehabilitation process as an adjunct therapy. Increasing the number of exercises for neurological patients led to better results on clinical scales, which corresponds to improved hand function, independence, and functional autonomy, or increased motivation for rehabilitation. Different solutions should be sought to reduce digital exclusion and encourage older people to diversify their neurological rehabilitation.

Author Contributions: Conceptualization, K.M., I.Z. and E.M.; methodology, I.Z. and K.M.; software, I.Z.; validation, J.R., J.G. and P.K.; formal analysis, E.M.; investigation, K.M.; resources I.Z. and K.M.; data curation, I.Z. and K.M.; writing—original draft preparation, K.M. and J.R.; writing—review and editing, K.M. and I.Z.; visualization, K.M.; supervision, E.M.; project administration, K.M.; funding acquisition, E.M. All authors have read and agreed to the published version of the manuscript.

Funding: Funding from a grant by the National Centre for Research and Development (grant number LIDER/50/0203/L-11/19/NCBR/2020) made this project possible.

Institutional Review Board Statement: The Bioethics Committee of the Medical University of Łódź approved the study for the project "Single-use and personalizable devices for hand rehabilitation" (LIDER/50/0203/L-11/19/NCBR/2020) (RNN/281/20/KE). The study was conducted in accordance with the Declaration of Helsinki.

Informed Consent Statement: Informed consent was obtained from all subjects involved in the study.

Data Availability Statement: The article contains all of the data.

Conflicts of Interest: The authors declare no conflicts of interest.

References

1. Kim, J.; Thayabaranathan, T.; Donnan, G.A.; Howard, G.; Howard, V.J.; Rothwell, P.M.; Feigin, V.; Norrving, B.; Owolabi, M. Pandian, J.; et al. Global Stroke Statistics 2019. *Int. J. Stroke* **2020**, *15*, 819–838. [CrossRef]
2. Bertani, R.; Melegari, C.; De Cola, M.C.; Bramanti, A.; Bramanti, P.; Calabro, R.S. Effects of robot-assisted upper limb rehabilitation in stroke patients: A systematic review with meta-analysis. *Neurol. Sci.* **2017**, *38*, 1561–1569. [CrossRef]
3. Singh, R.J.; Chen, S.; Ganesh, A.; Hill, M.D. Long-term neurological, vascular, and mortality outcomes after stroke. *Int. J. Stroke* **2018**, *13*, 787–796. [CrossRef] [PubMed]
4. Dembovski, A.; Amitai, Y.; Levy-Tzedek, S. A Socially Assistive Robot for Stroke Patients: Acceptance, Needs, and Concerns of Patients and Informal Caregivers. *Front. Rehabil. Sci.* **2021**, *2*, 793233. [CrossRef] [PubMed]
5. Franceschini, M.; Ceravolo, M.G.; Agosti, M.; Cavallini, P.; Bonassi, S.; Dall'Armi, V.; Massucci, M.; Schifini, F.; Sale, P. Clinical relevance of action observation in upper-limb stroke rehabilitation: A possible role in recovery of functional dexterity. A randomized clinical trial. *Neurorehabilit. Neural Repair* **2012**, *26*, 456–462. [CrossRef] [PubMed]
6. Yin, P.B.; Kitazawa, S. Long-lasting aftereffects of prism adaptation in the monkey. *Exp. Brain Res.* **2001**, *141*, 250–253. [CrossRef]
7. Kwakkel, G.; Kollen, B.; Lindeman, E. Understanding the pattern of functional recovery after stroke: Facts and theories. *Restor Neurol. Neurosci.* **2004**, *22*, 281–299. [CrossRef]
8. Cauraugh, J.H.; Kim, S.B. Chronic stroke motor recovery: Duration of active neuromuscular stimulation. *J. Neurol. Sci.* **2003**, *215* 13–19. [CrossRef]
9. Wist, S.; Clivaz, J.; Sattelmayer, M. Muscle strengthening for hemiparesis after stroke: A meta-analysis. *Ann. Phys. Rehabil. Med* **2016**, *59*, 114–124. [CrossRef]
10. Bohannon, R.W. Muscle strength and muscle training after stroke. *J. Rehabil. Med.* **2007**, *39*, 14–20. [CrossRef]
11. Rabelo, M.; Nunes, G.S.; da Costa Amante, N.M.; de Noronha, M.; Fachin-Martins, E. Reliability of muscle strength assessment in chronic post-stroke hemiparesis: A systematic review and meta-analysis. *Top. Stroke Rehabil.* **2016**, *23*, 26–36. [CrossRef]
12. Mehta, S.; Pereira, S.; Viana, R.; Mays, R.; McIntyre, A.; Janzen, S.; Teasell, R.W. Resistance training for gait speed and total distance walked during the chronic stage of stroke: A meta-analysis. *Top. Stroke Rehabil.* **2012**, *19*, 471–478. [CrossRef]
13. Owen, M.; Ingo, C.; Dewald, J.P. Upper extremity motor impairments and microstructural changes in bulbospinal pathways in chronic hemiparetic stroke. *Front. Neurol.* **2017**, *8*, 257. [CrossRef]
14. de-la-Torre, R.; Ona, E.D.; Balaguer, C.; Jardon, A. Robot-Aided Systems for Improving the Assessment of Upper Limb Spasticity: A Systematic Review. *Sensors* **2020**, *20*, 5251. [CrossRef] [PubMed]
15. Sheng, B.; Zhang, Y.; Meng, W.; Deng, C.; Xie, S. Bilateral robots for upper-limb stroke rehabilitation: State of the art and future prospects. *Med. Eng. Phys.* **2016**, *38*, 587–606. [CrossRef] [PubMed]
16. Sale, P.; Franceschini, M.; Mazzoleni, S.; Palma, E.; Agosti, M.; Posteraro, F. Effects of upper limb robot-assisted therapy on motor recovery in subacute stroke patients. *J. Neuroeng. Rehabil.* **2014**, *11*, 104. [CrossRef] [PubMed]
17. Li, L.; Tyson, S.; Weightman, A. Professionals' Views and Experiences of Using Rehabilitation Robotics with Stroke Survivors: A Mixed Methods Survey. *Front. Med. Technol.* **2021**, *3*, 780090. [CrossRef]

18. Maille, B.; Wilkin, M.; Million, M.; Resseguier, N.; Franceschi, F.; Koutbi-Franceschi, L.; Hourdain, J.; Martinez, E.; Zabern, M.; Gardella, C.; et al. Smartwatch Electrocardiogram and Artificial Intelligence for Assessing Cardiac-Rhythm Safety of Drug Therapy in the COVID-19 Pandemic. The QT-logs study. *Int. J. Cardiol.* **2021**, *331*, 333–339. [CrossRef]
19. Martinato, M.; Lorenzoni, G.; Zanchi, T.; Bergamin, A.; Buratin, A.; Azzolina, D.; Gregori, D. Usability and Accuracy of a Smartwatch for the Assessment of Physical Activity in the Elderly Population: Observational Study. *JMIR mHealth uHealth* **2021**, *9*, e20966. [CrossRef]
20. Fan, J.; Liu, Q.; Dai, H.; Zhou, D.; Guo, Y.; Xu, J.; Wang, L.; Hu, P.; Jiang, J.; Lin, X.; et al. Daily Physical Activity Measured by Wearable Smartwatch for Patients Undergoing Transcatheter Aortic Valve Replacement: Insights from the SMART TAVR Study. *Circ. Cardiovasc. Qual. Outcomes* **2024**, *17*, e010066. [CrossRef]
21. Burns, S.P.; Terblanche, M.; Perea, J.; Lillard, H.; DeLaPena, C.; Grinage, N.; MacKinen, A.; Cox, E.E. mHealth Intervention Applications for Adults Living with the Effects of Stroke: A Scoping Review. *Arch. Rehabil. Res. Clin. Transl.* **2021**, *3*, 100095. [CrossRef] [PubMed]
22. Torriani-Pasin, C.; Demers, M.; Polese, J.C.; Bishop, L.; Wade, E.; Hempel, S.; Winstein, C. mHealth technologies used to capture walking and arm use behavior in adult stroke survivors: A scoping review beyond measurement properties. *Disabil. Rehabil.* **2022**, *44*, 6094–6106. [CrossRef] [PubMed]
23. Costa, P.H.V.; de Jesus, T.P.D.; Winstein, C.; Torriani-Pasin, C.; Polese, J.C. An investigation into the validity and reliability of mHealth devices for counting steps in chronic stroke survivors. *Clin. Rehabil.* **2020**, *34*, 394–403. [CrossRef] [PubMed]
24. Alanzi, T.; Rehman, S.U.; Khan, M.A.; Istepanian, R.S.H. The evolution and mapping trends of mobile health (m-Health): A bibliometric analysis (1997–2023). *nHealth* **2024**, *10*, 23. [CrossRef]
25. Hamine, S.; Gerth-Guyette, E.; Faulx, D.; Green, B.B.; Ginsburg, A.S. Impact of mHealth chronic disease management on treatment adherence and patient outcomes: A systematic review. *J. Med. Internet Res.* **2015**, *17*, e52. [CrossRef]
26. World Health Organization. *WHO Guideline: Recommendations on Digital Interventions for Health System Strengthening: Web Supplement 2: Summary of Findings and GRADE Tables*; World Health Organization: Geneva, Switzerland, 2019.
27. Adcock, A.K.; Haggerty, T.; Crawford, A.; Espinosa, C. mHealth impact on secondary stroke prevention: A scoping review of randomized controlled trials among stroke survivors between 2010–2020. *mHealth* **2022**, *8*, 19. [CrossRef]
28. Khirasaria, R.; Singh, V.; Batta, A. Exploring digital therapeutics: The next paradigm of modern health-care industry. *Perspect. Clin. Res.* **2020**, *11*, 54–58. [CrossRef]
29. Rakhshan, M.; Najafi, H.; Valizadeh, G.A. Lifestyle of Patients with Atrial Fibrillation Following Self-Management Interventions: A Randomized Clinical Trial. *J. Caring Sci.* **2019**, *8*, 83–88. [CrossRef]
30. Whitehead, L.; Seaton, P. The Effectiveness of Self-Management Mobile Phone and Tablet Apps in Long-term Condition Management: A Systematic Review. *J. Med. Internet Res.* **2016**, *18*, e97. [CrossRef]
31. Boukhennoufa, I.; Zhai, X.; Utti, V.; Jackson, J.; McDonald-Maier, K.D. Wearable sensors and machine learning in post-stroke rehabilitation assessment: A systematic review. *Biomed. Signal Process. Control* **2022**, *71*, 103197. [CrossRef]
32. Zubrycki, I.; Prączko-Pawlak, E.; Dominik, I. Sensing System for Plegic or Paretic Hands Self-Training Motivation. *Sensors* **2022**, *22*, 2414. [CrossRef]
33. Nijland, R.; Kwakkel, G.; Bakers, J.; van Wegen, E. Constraint-induced movement therapy for the upper paretic limb in acute or sub-acute stroke: A systematic review. *Int. J. Stroke* **2011**, *6*, 425–433. [CrossRef]
34. Nijland, R.H.; van Wegen, E.E.; Harmeling-van der Wel, B.C.; Kwakkel, G. Presence of finger extension and shoulder abduction within 72 hours after stroke predicts functional recovery: Early prediction of functional outcome after stroke: The EPOS cohort study. *Stroke* **2010**, *41*, 745–750. [CrossRef] [PubMed]
35. Lundquist, C.B.; Maribo, T. The Fugl–Meyer assessment of the upper extremity: Reliability, responsiveness and validity of the Danish version. *Disabil. Rehabil.* **2017**, *39*, 934–939. [CrossRef] [PubMed]
36. Yoshida, T.; Otaka, Y.; Kitamura, S.; Ushizawa, K.; Kumagai, M.; Kurihara, Y.; Yaeda, J.; Osu, R. Development and validation of new evaluation scale for measuring stroke patients' motivation for rehabilitation in rehabilitation wards. *PLoS ONE* **2022**, *17*, e0265214. [CrossRef] [PubMed]
37. Maeda, N.; Urabe, Y.; Murakami, M.; Itotani, K.; Kato, J. Discriminant analysis for predictor of falls in stroke patients by using the Berg Balance Scale. *Singap. Med. J.* **2015**, *56*, 280. [CrossRef]
38. Murphy, T.H.; Corbett, D. Plasticity during stroke recovery: From synapse to behaviour. *Nat. Rev. Neurosci.* **2009**, *10*, 861–872. [CrossRef]
39. Woldag, H.; Hummelsheim, H. Evidence-based physiotherapeutic concepts for improving arm and hand function in stroke patients: A review. *J. Neurol.* **2002**, *249*, 518–528. [CrossRef]
40. Chung, B.P.H.; Chiang, W.K.H.; Lau, H.; Lau, T.F.O.; Lai, C.W.K.; Sit, C.S.Y.; Chan, K.Y.; Yeung, C.Y.; Lo, T.M.; Hui, E. Pilot study on comparisons between the effectiveness of mobile video-guided and paper-based home exercise programs on improving exercise

adherence, self-efficacy for exercise and functional outcomes of patients with stroke with 3-month follow-up: A single-blin randomized controlled trial. *Hong Kong Physiother. J.* **2020**, *40*, 63–73.
41. Kim, D.-W.; Park, J.E.; Kim, M.-J.; Byun, S.H.; Jung, C.I.; Jeong, H.M.; Woo, S.R.; Lee, K.H.; Lee, M.H.; Jung, J.-W. Automati assessment of upper extremity function and mobile application for self-administered stroke rehabilitation. *IEEE Trans. Neura Syst. Rehabil. Eng.* **2024**, *32*, 652–661. [CrossRef]
42. Ballard, K.J.; Etter, N.M.; Shen, S.; Monroe, P.; Tien Tan, C. Feasibility of automatic speech recognition for providing feedbac during tablet-based treatment for apraxia of speech plus aphasia. *Am. J. Speech-Lang. Pathol.* **2019**, *28*, 818–834. [CrossRef] [PubMed]
43. Seifert, A. The digital exclusion of older adults during the COVID-19 pandemic. *J. Gerontol. Soc. Work* **2020**, *63*, 674–676. [CrossRef] [PubMed]
44. Lu, X.; Yao, Y.; Jin, Y. Digital exclusion and functional dependence in older people: Findings from five longitudinal cohort studie *eClinicalMedicine* **2022**, *54*, 101708. [CrossRef] [PubMed]
45. Hunsaker, A.; Hargittai, E. A review of Internet use among older adults. *New Media Soc.* **2018**, *20*, 3937–3954. [CrossRef]
46. Eurostat. Individuals' Level of Digital Skills (From 2021 Onwards). 2024. Available online: https://ec.europa.eu/eurostat databrowser/view/ISOC_SK_DSKL_I21/default/table (accessed on 18 August 2025).
47. Nakagomi, A.; Shiba, K.; Kawachi, I.; Ide, K.; Nagamine, Y.; Kondo, N.; Hanazato, M.; Kondo, K. Internet use and subsequen health and well-being in older adults: An outcome-wide analysis. *Comput. Hum. Behav.* **2022**, *130*, 107156. [CrossRef]
48. Xavier, A.J.; d'Orsi, E.; de Oliveira, C.M.; Orrell, M.; Demakakos, P.; Biddulph, J.P.; Marmot, M.G. English Longitudinal Study o Aging: Can Internet/E-mail use reduce cognitive decline? *J. Gerontol. Ser. A Biomed. Sci. Med. Sci.* **2014**, *69*, 1117–1121. [CrossRef]
49. Choi, N.G.; DiNitto, D.M. Internet use among older adults: Association with health needs, psychological capital, and socia capital. *J. Med. Internet Res.* **2013**, *15*, e2333. [CrossRef]
50. Greer, B.; Robotham, D.; Simblett, S.; Curtis, H.; Griffiths, H.; Wykes, T. Digital exclusion among mental health service users Qualitative investigation. *J. Med. Internet Res.* **2019**, *21*, e11696. [CrossRef]
51. Zapletal, A.; Wells, T.; Russell, E.; Skinner, M.W. On the triple exclusion of older adults during COVID-19: Technology, digita literacy and social isolation. *Soc. Sci. Humanit. Open* **2023**, *8*, 100511. [CrossRef]
52. Carmichael, S.T. The 3 Rs of stroke biology: Radial, relayed, and regenerative. *Neurotherapeutics* **2016**, *13*, 348–359. [CrossRef]
53. Bernardo-Castro, S.; Sousa, J.A.; Brás, A.; Cecília, C.; Rodrigues, B.; Almendra, L.; Machado, C.; Santo, G.; Silva, F.; Ferreira, L Pathophysiology of blood–brain barrier permeability throughout the different stages of ischemic stroke and its implication on hemorrhagic transformation and recovery. *Front. Neurol.* **2020**, *11*, 594672. [CrossRef] [PubMed]
54. Powers, W.J.; Rabinstein, A.A.; Ackerson, T.; Adeoye, O.M.; Bambakidis, N.C.; Becker, K.; Biller, J.; Brown, M.; Demaerschalk B.M.; Hoh, B. Guidelines for the early management of patients with acute ischemic stroke: 2019 update to the 2018 guidelines for the early management of acute ischemic stroke: A guideline for healthcare professionals from the American Heart Association/American Stroke Association. *Stroke* **2019**, *50*, e344–e418. [PubMed]
55. Cauraugh, J.H.; Kim, S.-B.; Summers, J.J. Chronic stroke longitudinal motor improvements: Cumulative learning evidence found in the upper extremity. *Cerebrovasc. Dis.* **2008**, *25*, 115–121. [CrossRef] [PubMed]
56. Peng, R.H.-T.; He, D.; James, S.A.; Williamson, J.N.; Skadden, C.; Jain, S.; Hassaneen, W.; Miranpuri, A.; Kaur, A.; Sarol, J.N Determining the effects of targeted high-definition transcranial direct current stimulation on reducing post-stroke upper limb motor impairments—A randomized cross-over study. *Trials* **2024**, *25*, 34. [CrossRef]
57. Kinoshita, T.; Yoshikawa, T.; Nishimura, Y.; Kamijo, Y.-I.; Arakawa, H.; Nakamura, T.; Hashizaki, T.; Hoekstra, S.P.; Tajima, F Mobilization within 24 hours of new-onset stroke enhances the rate of home discharge at 6-months follow-up: A prospective cohort study. *Int. J. Neurosci.* **2021**, *131*, 1097–1106. [CrossRef]
58. Nguyen, P.T.; Chou, L.-W.; Hsieh, Y.-L. Proprioceptive neuromuscular facilitation-based physical therapy on the improvement of balance and gait in patients with chronic stroke: A systematic review and meta-analysis. *Life* **2022**, *12*, 882. [CrossRef]
59. Chang, W.H.; Kim, Y.-H. Robot-assisted therapy in stroke rehabilitation. *J. Stroke* **2013**, *15*, 174. [CrossRef]
60. Cho, K.H.; Hong, M.-R.; Song, W.-K. Upper limb robotic rehabilitation for chronic stroke survivors: A single-group preliminary study. *J. Phys. Ther. Sci.* **2018**, *30*, 580–583. [CrossRef]
61. Devittori, G.; Ranzani, R.; Dinacci, D.; Romiti, D.; Califfi, A.; Petrillo, C.; Rossi, P.; Gassert, R.; Lambercy, O. Automatic and personalized adaptation of therapy parameters for unsupervised robot-assisted rehabilitation: A pilot evaluation. In Proceedings of the 2022 International Conference on Rehabilitation Robotics (ICORR), Rotterdam, The Netherlands, 25–29 July 2022; pp. 1–6.
62. Toh, F.M.; Lam, W.W.; Gonzalez, P.C.; Fong, K.N. 'Smart reminder': A feasibility pilot study on the effects of a wearable device treatment on the hemiplegic upper limb in persons with stroke. *J. Telemed. Telecare* **2024**, *31*, 796–806. [CrossRef]
63. Han, S.; Wang, H.; Yu, H. Human–robot interaction evaluation-based AAN control for upper limb rehabilitation robots driven by series elastic actuators. *IEEE Trans. Robot.* **2023**, *39*, 3437–3451. [CrossRef]

4. Li, Z.; Su, C.-Y.; Wang, L.; Chen, Z.; Chai, T. Nonlinear disturbance observer-based control design for a robotic exoskeleton incorporating fuzzy approximation. *IEEE Trans. Ind. Electron.* **2015**, *62*, 5763–5775. [CrossRef]
5. Chae, S.H.; Kim, Y.; Lee, K.-S.; Park, H.-S. Development and clinical evaluation of a web-based upper limb home rehabilitation system using a smartwatch and machine learning model for chronic stroke survivors: Prospective comparative study. *JMIR mHealth uHealth* **2020**, *8*, e17216. [CrossRef] [PubMed]
6. Nathan, D.E.; Johnson, M.J. Design of a grasp assistive glove for ADL-focused, robotic assisted therapy after stroke. In Proceedings of the 2007 IEEE 10th International Conference on Rehabilitation Robotics, Noordwijk, The Netherlands, 13–15 June 2007; pp. 943–950.
7. Maceira-Elvira, P.; Popa, T.; Schmid, A.C.; Hummel, F.C. Wearable technology in stroke rehabilitation: Towards improved diagnosis and treatment of upper-limb motor impairment. *J. Neuroeng. Rehabil.* **2019**, *16*, 142. [CrossRef] [PubMed]
8. Cheong, M.J.; Kang, Y.; Kang, H.W. Psychosocial factors related to stroke patients' rehabilitation motivation: A scoping review and Meta-Analysis focused on South Korea. *Healthcare* **2021**, *9*, 1211. [CrossRef] [PubMed]
9. Kang, H.-J.; Kwon, S.; Youn, S.-C. The convergent influence of perceived stress and the empowerment on rehabilitation motive of stroke patients. *J. Digit. Converg.* **2016**, *14*, 291–303. [CrossRef]
0. Cheong, M.J.; Jeon, B.; Noh, S.E. A protocol for systematic review and meta-analysis on psychosocial factors related to rehabilitation motivation of stroke patients. *Medicine* **2020**, *99*, e23727. [CrossRef]
1. Gladstone, D.J.; Danells, C.J.; Black, S.E. The fugl-meyer assessment of motor recovery after stroke: A critical review of its measurement properties. *Neurorehabilit. Neural Repair* **2002**, *16*, 232–240. [CrossRef]
2. Beninato, M.; Gill-Body, K.M.; Salles, S.; Stark, P.C.; Black-Schaffer, R.M.; Stein, J. Determination of the minimal clinically important difference in the FIM instrument in patients with stroke. *Arch. Phys. Med. Rehabil.* **2006**, *87*, 32–39. [CrossRef]
3. Page, P. Beyond statistical significance: Clinical interpretation of rehabilitation research literature. *Int. J. Sports Phys. Ther.* **2014**, *9*, 726–736.
4. Sriram, V.M.; Gururaj, G.; Hyder, A.A. Public–private implementation of integrated emergency response services: Case study of GVK Emergency Management and Research Institute in Karnataka, India. *Surgery* **2017**, *162*, S63–S76. [CrossRef]
5. Xuefang, L.; Guihua, W.; Fengru, M. The effect of early cognitive training and rehabilitation for patients with cognitive dysfunction in stroke. *Int. J. Methods Psychiatr. Res.* **2021**, *30*, e1882. [CrossRef]
6. Hussain, S.; Jamwal, P.K.; Vliet, P.V.; Brown, N.A. Robot assisted ankle neuro-rehabilitation: State of the art and future challenges. *Expert Rev. Neurother.* **2021**, *21*, 111–121. [CrossRef]

sensors

MDPI

Article

Narrowband Theta Investigations for Detecting Cognitive Mental Load

Silviu Ionita [1,*] and Daniela Andreea Coman [2]

1 Department of Electronics, Computers and Electrical Engineering, National University of Science and Technology POLITEHNICA Bucharest, 110040 Pitesti, Arges, Romania

2 Ecological College 'Prof. Univ. Dr. Alexandru Ionescu', Intrarea Teilor, No 4, 110029 Pitesti, Arges, Romania; daniela.coman2204@upb.ro

* Correspondence: silviu.ionita@upb.ro

Abstract: The way in which EEG signals reflect mental tasks that vary in duration and intensity is a key topic in the investigation of neural processes concerning neuroscience in general and BCI technologies in particular. More recent research has reinforced historical studies that highlighted theta band activity in relation to cognitive performance. In our study, we propose a comparative analysis of experiments with cognitive load imposed by arithmetic calculations performed mentally. The analysis of EEG signals captured with 64 electrodes is performed on low theta components extracted by narrowband filtering. As main signal discriminators, we introduced an original measure inspired by the integral of the curve of a function—specifically the signal function over the period corresponding to the filter band. Another measure of the signal considered as a discriminator is energy. In this research, it was used just for model comparison. A cognitive load detection algorithm based on these signal metrics was developed and tested on original experimental data. The results present EEG activity during mental tasks and show the behavioral pattern across 64 channels. The most precise and specific EEG channels for discriminating cognitive tasks induced by arithmetic tests are also identified.

Keywords: EEG signal processing; signal metrics; mental state discrimination

1. Introduction

Cognitive functions are based on complex brain activity in multiple processes such as sensation and perception, learning, thinking, reasoning, and problem solving, but also imagination and creativity. Thus, a multitude of recognized responsible neuronal areas work cooperatively conjugately or alternatively, in parallel and serially, and this is how we see the effect of the brain's electrical activity at standard measurement points. Using scalp EEG mapping we can investigate the dynamics of electrical activity in real time in a non-invasive and cost-effective way. The choice of frequency domain for EEG signal analysis is based on evidence from neuroscience as well as practical signal processing considerations. Thus, the theta band (4–7 Hz) is particularly interesting because it involves the existence of several functionally independent activities related to arousal, motivation, cognitive flexibility, and memory-related processes [1]. For the investigation of cognitive mental tasks that involve a state of consciousness, attention, and concentration, the interest in theta waves is precisely related to their specificity in the opposite states, i.e., deep relaxation and sleep [2], as well as in the study of attention deficit [1]. Thus, in our study we chose the theta band considering that it is potentially more precise and specific to cognitive states involving attention, concentration, and working with memory.

The interest in narrowband theta investigations is also motivated by recent studies, which report, for example, that 4 Hz oscillations signify increased motivation (which induces attention), which is reflected by the intensification of the exchange of information between the ACC (anterior cingulate cortex) and the VTA (ventral tegmental area). An increase in the 4 Hz signal has been demonstrated during anticipatory decision making and feedback processing and in the manifestation of behavioral flexibility. Local field potential measurements have shown that in the ACC and VTA, there are peaks of spectral power between 3 and 5 Hz [1]. Additionally, another argument in favor of narrowband investigations is of a practical nature regarding the increased specificity of the analysis of a phenomenon observed strictly on a certain frequency. It will also avoid frequency analysis with the classic FFT technique, applying narrowband filtering instead.

However, the problem of detecting a certain type of cognitive task consists in discriminating against a specific mental state based on the behavior of EEG signals. Thus, the brain's response to a specific imposed cognitive task must be discriminated against the basic electrical activity related to other nonspecific processes. But this is not simple, for the following reasons: (1) the discontinuity and relative latency of the brain's response through electrical signals; (2) individual physiological peculiarities that diversify the behavioral pattern of brain waves from individual to individual, depending on several factors (age, gender, education, health status, etc.); (3) the insufficiency of models and detection criteria used in order to classify mental states with very high accuracy; (4) the presence of artifacts in EEG signals; and finally (5) the problem of initial calibration to determine a reference state for mental task detection. Therefore, the identification and recognition of the occurrence of the specific cognitive task is the main task in our research. For this purpose, we proposed a type of mental task of the arithmetic type presented visually, which the subject must solve in the mind, excluding other voluntary motor activities, such as writing and speaking. The actual work task consists of mental numerical calculation operations that are applied continuously, with breaks, respectively, within a series of tests. During arithmetic tasks, a suite of neural processes related to the perception of numbers, the manipulation of numerical quantities, and the decision on the result are carried out, processes that involve memory, attention, and algorithmic and logical processing [3]. The purpose of this paper is to present original results, as a contribution to the methods of analyzing EEG signals for the detection of brain activity during mental arithmetic tasks. The objective of this research is to aim towards BCI technologies for the automatic detection of cognitive brain activity.

2. Methodology

The dynamics of the electrical activity of the brain subjected to cognitive tasks involve multiple neural areas and complex signal behavior. As a general goal, we want to detect the brain state during cognitive tasks with non-invasive techniques incorporated into BCI interfaces that are as simple as possible. The working methodology for discriminating certain mental tasks in relation to the background (baseline) activity of the brain includes the following steps: (1) performing experiments with the application of specific tests to induce the specific cognitive mental state; (2) acquiring and exploring EEG signals at a sufficient number of points on the surface of the head; (3) establishing relevant signal measures (metrics) for real-time analysis to detect the cognitive task; (4) choosing task discrimination/recognition criteria in relation to a reference mental state; (5) calibrating the system to establish the reference state.

This paper presents a new way of investigating EEG signals and develops an algorithm that can distinguish as precisely as possible the brain activity specific to arithmetic calculation, without the use of machine learning and deep learning methods. Our approach is based on calibrating the system correctly during the experiment on the test subject. Thus, the uniqueness of any subject is considered, and this allows the application of the method to different subjects by individual recalibration based on the EEG acquisition even in the current state preceding the task. Unlike approaches based on machine learning, this algorithm applies an analytical approach to analyzing signals in real time, without requiring large volumes of data for training. In contrast to the shortcomings of machine learning-based techniques, the proposed method has the following advantages:

- It does not require large amounts of preprocessed, labeled data;

- It does not depend on models trained on certain groups of subjects, performed under laboratory conditions;

- It is based on a transparent, interpretable detection model and can therefore be controlled through its parameters that are explicit;

- It provides better real-time responses with reduced computing resources;

- It provides greater confidence in conditions of noise, motion, or other biological and non-biological artifacts.

Inter-subject variability is a critical factor influencing the performance of mental load detection models and especially limits machine learning-based recognition algorithms. This obstacle led us to approach an analytical model detection method instead and to limit ourselves to investigating a single subject through multiple tests.

2.1. Test Design

For experimentation, we proposed a number of cognitive stimulation tests consisting of mental arithmetic tasks. The tests consisted of arithmetic calculation exercises, displayed on the screen with a predetermined time limit. In order to maintain the subject's attention and concentration on the main task, the calculation operations consisted of successive and recursive subtractions and additions, starting from different numbers, with a subtraction/addition rate of 2, 3, 4, 5, or 6 units (for example: $100 - 2 - 2 - \ldots$, $60 + 3 + 3 + \ldots$, $32 + 4 + 4 + \ldots$, $41 + 5 + 5 + \ldots$, or $41 + 6 + 6 + \ldots$). The datasets collected correspond to the following types of tests:

- 6 tests without task, with eyes open (looking at a white display), called TW1 to TW6.
- 6 no-load, eyes-closed, relaxed tests, called T01 to T06.
- 6 continuous arithmetic task tests, called TC2, to TC7.
- 6 alternating arithmetic task tests, designated TI5 to TI10.

Each task test included a 10 s break at the beginning and a break of at least 5 s at the end. The intermittent task tests were organized with three calculation rounds with 10 s breaks between them, while the continuous task tests had five successive calculation rounds without a break between them, as illustrated in Figure 1.

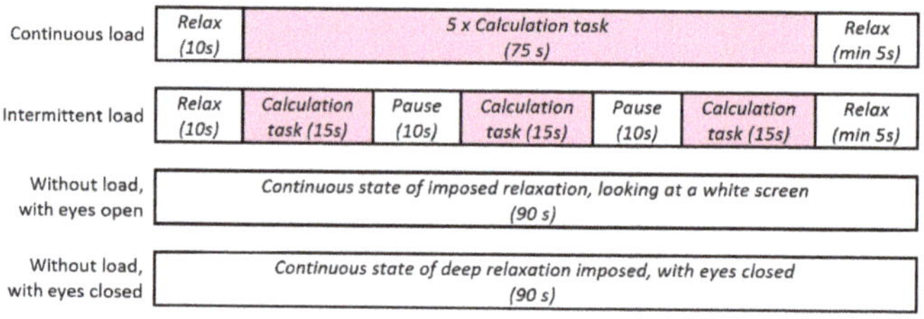

Figure 1. Test structure.

2.2. EEG Exploration

Exploration of the electrical activity of the brain in the experiments was carried out by acquiring EEG signals using the Biosemi Active Two system, configured with 64 channels in monopolar mounting, positioned and labeled according to the international standard "10-20" [Biosemi EEG ECG EMG BSPM NEURO amplifier electrodes]. The equipment used provides a large amount of data from the 64 measurement points that provide good spatial resolution. The EEG signals are sampled at a frequency of 8192 Hz, which allows the acquisition of neuronal impulses on the scalp surface with good temporal resolution. The raw original signals were acquired in the frequency band set to 0.16 Hz to 40 Hz, digitally converted to 24 bits and stored in files in the bdf (Binary Data File) format. An experimental instance and the map of the measurement points are shown in Figure 2.

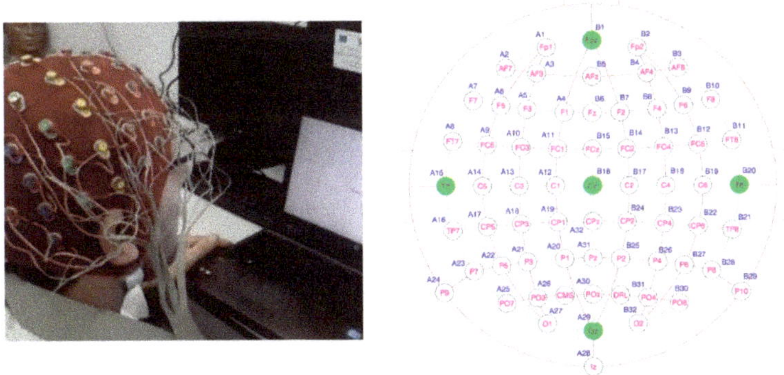

Figure 2. Experimental setup. The green points are used as references points to measure the brain activity.

The experiment involved an adult subject, 58 years old, male, with professional activity in the field of engineering. The subject participated in 18 consecutive sessions, each lasting approximately 1.5 minutes, totaling approximately one and a half hours of participation, including technical breaks.

As an additional measure of protection against possible electromagnetic disturbances during the acquisition, the subject was placed together with the equipment in a metallic shielding enclosure. No device powered by a switching power supply was located inside, as all the devices involved there were powered by batteries. Data transmission to the external process computer as well as acquisition control were performed via optical fiber, through the specific interface from Biosemi. The experimental procedure included the preliminary stage of subject preparation and the application of the measurement electrodes. The subject was previously instructed on the structure of the tests and the type of arithmetic tasks to be performed. The tests described above were visually displayed with PowerPoint, triggered by the subject by pressing a key—the only motor action performed by him. After one second, a short sound signal was emitted and the external operator commanded the start of the acquisition on the process computer. At the end of the test, a specific acoustic signal would announce the stop of the recording. There was no automatic triggering and stopping of the tests and thus the duration of the recordings may have differed slightly from one test to another, but this did not affect the integrity and structure of the useful data. Usually there was a small variable latency when stopping the recording, which slightly affected the final quiet period. During the tests, the subject complied with the preliminary instructions: to be as relaxed as possible, not to move, to blink as rarely as possible, to keep his gaze fixed on the center of the screen, and to control his thoughts and mental state in accordance with the task—that is, to be absolutely focused on the calculations when they appear, respectively, and to relax mentally as much as possible during the break periods. The relaxation and break periods are spent with the eyes open, without natural ambient light, except from the white background displayed by the PowerPoint application during the test. We highlight the fact that in these tests, the relaxation periods, breaks, and periods of mental load are part of the same recording, which limits the effects of subject variability. This supports the proposed detection method by bringing the relaxation period used as a reference for calibration as close as possible to the subject's current mental state and physiological condition. In contrast, machine learning-based reference models are not actually personalized and are susceptible to failure.

3. Principle of the Method

In this section we describe the last three points of the proposed working method for signal processing and analysis, which concern the following: signal metrics, mental task discrimination criteria, and the calibration method for the reference state Section 3.1.

3.1. Signal Metrics

The considered metrics usually determine the signal analysis method. In EEG, parameters such as signal energy, number of zero crossings, or other transient signal behaviors are used in the time domain analysis. Parameters related to signal frequency, such as spectral power and its distribution, which are typically based on Fourier analysis and transformation, are used in the frequency domain analysis. Also, combined time–frequency methods provide specific distributions that are useful in EEG interpretation. Finally, the probabilistic behavior of signals can be quantified with known statistical parameters within the framework of statistical analysis methods. These analysis techniques, which are widely used in EEG studies, constitute the majority of reports in the literature dedicated to the field. We mention here some of those that address the issue of recognizing electrical activity of the brain in the presence of mental stress induced by mathematical tasks. Thus, in references [4,5] the use of signal energy and statistical parameters as metrics to detect arithmetic mental load is reported, and the analysis in frequency and time–frequency domains is addressed in [6,7]. The use of statistical measures together with machine learning techniques is reported in [8,9], while several works address spectral analysis based on FFT, the spectral power distribution indicator, including in combination with statistical indicators [10–14]. We also mention here a previous work by the authors of this research [15], in which we reported some results obtained with the statistical correlation method and the spectral analysis method based on FFT evaluation. On the other hand, alternative brain scanning methods that do not use EEG signals, such as functional magnetic resonance imaging (fMRI) and functional near-infrared spectroscopy (fNIRS), use specific image analysis techniques [16]. In our study we introduce as a measure for the analysis a signal parameter consisting of the length of the signal curve over a period. Since the period of EEG signals is variable in the dedicated analysis bands, we build our metric for a narrowband signal that we obtain with a suitable bandpass filter (BPF), with the median frequency $F_{med_{BPF}}$. Thus, the filtered signal for analysis will have a constant period $T_{med} = 1/F_{med_{BPF}}$ and by sampling with the frequency F_s, one period will contain $n = T_{med} \cdot F_s$ signal discrete points. For the discretized signal $S(t_k)$, $k = 1, \ldots n$ with the sampling frequency F_s, we will accept for the beginning the expression for calculating the length of the signal curve over the period p, as follows:

$$Lsc(p) = \sum_{k=1}^{n} \sqrt{(\Delta_k S)^2 + \left(\frac{1}{F_s}\right)^2} \tag{1}$$

Even though the relation is not dimensionally homogeneous, it expresses a sum of elementary Euclidean distances and therefore the path traveled by the signal in the signal–time plane during a period. Since $\Delta t = 1/F_s$ is the (constant) time step of discretization, the relation can be reduced to the following form:

$$Lsc(p) = \Delta t \sum_{k=1}^{n} \sqrt{\left(\frac{\Delta_k S}{\Delta t}\right)^2 + 1} \quad (2)$$

Lsc expresses the length of a path parameterized in R2, where the parameter is the time variable itself, which can be evaluated with the discrete formula of the first-order curvilinear integral. However, we would prefer to normalize this parameter by referring to T_{med}, successively obtaining the following relations:

$$Lscn(p) = \frac{\Delta t}{T_{med}} \sum_{k=1}^{n} \sqrt{\left(\frac{\Delta_k S}{\Delta t}\right)^2 + 1} = \frac{F_{med\,BPF}}{F_s} \sum_{k=1}^{n} \sqrt{\left(\frac{\Delta_k S}{\Delta t}\right)^2 + 1} = \frac{1}{n} \sum_{k=1}^{n} \sqrt{\left(\frac{\Delta_k S}{\Delta t}\right)^2 + 1} \quad (3)$$

In this form, the parameter length of the signal curve during a period, is equal to 1 at the limit, which represents the minimum value that is reached for the constant signal. The parameter *Lsc* depends on quantitative characteristics of the signal—amplitude and dynamics but is also sensitive to the shape of the signal affected by transient local variations. However, it is not influenced by the level (bias) of the signal, which gives it immunity to the non-stationary behavior of signals. It is a good indicator of the signal energy provided by the signal dynamics and not by its level. Finally, it is specific only for narrowband filtered signals and thus for a nominal frequency analyzed. Other practical benefits of the proposed signal parameter are related to the relatively reduced processing effort, which no longer involves the calculation of the Fourier transform for laborious spectral analyses in wider frequency bands. The signal energy for a period with n samples is a measure with the absolute value given by the following equation:

$$Ea(p) = \sum_{k=1}^{n} (S(t_k))^2 \quad (4)$$

Unlike *Lsc*, the energy also depends on the signal bias in the period p and will be considered as an additional criterion for discriminating mental tasks strictly in the narrow working band. However, the current signal level may also depend on other causes not specific to the mental task under study. Therefore, we will use the relative value of the energy calculated in relation to the average signal over the current period p, denoted by $\left(\overline{S(t_k)}\right)_p$, according to the following relationship:

$$Er(p) = \sum_{k=1}^{n} \left(S(t_k) - \left(\overline{S(t_k)}\right)_p\right)^2 \quad (5)$$

3.2. Detection Criteria and Conditions

Building mental load detection criteria takes into account the signal measures discussed above for the calculation of detection thresholds and the formation of discrimination/recognition conditions of the mental state for each measured EEG channel $i = 1, \ldots 64$. The calculation of detection thresholds is the subject of the system calibration operation, preceding the acquisition of signals in the cognitive load experiments. The basic idea of the mental load detection algorithm is the dynamic processing of the acquired data and the comparison of the discrimination characteristics with detection thresholds calculated on a portion of the beginning of the signals, within a time interval allocated for calibration. This solution does not use machine learning techniques that require large volumes of training data and the performance of many EEG signal acquisition experiments. Unlike the pattern recognition technique which functions by referring to a model learned from multiple examples, the proposed method is limited to the preliminary processing of a signal portion with duration t_{calib} from the beginning of each EEG signal captured from the subject in a voluntary state of mental rest (relaxation). Therefore, the detection thresholds are defined based on the averaging of the signal characteristic (*Lscn* or *Er*) in the window with a set number of periods $p = 1, \ldots, w$, which moves incrementally by one period throughout the calibration duration t_{calib}, finally selecting the maximum value found, as follows:

$$Tresh1(i) = \max_{t_{calib}}\left(\left(\overline{Lscn(p)}\right)_{p=1,w}\right), \tag{6}$$

and

$$Tresh2(i) = \max_{t_{calib}}\left(\left(\overline{Er(p)}\right)_{p=1,w}\right), \tag{7}$$

where w is the number of signal periods that defines the width of the averaging window for the signal characteristic being evaluated. The use of detection thresholds is conducted with the following relations:

$$\left(\left(\overline{Lscn(p)}\right)_{p=1,w}\right) > Tresh1(i), \tag{8}$$

$$\left(\left(\overline{Er(p)}\right)_{p=1,w}\right) > Tresh2(i), \tag{9}$$

applied iteratively with a step of one period to calculate the current values of the averaged signal measures if the current time $t > t_{calib}$. Thus, after the calibration period, following the processing of the signals on each EEG channel i in successive windows with w periods that move incrementally with a step of one period, current values of the averaged signal measures are obtained, which are compared with the threshold values determined during calibration according to relations (8) and (9). The classification of the current mental state associated with the presence or absence of mental load is therefore made based on the threshold limit conditions. If one of the above conditions is true, then it is considered that the mental load has been detected according to the respective criteria, and the presence of this state will be signaled.

3.3. Detection Algorithm

The detection of cognitive mental load in the low theta band begins with the processing of EEG signals by filtering. For this purpose, two filters were designed: the first, a lowpass filter (LPF) with a cutoff frequency of 2 Hz to extract slow components from the raw EEG signals, and the second, a bandpass filter (BPF) for the narrow band (4–5 Hz) of the low theta wave domain. These are high-order FIR digital filters. The first filter has the role of providing a signal with a slow variation below 2 Hz that will be subtracted from the raw signal to reduce the effect of level drift. The second filter provides the signal component in the narrow frequency band of interest for analysis.

Artifact removal is a generally necessary step for analysis in wider frequency bands. In the case of narrowband analysis, even after eliminating the effects of low-frequency components, the problem arises of eliminating spike-type disturbances that are generally more visible in raw data when the sampling frequency is high. Usually, resampling the signal with half the initial frequency reduces these signal spikes acceptably. In our case, the signals are sampled with $F_s = 8192$ Hz, which is of high value, and we do not want to lose this advantage. Therefore, we proposed an algorithm for treating spike-type disturbances using a condition for their detection and a rule of replacement and not of elimination itself. The working principle of the designed algorithm is stated as follows: if the signal peak in the current analysis period exceeds a threshold set in relation to the average of the signal peaks in the previous signal window, then the current signal period is considered a disturbance and is eliminated by replacement. Elimination by replacement ensures a local signal uniformity as an effect of replacing the current signal period, as well as a number of neighboring periods, with the average of the signals in the previous window. The working steps of the proposed algorithm for treating peak disturbances are structured as follows:

{1} The artifact detection condition is defined by the signal peak criterion (SPC):

$$SPC = \frac{\mathrm{Speak(p)} - \left(\overline{\mathrm{Speak}(p)}\right)_{p=p-np,\ldots,p-1}}{\left(\overline{\mathrm{Speak}(p)}\right)_{p=p-np,\ldots,p-1}} > Tresh, \quad (10)$$

where np is the number of periods considered in the window preceding the current signal period p, and $Tresh$ is the value set for artifact detection.

$$\left(\overline{\mathrm{Ssp}(p)}\right)_{p=p-np,\ldots,p-1} \quad (11)$$

{2} If condition (10) is true, the signal segment corresponding to period p, Ssp(p), respectively, is considered an artifact and is eliminated. The elimination rule is applied as follows: replace the artifact signal segment Ssp(p) as well as the neighboring segments Ssp(p − 1), Ssp(p + 1), Ssp(p + 2) with the average value of the signal in the window preceding the artifact.

Now, the entire algorithm for cognitive load detection can be run according to the following steps:

(1) Starting the acquisition of raw EEG data on 64 channels (in the 20-10 system).
(2) Starting data processing after a stabilization time interval (t_{start} = 0...2 s).
(3) Data normalization (equivalent to signal conditioning).
(4) Applying the correction filter to reduce the slow variation of the signals (below 2 Hz);
(5) Narrowband filtering (BPF application) and data retention after 1 s.
(6) Calculation of the average period of the filtered signal based on the average frequency of the BPF passband: $T_{med} = 1/F_{med_{BPF}}$.
(7) Calculation of the number of signal samples from an average period: $n = T_{med} \cdot F_s$, where F_s is the sampling frequency of the EEG signals (8192 Hz).
(8) The current signal is dynamically segmented into frames equal to the average period—containing n samples: $Ssp(p) = (S_k)_p$, for k = 1, ..., n and p = 1, ..., Np, where Np is the number of periods in whole signal.
(9) Application of an algorithm for automatic artifact removal.
(10) The signal measures are iteratively calculated for each period p equal to $Tmed$, respectively, $Lscn(p)$ with relation (3) and $Er(p)$ with relation (5).
(11) The calculated characteristics are averaged over a sliding window containing w signal periods: $\overline{Lscn(p)}_{p=1,w}$, respectively, $\overline{Er(p)}_{p=1,w}$. The width of the signal window for averaging is chosen as w = 3...20 periods.
(12) The detection thresholds are calculated as the maximum value of the averages of the characteristic over the established calibration period t_{calib}, for each channel i = 1, ..., 64 measured, with the relations (6) and (7). The calibration period is at least 10 s, at the beginning of the EEG signal acquisition session; a state of imposed mental rest is mandatory, usually with eyes open.

(13) After the calibration period has elapsed, the mental task discrimination conditions are evaluated on successive signal windows with width w, in the form of the criteria expressed by the relational expressions (8) and/or (9).

This algorithm was implemented and tested using MATLAB (version 2023b), including the Signal Processing Toolbox, as well as the additional library FieldTrip [17], for reading BDF format data recorded with the Biosemi equipment. In our study, we used this algorithm in an application program to investigate the already recorded data, working offline with the EEG acquisition equipment. However, the program is designed modularly so that it can be integrated with the specific acquisition equipment SDK (from Biosemi, in our case) and thus exploit the real-time mental load detection algorithm capacity.

We applied the cognitive load detection algorithm on the data recorded, with the following parameters set:

- Narrow analysis bandwidth 4–5 Hz;
- Average window size w = 10 periods;
- Calibration duration t_{calib} =10 s;
- Signal metrics used *Lscn*, and *Er* only for some comparisons.

In the data preprocessing stage, steps (3)–(5) are effectively considered. Thus, in the offline working mode, in step (3), the data were read using the ft_read_header and ft_read_data function pair from the FieldTrip toolbox, after which they were normalized using the z-score method, in the range [−1, 1]. Then, in step (4) the lowpass filter was effectively applied in the baseline correction and also to exclude certain biological and non-biological artifacts. The lowpass filter is of the digital IIR Butterworth type with a pass frequency of 2 Hz and a cutoff frequency of 2.25 Hz. It extracts the slow signal, which is then subtracted from the raw signal. In step (5), narrowband filtering specific for mental load detection is applied. A high-order FIR digital filter, more precisely 4000, with a narrow passband from 4 to 5 Hz was used. This results in the signal to be analyzed for mental load detection following steps (6)–(12). In step (13), the calibration is already completed, and the algorithm continues its execution cyclically, on successive signal windows with the application of the atypical peak artifact elimination model, according to Equations (10) and (11) and the testing of the load conditions with Equations (8) and (9). The answer consists of the number of occurrences of the detected cognitive load, which are counted and displayed graphically for all EEG channels.

4. Results and Discussions

To prove the proposed concept for narrowband cognitive task detection, we exploited the open-access Physionet international database Electroencephalograms during Mental Arithmetic Task Performance [https://www.mdpi.com/2306-5729/4/1/14, accessed on 1 March 2025]. This provides a sample of 34 valid recordings selected from an initial experimental sample of 66 young participants aged 16 to 24 years, both male and female, who were subjected to mental arithmetic tests based on serial subtraction. The data are provided from a 19-channel EEG system in the 20-10 system, with the following EEG channels: Fp1, Fp2, F3, F4, F7, F8, T3, T4, C3, C4, T5, T6, P3, P4, O1, O2, Fz, Cz, and Pz. By processing the data, we generated two datasets for each EEG channel: the first from the no-load recordings during a relaxation period with eyes closed (60 s) and the second from the recordings with the computational load applied (the next 60 s), for the entire sample of participants. To evaluate the effect of the proposed task detector, we applied the standard statistical *t*-test. The test hypotheses concern the significance of the difference between the statistical means of the two datasets containing the number of activations (cognitive task detections) on each EEG channel, obtained from each participant, the first set without the cognitive task, and the second with the application of the mental task. Table 1 presents the results of the *t*-test for two confidence levels $\alpha = 0.05$, respectively, and 0.01 with the validation of the hypothesis H1—"the difference between the means is significant". The true value for this hypothesis occurs if $|t| >$ the critical value from the *t*-table, which means that the respective EEG channel could be reliable for the detection of the cognitive task. The critical values in the *t*-test table for the parameter degree of freedom df = 33 were calculated by linear interpolation between the values available in the *t*-test table that correspond to the neighboring values df = 30 and df = 40.

Table 1. The significance of cognitive load detection.

EEG Channel		*t*-Test Absolute Value	*p*-Value	Decision on Hypothesis H_1 *	
No	Name			$\alpha = 0.05$	$\alpha = 0.01$
1	Fp1	4.133	0.0002	TRUE	TRUE
2	Fp2	2.228	0.0915	TRUE	FALSE
3	F3	4.045	0.0015	TRUE	TRUE
4	F4	2.577	0.0173	TRUE	FALSE
5	F7	1.010	0.4759	FALSE	FALSE
6	F8	1.593	0.1305	FALSE	FALSE
7	T3/T7	1.684	0.1428	FALSE	FALSE
8	T4/T8	0.949	0.3685	FALSE	FALSE
9	C3	0.699	0.5805	FALSE	FALSE
10	C4	3.282	0.0035	TRUE	TRUE
11	T5/P7	1.280	0.3209	FALSE	FALSE
12	T6/P8	1.972	0.0567	FALSE	FALSE
13	P3	3.453	0.0009	TRUE	TRUE
14	P4	0.785	0.4568	FALSE	FALSE
15	O1	0.627	0.6080	FALSE	FALSE
16	O2	1.603	0.0720	FALSE	FALSE
17	Fz	0.459	0.6355	FALSE	FALSE
18	Cz	0.000	0.9858	FALSE	FALSE
19	Pz	0.812	0.3954	FALSE	FALSE

* Critical values from t-table: 2.0317 for $\alpha = 0.05$ and 2.7272 for $\alpha = 0.01$.

Therefore, the EEG channels sensitive to the detection of cognitive computational load are Fp1, Fp2, F3, F4, C4, and P3 with the 95% confidence level, and Fp1, F3, C4, and P3 with the 99% confidence level, respectively. For a lower level of accepted confidence, for example 80%, obviously more EEG signals become potentially eligible for the detection of cognitive load, as follows: Fp1, Fp2, F3, F4, F8, T3, C4, T6, P3, and O2. For all channels found to be reliable, the results are statistically significant, with the calculated *p*-value being less than 0.02. A summary statistical representation with a box plot can be seen in Figure 3. It is observed that, in general, the eligible channels with a high confidence level do not contain data with outliers, those marked with a circle in Figure 3.

In relation to what was found in this analysis, we mention that the channels found to be sensitive to the cognitive computational task are among those found with other conventional signal metrics, or novel combinations thereof. A synthetic review of the results reported in the literature can be found in the paper [15]. We synthetically highlight the particularities of performing the experiments in the Physionet database [18], as follows:

- The sampling frequency of the signals is 500 Hz.
- The 19 EEG signals captured in the 0.5–45 Hz frequency band were recorded and previously cleaned of artifacts.
- The computational task was communicated to each participant verbally by acoustic means.
- The participants were in the reference state (relaxation without cognitive load) with eyes closed.
- The computational task was processed continuously without voluntary interruptions.

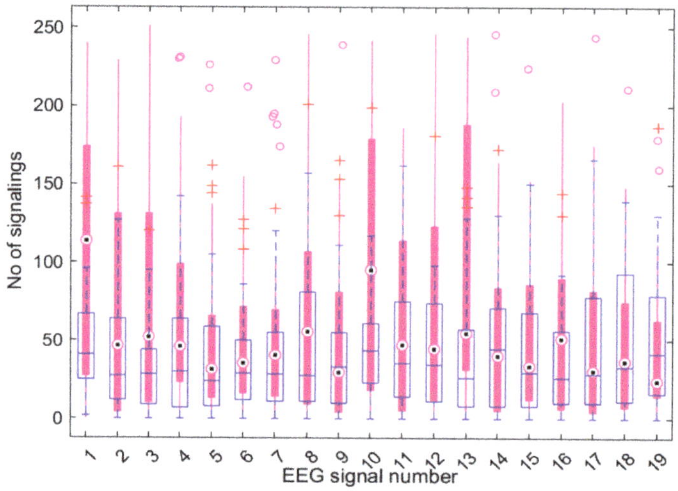

Figure 3. Statistical activity on EEG channels with box plot elements. Empty boxes and blue markers are for data without cognitive load, and filled boxes with red markers belong to data with mental computational load. Magenta circles mark outliers for cognitive load tests. Red + symbols mark outliers for tests without cognitive load. The thin lines in the extension of the boxes denote the range of values.

Our own experiment comes with particularities that complete and add more information, as follows:

- The signal sampling frequency is 8192 Hz.
- The number of electrodes used for measurements is 64 in the 10-10 system, which provides a higher EEG mapping resolution; at least, this is expected.
- The task detection algorithm is designed to work on-line with the subject, in real time as much as possible; so we avoided using an artifact removal technique that requires intensive computing resources (ICA for example). We applied our own simpler algorithm (see in Section 3.3), which was close to the wavelet-based principle. In addition, we applied a rejection of slow components below 2 Hz by extracting them with the lowpass filter, followed by subtracting these components from the raw signal. Moreover, the narrowband working principle of the proposed method has the advantage of eliminating some biological and non-biological artifacts.
- During the experiments, the computational task is exclusively communicated to the subject visually by displaying it on the screen.
- The experimental sample includes six repeated measurements of a single participant under three test conditions: (i) without imposed cognitive load, (ii) with continuously applied cognitive load, and (iii) with intermittently applied cognitive load, with precisely determined breaks. We argue this approach as follows:

(a) A multitude of variables that differentiate subjects in an experiment are eliminated, in relation to the following: age, gender, level of education, cognitive abilities, emotional control, attitude towards the experiment itself and the degree of involvement, some physiological, psychological, and general health characteristics, etc.

(b) A single subject trained and appropriately motivated has better controlled behavior during the experiments, which gives a higher degree of confidence in the results.

In the experiment, the tests were classified and named as follows:

- Tests for the reference state, without cognitive load TW1 to TW6,
- Tests with continuously applied cognitive load TC2 to TC7,
- Tests with intermittently applied cognitive load TI5to TI10.

The *t*-test works quite well when the sample size is small, so in our case we applied it twice on paired data samples: the first time for continuous load versus no load, and the second time for intermittent load versus no load. For both cases, the EEG activity on all 64 channels is statistically represented in Figure 4a,b.

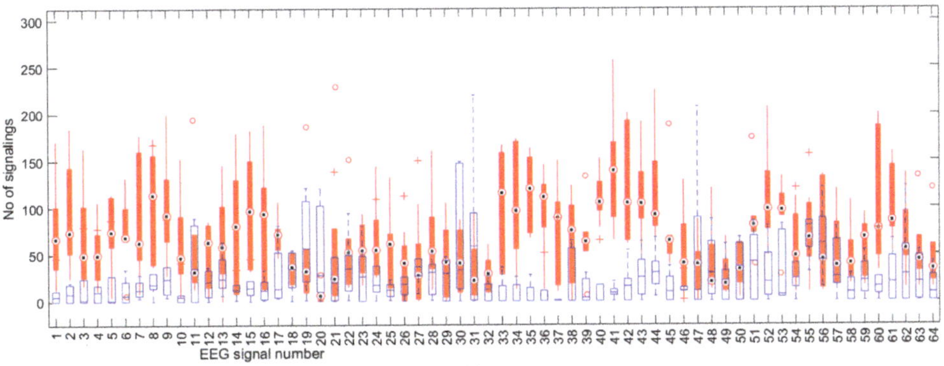

(**a**)

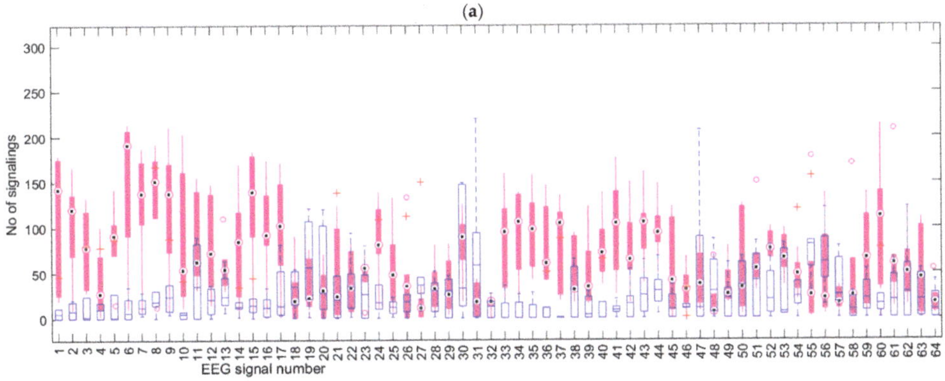

(**b**)

Figure 4. Statistical activity on 64 EEG channels: (**a**) for continuous load charge with red filled boxes and (**b**) for intermittent load charge with magenta filled boxes, both comparatively with the no-load state drawn with blue empty boxes. Magenta circles mark outliers for cognitive load tests. Red + symbols mark outliers for tests without cognitive load. The continuous and dashed thin lines in the extension of the boxes denote the range of values.

At a glance we see a fairly correct statistical distribution, with few outliers and median values significantly detached in several EEG channels. We applied the *t*-test for three confidence levels α: 0.05, 0.02, and 0.01. Table 2 presents the results that verify the alternative hypothesis H1 for the continuous cognitive task. Table 3 presents the results for the intermittent load tests.

Table 2. Significance of detection for continuous cognitive load versus no load.

EEG Channel		*t*-Test Absolute Value	*p*-Value	Decision on Hypothesis H_1 *		
No	Name			$\alpha = 0.05$	$\alpha = 0.02$	$\alpha = 0.01$
1	Fp1	2.755	0.0469	TRUE	FALSE	FALSE
2	AF7	3.691	0.0210	TRUE	TRUE	FALSE
5	F3	3.794	0.0646	TRUE	TRUE	FALSE
6	F5	3.410	0.0129	TRUE	TRUE	FALSE
7	F7	3.015	0.0434	TRUE	FALSE	FALSE
8	FT7	3.170	0.1514	TRUE	FALSE	FALSE
9	FC5	3.285	0.0457	TRUE	FALSE	FALSE
10	FC3	2.880	0.0697	TRUE	FALSE	FALSE
12	C1	2.624	0.0675	TRUE	FALSE	FALSE
14	C5	2.875	0.0709	TRUE	FALSE	FALSE
15	T7	3.188	0.0224	TRUE	FALSE	FALSE
16	TP7	2.752	0.0435	TRUE	FALSE	FALSE
17	CP5	2.577	0.0569	TRUE	FALSE	FALSE
25	PO7	2.669	0.0612	TRUE	FALSE	FALSE
33	Fpz	3.636	0.0136	TRUE	TRUE	FALSE
34	Fp2	3.516	0.0161	TRUE	TRUE	FALSE
35	AF8	5.683	0.0011	TRUE	TRUE	TRUE
36	AF4	4.528	0.0053	TRUE	TRUE	TRUE
39	F2	2.912	0.0230	TRUE	FALSE	FALSE
40	F4	11.777	0.0004	TRUE	TRUE	TRUE
41	F6	5.073	0.0048	TRUE	TRUE	TRUE
42	F8	3.768	0.0091	TRUE	TRUE	FALSE
43	FT8	6.271	0.0044	TRUE	TRUE	TRUE
44	FC6	3.342	0.0145	TRUE	FALSE	FALSE
45	FC4	2.968	0.0315	TRUE	FALSE	FALSE
52	T8	3.7367	0.0126	TRUE	TRUE	FALSE
53	TP8	4.3212	0.0052	TRUE	TRUE	TRUE
58	P4	2.7750	0.0288	TRUE	FALSE	FALSE
60	P8	2.6361	0.0516	TRUE	FALSE	FALSE
61	P10	5.4085	0.0036	TRUE	TRUE	TRUE

* Critical values from t-table: 2.5706 for $\alpha = 0.05$, 3.3650 for $\alpha = 0.02$, and 4.0321 for $\alpha = 0.01$.

The results show that for both modes of load application (continuous or intermittent), even at a high confidence level of 99%, the detector was able to discriminate cognitive activity induced by the mental calculation task from background brain activity, without the task, with eyes open. This is possible for a few EEG measurement channels located over recognized portions of the cortex with responsibilities in numerical calculation skills. It is evident that the significant EEG channels are increasingly numerous, as the accepted confidence level decreases. We note that from the point of view of statistical significance, some channels do not meet the $p < 0.05$ condition, such as FT7, FC3, C1, C5, CP5, and PO7 in Table 2 and FC1, F2, FC4, P10, and PO7 in Table 3. At this stage, they are not considered. Table 4 shows the significant channels that are successively added from bottom to top to the initial set found for the highest confidence level.

Table 3. Significance of detection for intermittent cognitive load versus no load.

EEG Channel		*t*-Test Absolute Value	*p*-Value	Decision on Hypothesis H_1 *		
No	Name			$\alpha = 0.05$	$\alpha = 0.02$	$\alpha = 0.01$
1	Fp1	3.293	0.0184	TRUE	FALSE	FALSE
2	AF7	4.735	0.0092	TRUE	TRUE	TRUE
5	F3	3.000	0.0289	TRUE	FALSE	FALSE
6	F5	4.396	0.0081	TRUE	TRUE	TRUE
7	F7	4.421	0.0075	TRUE	TRUE	TRUE
11	FC1	6.136	0.0986	TRUE	TRUE	TRUE
12	C1	2.650	0.0375	TRUE	FALSE	FALSE
15	T7	3.962	0.0100	TRUE	TRUE	FALSE
16	TP7	3.399	0.0143	TRUE	TRUE	FALSE
25	PO7	2.705	0.0661	TRUE	FALSE	FALSE
33	Fpz	3.601	0.0139	TRUE	TRUE	FALSE
34	Fp2	4.350	0.0072	TRUE	TRUE	TRUE
35	AF8	5.291	0.0035	TRUE	TRUE	TRUE
36	AF4	5.098	0.0151	TRUE	TRUE	TRUE
39	F2	2.645	0.0774	TRUE	FALSE	FALSE
40	F4	9.747	0.0120	TRUE	TRUE	TRUE
41	F6	4.694	0.0108	TRUE	TRUE	TRUE
42	F8	2.717	0.0284	TRUE	FALSE	FALSE
43	FT8	5.204	0.0034	TRUE	TRUE	TRUE
44	FC6	5.058	0.0044	TRUE	TRUE	TRUE
45	FC4	2.661	0.1205	TRUE	FALSE	FALSE
52	T8	3.691	0.0156	TRUE	TRUE	FALSE
61	P10	2.608	0.1044	TRUE	FALSE	FALSE

* Critical values from t-table: 2.5706 for $\alpha = 0.05$, 3.3650 for $\alpha = 0.02$, and 4.0321 for $\alpha = 0.01$.

Table 4. EEG channels that become significant with decreasing confidence level.

Level of Confidence	Cognitive Load		
	Continuous	Intermittent	Physionet
95%	Fp1, F7, FT7, FC5, FC3, C1, C5, T7, TP7, CP5, PO7, F2, FC6, FC4, P4, P8	Fp1, F3, C1, PO7, F8, FC4, P10	Fp1, Fp2, F3, F4, C4, P3
98%	AF7, F3, F5, Fpz, Fp2, F8, T8	T7, TP7, Fpz, T8	
99%	AF8, AF4, F4, F6, FT8, TP8, P10	AF7, F5, F7, Fp2, AF8, AF4, F4, F6, FT8, FC6	Fp1, F3, C4, P3

The EEG channels that stand out from the background in the presence of cognitive load cover the prefrontal region that governs executive operations for mental control responsible for working memory and attention. Both processes are involved in arithmetic calculation tasks in specific tests with serial subtraction or addition operations that are equivalent to counting backward or forward by an arbitrary step, starting from a specified number.

The methodology used is the comparative analysis of the results of the two-step test process quantifying the following indicators:

(i) The activity of each EEG channel in the absence of the load, by the number of validations of the detection condition with the calibration reference threshold calculated in the first 10 s.

(ii) The activity of each EEG channel in the presence of the cognitive load, by the number of validations of the detection condition with the calibration reference threshold calculated in the first 10 s.

The first indicator, from step (i), gives us information about the activity of the EEG channels caused by causes other than the imposed cognitive load. In a sense, it shows us how stable the imposed (relaxed) state is in non-load tests and gives us information about the background brain activity on each EEG channel. Basically, it is necessary to discriminate the cognitive load state from the background state (generated by other causes).

The second indicator, from step (ii), provides the quantitative response on each channel in the presence of the task, but without excluding false positive responses generated by other causes.

In Figure 5 we provide as an example the detected activity of each channel for the reference no-task test with eyes-open T1. In Figure 6 the evolution of the cumulative activity of the EEG channels during the test is shown, which reflects the fluctuation of the stability of the (relaxation) state imposed during the test. It is observed that most of the EEG channels are active in all areas of the head and, cumulatively, they manifest themselves throughout the test, which proves that the specific relaxation state imposed is not exactly stable in the sense of uniformity. This fact can be attributed to background neural processes, as well as to involuntary mental states. From the point of view of the specific cognitive mental task, these represent responses in the false positive category. The most active and fluctuating signals in the relaxed states were detected in the parietal and occipital areas, in both cerebral hemispheres. The least active channels are detected in the frontal and prefrontal areas and only a few in the central and parietal and occipital regions.

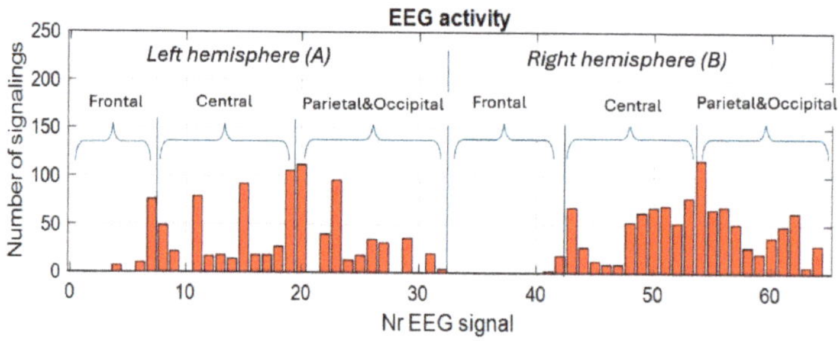

Figure 5. Activity on EEG channels for the no-cognitive-task test with eyes open (TW1).

In the case of the tests without load with eyes closed, the activity on the channels has a different appearance than that in the test with eyes open. The study of these experiments will be addressed separately in a future paper. Next, we approach the second step for evaluating the activity on the EEG channels in the presence of the imposed cognitive load. For exemplification, the quantitative graphs with the number of activations on each channel cumulated during the tests with the load are shown in Figure 7 for a few tests with continuous load and in Figure 8 for some tests with an intermittent load.

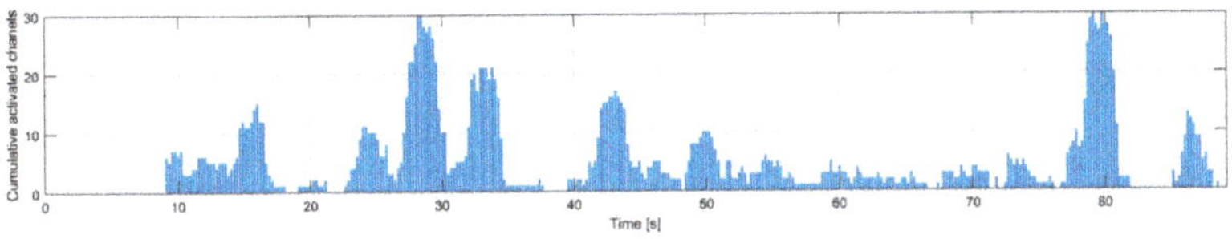

Figure 6. Cumulative activity on all EEG channels during the TW1 test. Denotes the fluctuation of the background state of the brain and due to other causes.

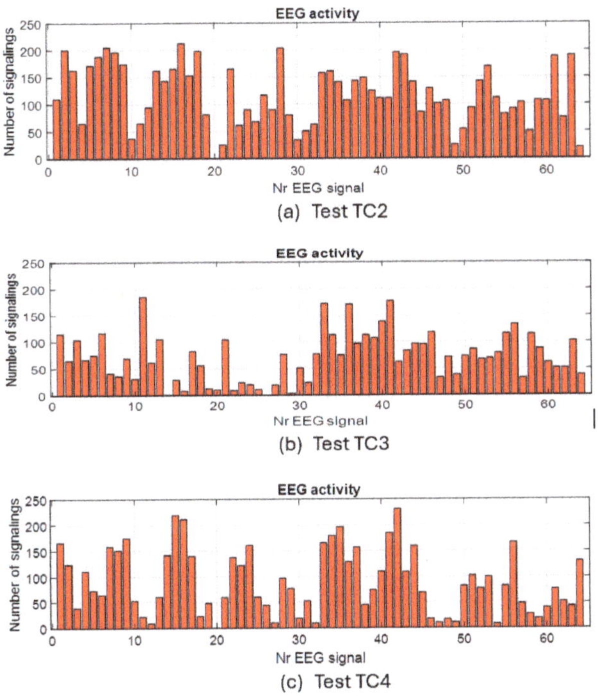

Figure 7. Activity on EEG channels for continuous cognitive task tests.

The main objective is to identify active EEG channels that, on the one hand, are specific and sensitive to the imposed cognitive load and, on the other hand, reflect with maximum precision the presence of cognitive load. This problem has been addressed in the literature with the aim of optimizing the number of electrodes used for signal capture [6,13]. A first level of validation of the relevant detection channels was achieved with the *t*-test, which confirmed the specificity of some channels. Now we bring the issue of real-time detection; in this case we need to analyze the accuracy and sensitivity of detection. Here are the dynamics of the application of the cognitive task matters, to see the response of the detector in relation to the task profile during the test.

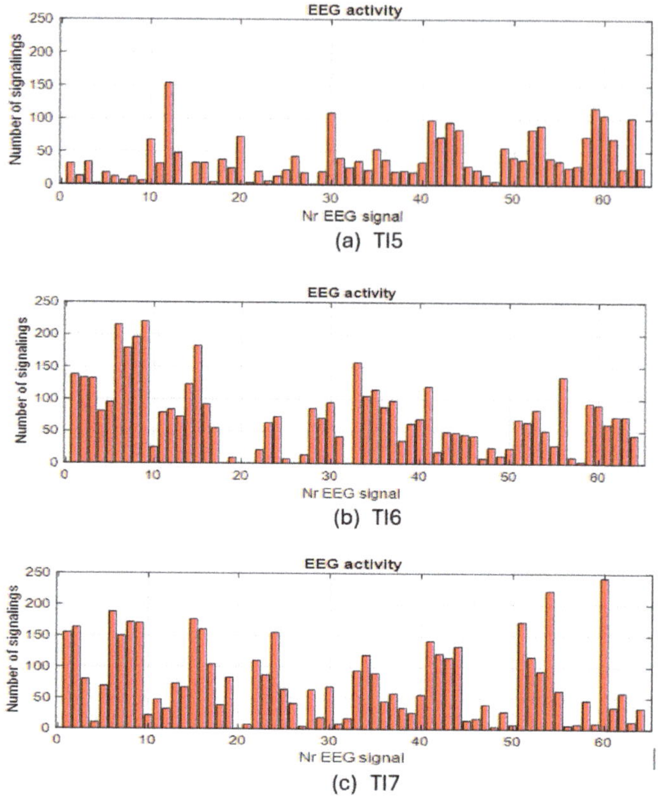

Figure 8. Activity on EEG channels for intermittent cognitive task tests.

The confidence in the algorithm's ability to discriminate mental load is assessed with the set of known criteria, defined as follows:

$$Accuracy = \frac{TP + TN}{TP + FP + TN + FN} \tag{12}$$

$$Precision = \frac{TP}{TP + FP} \tag{13}$$

$$Sensitivity = \frac{TP}{TP + FN} \tag{14}$$

$$Specificity = \frac{TN}{TN + FP} \tag{15}$$

If we merge relations (14) and (15) with (12), we obtain the accuracy in the following suggestive form:

$$Accuracy = \frac{TP + TN}{\frac{TP}{Senzitivity} + \frac{TN}{Specificity}} \tag{16}$$

We mention that these indicators are based on the probabilistic quantities that quantify the detector response: true positive (TP), false positive (FP), true negative (TN), and true positive (TP). In principle, they depend on the number and timing of response occurrences due to the fulfillment of conditional Equations (9) and (10). The ideal situation of maximum detection accuracy is when sensitivity and specificity simultaneously reach the maximum value of 1, and implicitly the precision will also be maximum. It is understood that the key factors are the rates of FP and FN. We applied a procedure to select EEG channels that meet the accuracy and precision parameters in discriminating the cognitive task to the greatest extent possible with the following steps:

(1) The channels classified as significant with the *t*-test are considered. These are those in Table 4. Statistically, they have been shown to be the most specific for the detection of cognitive load and provide a high degree of confidence. However, false positive responses are still possible, and this influences the detection precision.

(2) The confidence criteria are calculated with Equations (12)–(15), and precision is given priority. The highest values are eligible, the maximum being 1. In this stage, those channels with FP = 0 responses are identified, that is, those that have maximum precision and specificity. However, this situation is an ideal one; so the decision to choose a certain acceptable level of precision as well as sensitivity bears some discussion in the following.

The evaluation of false positive responses is conducted in relation to the temporal application profile of the cognitive task within the tests. Figure 9 shows the activity on channels 1 to 5 in the TI7 test with the intermittent task, where a general synchronization of the detector responses (red bars) with respect to the periods of application of the cognitive task (green lines) is observed. We recall that the statistical test validated channels 1, 2, and 5 at the 95% confidence level.

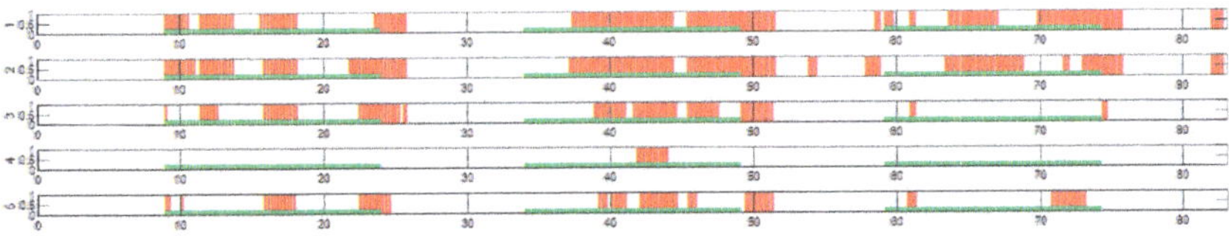

Figure 9. Response of EEG channels 1-5 in the presence of intermittent mental load captured from the analysis of the TI7 test. The red bars signify the detection of the load over time (represented in seconds on the abscissa), and the green lines indicate the intervals in which the cognitive load was applied.

The responses strictly overlapping with the task lines are the precise and specific ones. Other responses outside the task periods are also observed that are classified as false positive, and this disqualifies the channels from being precise and specific. Indeed, part of the false positive responses may be due to causes that could not be excluded by the reference test or during the calibration period, but some of them may also be due to the dynamics of the neural processes specific to the cognitive mental task. Thus, prolonged responses beyond the timing of the cognitive task (see channels 1, 2, 3, and 5) can be attributed to natural latencies of mental processing. Even other transient responses that occur recurrently during the pause periods between tasks could be attributed to cognitive aftereffects or nonspecific involuntary states (see channels 1 and 2). Under these circumstances, we could consider acceptable channels that show prolonged responses or recurrences within a certain time interval after the cognitive task has disappeared. We will call this time interval the *accepted latency*, and we will consider for it a cutoff value of 3 s. In this way, for example, channels 3 and 5 become accepted as precise and specific.

Another problem of detection is the continuity of responses, which is related to the sensitivity of the EEG channel to the specific cognitive task and which, implicitly, affects the accuracy of the detector. The issue of the sensitivity of the EEG channel is related to the number of true positive (TP) activations in relation to the imposed cognitive load; thus, the greater the number of TP responses or, conversely, the smaller the number of FN responses, the more sensitive the channel is. Figure 9 shows that channels 1 and 2 are more sensitive than the others and that channel 4 is the worst.

A good detector should have maximum precision and specificity, as high a sensitivity as possible, and this would also guarantee as high an accuracy as possible. In Figure 10 we have provided the result of the evaluation of the indicators discussed above, for three tests from both types of cognitive load.

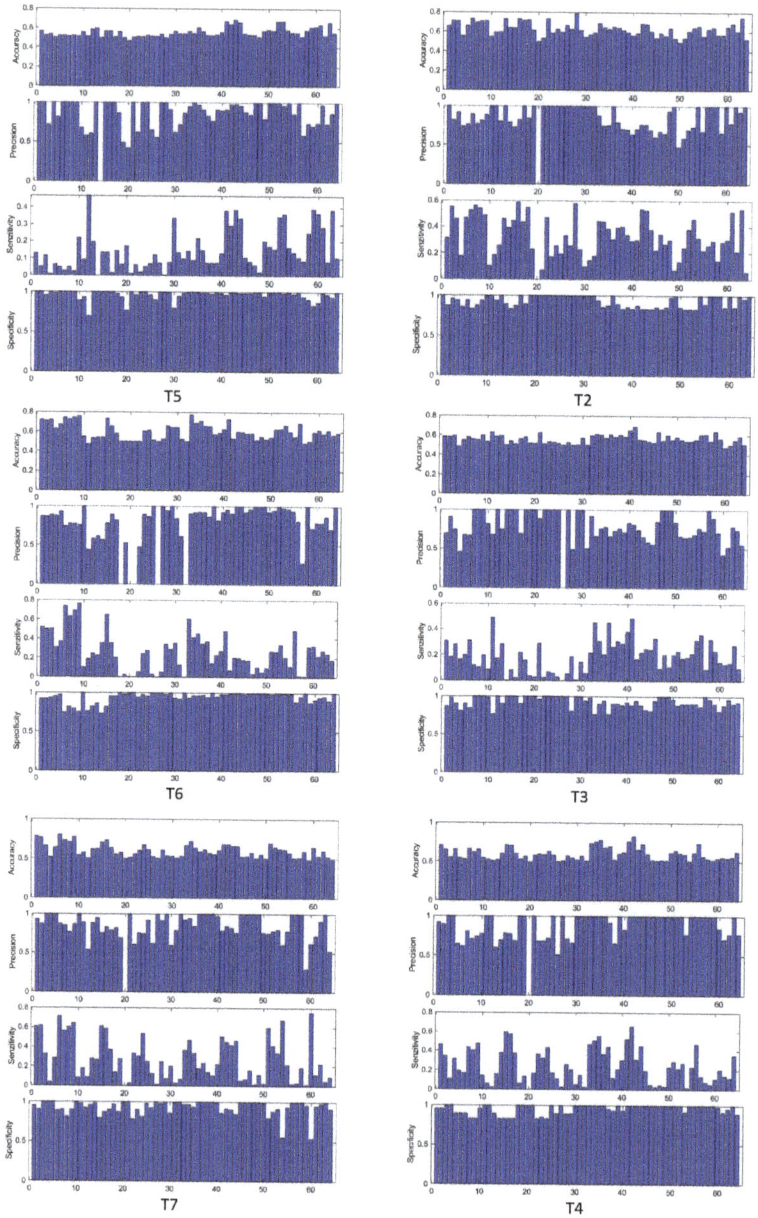

Figure 10. Accuracy, precision, sensitivity, and specificity indicators represented comparatively for all EEG channels in tests with intermittent load (left stack) and with continuous load (right stack).

Table 5 shows the numerical ranges for the performance criteria calculated for those specific EEG channels selected with the *t*-test for the highest confidence level (99%), for intermittent cognitive load applied.

Table 5. Values of performance indicators for tests with intermittent cognitive load.

EEG Channel		Precision	Specificity	Sensitivity	Accuracy
2	AF7	0.943–0.815	0.980–0.875	Max 0.550	0.713–0.581
6	F5	1–0.716	1–0.958	Max 0.500	0.707–0.555
7	F7	0.976–0.649	0.903–0.854	Max 0.500	0.660–0.544
34	Fp2	1–0.750	1–0.854	Max 0.500	0.720–0.645
35	AF8	1–0.754	1–0.875	Max 0.500	0.700–0.629
36	AF4	1–0.700	1–0.840	Max 0.500	0.685–0.652
40	F4	0.880–0.637	0.969–0.833	Max 0.500	0.750–0.563
41	F6	1–0.696	1–0.854	Max 0.500	0.760–0.594
43	FT8	0.890–0.637	0.833–0.800	Max 0.500	0.770–0.563
44	FC6	0.860–0.800	0.865–0.820	Max 0.600	0.670–0.530

These deterministic values are based on probabilistic values regarding the occurrence of the task detector response with respect to the task profile, which is strictly defined in time. But the neural dynamics are quite complex and there is no guarantee that the EEG signals should perfectly copy the cognitive task profile. Indeed, statistical tests show good detection specificity for certain signals, and this can even be seen visually in Figures 11–14.

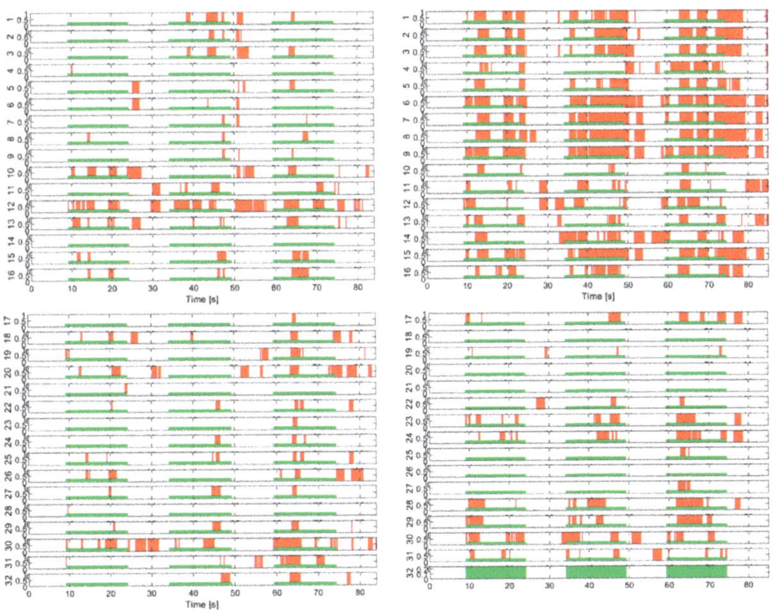

Figure 11. *Cont.*

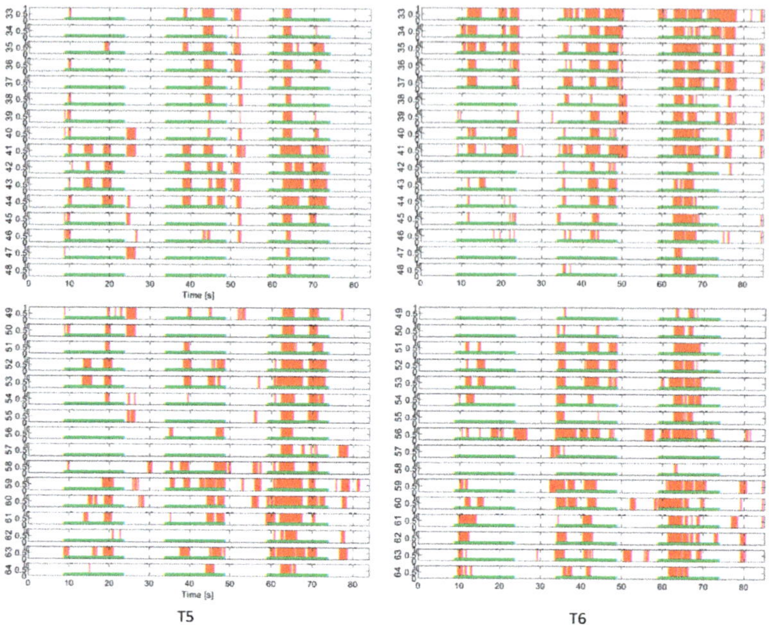

Figure 11. EEG channel activation patterns in T5 and T6 intermittent cognitive load tests. The light green areas indicate the periods of application of the cognitive load. The red areas indicate the detection of EEG activity in response to the load.

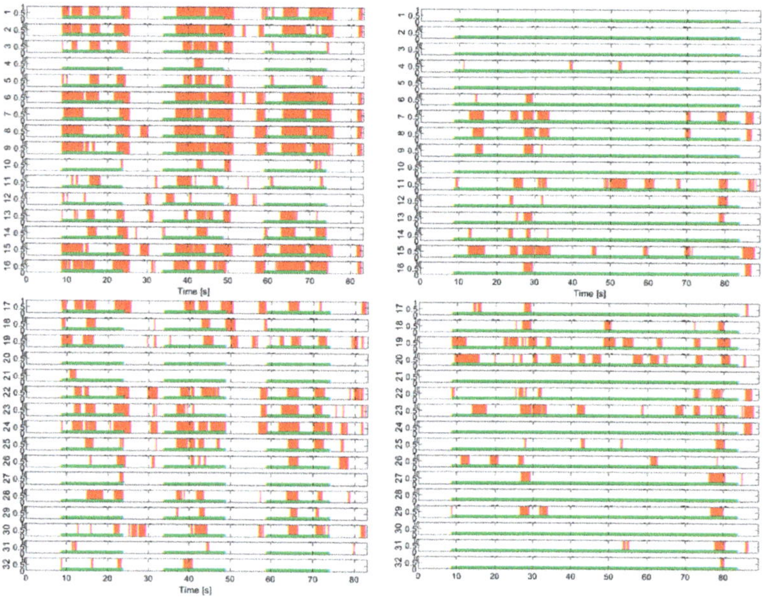

Figure 12. *Cont.*

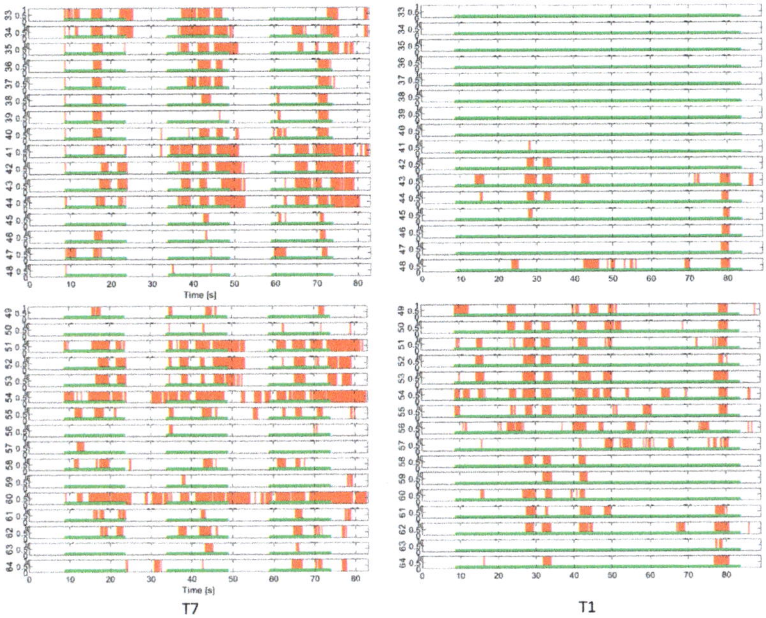

Figure 12. EEG channel activity presented in comparison between the T7 test—with intermittent cognitive task (left stack) and the reference test T1—relaxed state with eyes open (right stack).

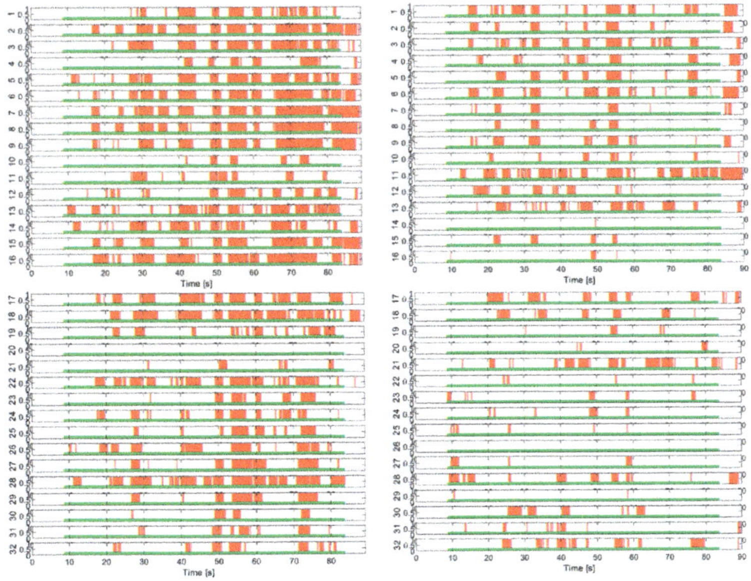

Figure 13. *Cont.*

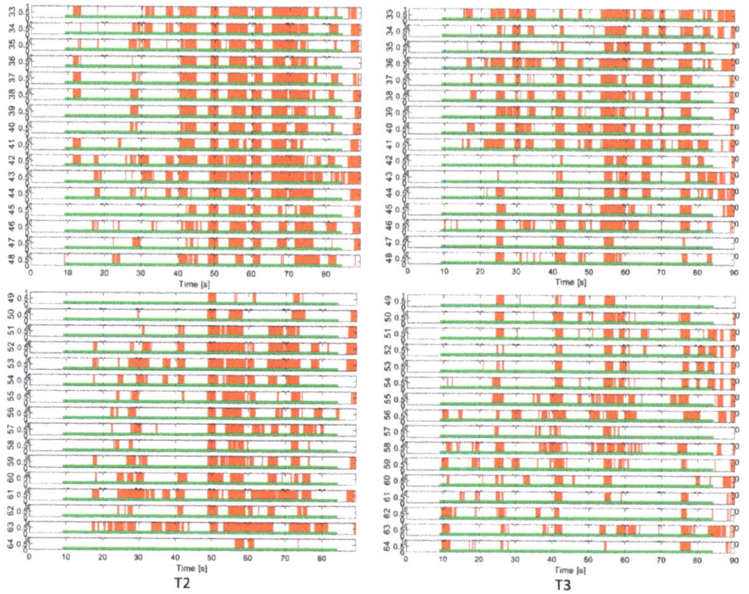

Figure 13. EEG activation patterns across channels in continuous cognitive load tests.

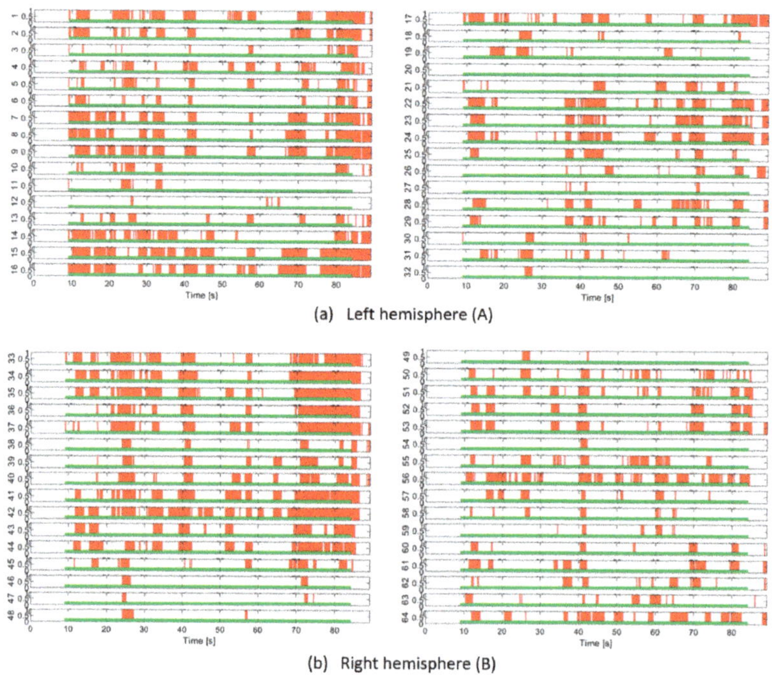

Figure 14. EEG activation patterns across channels for continuous cognitive load test T4.

Gathering the information revealed so far, we can make the following interpretations:

The EEG channels with high specificity (a confidence level of 98%) are located in cortical areas recognized for mental processes in the presence of cognitive tasks in general, and numerical ones in particular. Thus, in the frontal lobe, when the intermittent task is applied, the channels AF7, F5, F7, T7, and TP7 become active in the left hemisphere, and in the right hemisphere, Fpz, Fp2, AF8, AF4, F4, F6, FT8, T8, and FC6 become active. During tests with a continuously applied cognitive task, AF7, F5, and F3 were active in the left hemisphere, and TP8 and P10 were additionally activated in the right hemisphere. In the tests based on Physionet, the task was applied continuously, but as the number of measurement points was smaller, channels located in the same frontal areas were detected: Fp1 and F3 on the left, and Fp2 and F4 on the right, but in addition, the P3 channel was also detected in the left parietal, and C4 in the right central area.

This is remarkable in all tests to detect EEG activity in the frontal areas that govern executive operations for the mental control responsible for working memory and attention. Both processes are involved in arithmetic calculation tasks in specific tests with serial subtraction or addition operations that are equivalent to counting backwards or forwards by a certain step, starting from a specified number. The signals coming from the temporal and frontotemporal areas (T7, T8, FT8, TP7, and TP8) signify work with declarative memory. These do not manifest themselves in the same way in all tests, probably due to the variable mental effort. An interesting signal, detected only in the Physionet experiment, is P3 in the parietal region, where the existence of a so-called hub of computational abilities was recognized [19]. In our experiment this channel was not eligible according to statistical tests; in some tests it appears with low sensitivity and therefore has little activity. However, in tests with continuous load the activity of the opposite channel (in the right hemisphere) P4 is noted, but only for the 95% confidence level.

A remarkable fact is related to the differences in EEG activity in tests with intermittent load versus those with continuous load, where a certain balance appears in the left side of the frontotemporal area (including F7, T7, and TP7) in the case of intermittent load.

A more accurate decision on the choice of the most suitable EEG channels for a specific task can be made based on a larger experimental study. In any case, with the procedure described above, our study reveals distinct patterns of EEG activity on the selected channels, in correlation with the profile of the applied cognitive task. Thus, in Figure 11, we can clearly distinguish in a large part of the channels the gaps in EEG activity synchronized with the intermittent application of the mental task (tests T5 and T6). The T7 test is presented in Figure 12, the left stack, and in the right stack we can see the comparative EEG activity in the absence of the cognitive task in the T1 test. Also, in Figure 13 we see the EEG activity without regular gaps when the task is applied continuously in tests T2 and T3, respectively, in Figure 14 for the T4 test. In addition, in tests with continuous tasks we find an increase in the activation rate over time, as the mental task progresses, which suggests the effect of progressive brain loading.

These results are encouraging for our stated goal in the introduction of the paper, i.e., to detect cognitive load associated with arithmetic calculation without involving machine learning techniques and large datasets. The presented experiments proved that the detection of mental load based on an individual threshold—as a reference state, using a distinct signal metric and analyzing the signals in a specific narrow band—is feasible. The discussion of the results involves several panels.

First, the operation of the method was proven on the Physionet database and then on the datasets acquired through our own experiments. In both cases, the method proved capable of discriminating mental load in relation to the reference resting state despite the differences in equipment and test format. Regarding the performance of the load detector, we found that the duration of the calibration period positively influences the detection accuracy, but a duration that is too long may include disturbances in the individual's resting state, which was found in some recordings from Physionet where the last 40 s of rest before applying the mental load was taken for calibration. In our experiments, the subject undergoing tests was better controlled, in the sense of respecting the state imposed by the experimental protocol. In this case, this is an advantage of performing the tests on a single individual. The duration of the reference state imposed for calibration was only 10 s. Another parameter that influences the accuracy of the method is the size of the signal window in which the metric used for detection is averaged. The window comprises a specified number of signal periods over which the averaging is performed, and the size of this number is the subject of a compromise: a short window benefits real-time detection but degrades detection accuracy, and, conversely, a longer window increases accuracy but introduces a corresponding delay. We obtained the presented results using a signal frame containing 10 periods, which means about 2.2 s of response delay and the best detection accuracy of around 0.7 (as seen in Table 5). Increasing the frame length to 20 periods results in an inherent delay of over 4 s, but also an increase in accuracy to about 0.85.

Secondly, the relevance of the results from an experimental point of view is supported by the evident synchronization of the activation of some signals with the profile of the application of the cognitive task over time. Thus, our experiments were structured in such a way as to stimulate specific mental activity dynamically and intermittently in the narrow band chosen for analysis.

Third, the sustainability of the results from a neuroscience perspective comes from the statistical analysis of the experimental data which revealed a high level of confidence for certain signals with a confirmed role in the detection of mental load, as presented in Table 4.

5. Conclusions

In this paper, we presented the results of an original experimental study highlighting the EEG activity of the brain during the processing of a cognitive arithmetic task. This investigation is a complementary contribution to our previous work in the field, the results of which have already been reported [15]. In this study, we used our own mental task tests. The research methodology had two objectives: first, to create an EEG signal analysis algorithm for the detection of the specific cognitive task in real time, and second, to identify the most reliable EEG channels for the applied cognitive task. The study avoids the use of machine learning techniques that require large volumes of training data, which must be as diverse as possible—practically requiring the performance of numerous EEG experiments. Thus, instead of using pattern recognition through pre-trained models from multiple examples, the proposed method initially processes a short portion of the EEG signal in a state of imposed relaxation, to perform a calibration within the current monitoring, just before applying the cognitive task. This processing allows the establishment of reference threshold values for each EEG channel, to which the sequences of dynamically captured signals are subsequently related. The proposed signal metric is an original quantity represented by the length of the signal curve in portions equal to the signal period and which is related to the number of samples of the period. This metric is applied to the very narrow band of the filtered signal, with a width of 1 Hz. Thus, the proposed metric characterizes the signals not only from an energetic point of view, but also from the point of view of the shape of its function (curve). It does not give the signal energy itself, which can be evaluated as a separate measure, but depends on it. The use of the relative signal energy as a characteristic measure for task discrimination revealed similar results, with some small differences in the number of activations on certain channels. In summary, the main results of our research can be described as follows:

- We demonstrated narrowband EEG activity at low frequency in the theta wave domain for arithmetic cognitive tasks.
- We demonstrated the feasibility of an algorithm suitable for real-time detection of a cognitive task, using a particular signal metric—the length of the signal curve over a period, with detection criteria of the reference threshold type that are determined during the calibration stage, at the beginning of the test.
- We highlighted the EEG channels that provided the best detection performance indicators, in relation to the applied cognitive task.
- We highlighted the synchronization of responses to certain EEG channels with the temporal profile of cognitive task application; this is a remarkable fact, especially in tests with an intermittent task.

Finally, in relation to the issue of finding the most relevant and reliable EEG channels that respond to the specific cognitive task, our research led to pertinent results from a neuroscientific point of view and in agreement with other studies reported in the literature. The results reported in the literature differ, but all mention nearby channels in the same regions of the cortex. Our results reinforce some findings in the literature and, in addition, thanks to the 64 electrodes used, the additional signals AF3, AF4, and AF8 in the frontal region, FT8 from the frontotemporal region, FC6 from the right central frontal, and TP7 and TP8 from the temporal–parietal were revealed. These results are quite consistent with various reports cited in the field [4–10,15]. Our study also has some limitations. The first is related to the limited number of experiments and types of cognitive load tests applied. The second is related to the offline application, in a signal preprocessing stage, of a systematic procedure for eliminating artifacts. The subsequent research effort will be oriented towards systematizing the experiments and ensuring uniformity of the testing conditions to discriminate as precisely as possible different types of cognitive tasks. On the other hand, we consider the potential of the developed detection algorithm for investigating other mental states using different narrowband frequencies.

Author Contributions: Conceptualization, S.I. and D.A.C.; methodology, D.A.C. and S.I.; software, S.I.; validation, S.I. and D.A.C.; formal analysis, S.I. and D.A.C.; investigation, D.A.C.; resources, S.I.; data curation, D.A.C. and S.I.; writing—original draft preparation, S.I.; writing—review and editing, D.A.C. and S.I.; visualization, S.I.; supervision, S.I.; project administration, S.I. and D.A.C.; funding acquisition, S.I. All authors have read and agreed to the published version of the manuscript.

Funding: This research received no external funding.

Institutional Review Board Statement: The study was conducted in accordance with the Declaration of Helsinki, and approved by Ethics Committee of National University of Science and Technology POLITEHNICA Bucharest (Nr. 15/27.05.2025).

Informed Consent Statement: Written informed consent has been obtained from the subject involved to publish this paper.

Data Availability Statement: The data presented in this study are available on request from the corresponding author, due to the restriction of their use for commercial or non-academic purposes.

Conflicts of Interest: The authors declare no conflict of interest.

References

1. Schutter, D.J.; Kenemans, J.L. Theta-Beta Power Ratio. An Electrophysiological Signature of Motivation, Attention and Cognitive Control. In *The Oxford Handbook of EEG Frequency*; Oxford University Press: Cary, NC, USA, 2022; Chapter 15, pp. 352–376.
2. Lázár, A.S.; Lázár, Z.I.; Bódizs, R. Frequency Characteristics of Sleep. In *The Oxford Handbook of EEG Frequency*; Oxford University Press: Cary, NC, USA, 2022; Chapter 17; pp. 401–433.

3. Menon, V. Arithmetic in the Child and Adult Brain. In *The Oxford Handbook of Numerical Cognition*; Cohen Kadosh, R., Dowker, A., Eds.; Oxford University Press: Cary, NC, USA, 2015; pp. 503–530.
4. Fatimah, B.; Pramanick, D.; Shivashankaran, P. Automatic Detection of Mental Arithmetic Task and Its Difficulty Level Using EEG Signals. In Proceedings of the 2020 11th International Conference on Computing, Communication and Networking Technologies (ICCCNT), Kharagpur, India, 1–3 July 2020; IEEE: New York, NY, USA, 2020; pp. 1–6.
5. Fatimah, B.; Javali, A.; Ansar, H.; Harshitha, B.G.; Kumar, H. Mental Arithmetic Task Classification Using Fourier Decomposition Method. In Proceedings of the 2020 International Conference on Communication and Signal Processing (ICCSP), Melmaruvathur, India, 28–30 July 2020; IEEE: New York, NY, USA, 2020; pp. 46–50.
6. Attallah, O. An Effective Mental Stress State Detection and Evaluation System Using Minimum Number of Frontal Brain Electrodes. *Diagnostics* **2020**, *10*, 292. [CrossRef] [PubMed]
7. Ganguly, B.; Chatterjee, A.; Mehdi, W.; Sharma, S.; Garai, S. EEG Based Mental Arithmetic Task Classification Using a Stacked Long Short Term Memory Network for Brain-Computer Interfacing. In Proceedings of the 2020 IEEE VLSI Device Circuit and System (VLSI DCS), Kolkata, India, 18–19 July 2020; IEEE: New York, NY, USA, 2020; pp. 89–94.
8. Varshney, A.; Ghosh, S.K.; Padhy, S.; Tripathy, R.K.; Acharya, U.R. Automated Classification of Mental Arithmetic Tasks Using Recurrent Neural Network and Entropy Features Obtained from Multi-Channel EEG Signals. *Electronics* **2021**, *10*, 1079. [CrossRef]
9. Al-jumaili, S. Efficient Mental Arithmetic Classification Using Approximate Entropy Features and Machine Learning Classifiers. *Aurum J. Health Sci.* **2024**, *5*, 109–120.
10. Seleznov, I.; Zyma, I.; Kiyono, K.; Tukaev, S.; Popov, A.; Chernykh, M.; Shpenkov, O. Detrended Fluctuation, Coherence, and Spectral Power Analysis of Activation Rearrangement in EEG Dynamics During Cognitive Workload. *Front. Hum. Neurosci.* **2019**, *13*, 270. [CrossRef] [PubMed]
11. Saini, M.; Satija, U. State-of-the-Art Mental Tasks Classification Based on Electroencephalograms: A Review. *Physiol. Meas.* **2023**, *44*, 06TR01. [CrossRef] [PubMed]
12. So, W.K.Y.; Wong, S.W.H.; Mak, J.N.; Chan, R.H.M. An Evaluation of Mental Workload with Frontal EEG. *PLoS ONE* **2017**, *12*, e0174949. [CrossRef] [PubMed]
13. Hwang, T.; Kim, M.; Hwangbo, M.; Oh, E. Optimal Set of EEG Electrodes for Real-Time Cognitive Workload Monitoring. In Proceedings of the 18th IEEE International Symposium on Consumer Electronics (ISCE 2014), JeJu Island, Republic of Korea, 22–25 June 2014; IEEE: New York, NY, USA, 2014; pp. 1–2.
14. Wang, Q.; Sourina, O. Real-Time Mental Arithmetic Task Recognition From EEG Signals. *IEEE Trans. Neural Syst. Rehabil. Eng.* **2013**, *21*, 225–232. [CrossRef] [PubMed]
15. Coman, D.A.; Ionita, S.; Lita, I. Evaluation of EEG Signals by Spectral Peak Methods and Statistical Correlation for Mental State Discrimination Induced by Arithmetic Tasks. *Sensors* **2024**, *24*, 3316. [CrossRef] [PubMed]
16. Čeko, M.; Hirshfield, L.; Doherty, E.; Southwell, R.; D'Mello, S.K. Cortical cognitive processing during reading captured using functional-near infrared spectroscopy. *Sci. Rep.* **2024**, *14*, 19483. [CrossRef] [PubMed]
17. Oostenveld, R.; Fries, P.; Maris, E.; Schoffelen, J.-M. FieldTrip: Open Source Software for Advanced Analysis of MEG, EEG, and Invasive Electrophysiological Data. *Comput. Intell. Neurosci.* **2011**, *2011*, 156869. [CrossRef] [PubMed]
18. Zyma, I.; Tukaev, S.; Seleznov, I.; Kiyono, K.; Popov, A.; Chernykh, M.; Shpenkov, O. Electroencephalograms during Mental Arithmetic Task Performance. *Data* **2019**, *4*, 14. [CrossRef]
19. Mendez, M.F. *The Mental Status Examination Handbook*; Elsevier: Amsterdam, The Netherlands, 2021.

sensors

MDPI

Article

Early Findings on the Effectiveness of Novel Awakening Stimuli for Patients with Congenital Central Hypoventilation Syndrome

Silvia Rapella [1], Caterina Piazza [1], Francesco Morandi [2], Alessandro Carcano [2], Cinzia Arzilli [3], Niccolò Nassi [3], Igor Catalano [4], Francesca Formica [1] and Emilia Biffi [1,*]

1 Scientific Institute, IRCCS Eugenio Medea, 23842 Bosisio Parini, LC, Italy; silvia.rapella@lanostrafamiglia.it (S.R.); caterina.piazza@lanostrafamiglia.it (C.P.); francesca.formica@lanostrafamiglia.it (F.F.)
2 Italian Association for Congenital Central Hypoventilation Syndrome (AISICC), 50126 Florence, FI, Italy; morandifrancesco55@gmail.com (F.M.); carcaalex@gmail.com (A.C.)
3 Meyer Children's Hospital IRCCS, 50139 Florence, FI, Italy; arzillicinzia@hotmail.it (C.A.); niccolo.nassi@meyer.it (N.N.)
4 Pediatric Palliative Care, Pain Service, Department of Women's and Children's Health, University of Padua, 35128 Padua, PD, Italy; igor.catalano@vidas.it
* Correspondence: emilia.biffi@lanostrafamiglia.it; Tel.: +39-031-877862

Abstract: Congenital Central Hypoventilation Syndrome (CCHS) is a rare disorder that impairs autonomic breathing control, leading to alveolar hypoventilation and sometimes to central apnoea, predominantly during sleep. Patients typically require nocturnal ventilatory support and alarms to prevent life-threatening desaturation events. However, current alarm systems integrated into pulse oximeters do not provide adequate assistance at home. To address these limitations, we developed an assistive device with customizable multisensory stimulation that activates based on the severity and duration of desaturation episodes. In a multicenter clinical trial involving 4 children and 11 young adults with CCHS, we assessed the device's effectiveness and the role of arousals over three nights: one baseline and two test nights. The results showed that the device significantly improved awakening rates and enabled faster recovery from desaturations in young adults. However, no such improvements were observed in children compared to the baseline. Arousal events and sleep efficiency were unaffected by the device in both groups. These findings suggest that the device can enhance the safety and autonomy of young adults with CCHS but may be more effective in alerting caregivers in pediatric cases than directly waking children. Further studies are needed to refine its application across different age groups, given the limited sample size.

Keywords: congenital central hypoventilation syndrome; assistive device; desaturation episodes; arousal

1. Introduction

Congenital Central Hypoventilation Syndrome (CCHS), also referred to as Ondine's curse, is a rare genetic disease characterized by impaired breathing control associated with Autonomic Nervous System (ANS) dysfunction whose incidence is estimated at around 1/200,000 live births [1]. A definitive diagnosis of CCHS is made by confirming PHOX2B gene mutation; the majority of patients with CCHS have polyalanine repeat mutations (PARMs), while approximately 10% of patients are heterozygous for non-polyalanine repeat mutations (NPARMs) [2]. CCHS is mainly characterized by abnormally reduced or absent ventilatory responses to hypercapnia and hypoxia during sleep.

Since there is no definitive therapy for this disease, patients with CCHS are assisted, predominantly during sleep, using diaphragm pacing, non-invasive ventilation (NIV) or invasive ventilation with tracheostomy [1,3,4]. Furthermore, their blood oxygenation is monitored throughout the whole night by means of non-invasive pulse oximeters that measure peripheral blood oxygen saturation (SpO_2) according to the photoplethysmography principle, with a low-intensity infrared (IR) sensor usually located on a finger to assess potential decreases in oxygen levels in body tissues [5]. If low oxygen levels are detected by the pulse oximeter, the acoustic alarm integrated into the device signals the dangerous situation and wakes up the patient or alerts the caregiver [6]. The patient's awakening allows the recovery of the correct saturation level after a period of time that depends on the initial desaturation level. In contrast, without a wake-up stimulus or intervention, the CO_2 anesthesia can cause neurological damage and also lead to patient death. Currently, the only alarm systems available for patients with CCHS are those integrated into pulse oximeters; these alarms trigger every time the SpO_2 level falls below a safety threshold. Since patients may have reduced or an absent perception of audio alarms while asleep, a caregiver or a parent is needed all night long to serve as a supervisor and to take proper action if the situation worsens [7]. Sometimes oxygen saturation may fall below the threshold and return to normal levels within a few seconds while the patient is asleep, e.g., in case of sensor movement or an artefact in SpO_2 measurements. This situation, although it is no real danger for the patient, causes the alarm to sound, as the pulse oximeter does not take the time variable into account. Therefore, during the night, the pulse-oximeter alarm may activate several times for borderline situations and false alarms. This causes a tendency to lower the warning threshold values to not disturb the patient's or caregiver's sleep [8]. Another problem could be related to habituation: both patients and caregivers can become less responsive to frequent and repeated alarm stimuli. Thus, it is tough for young adults with CCHS to achieve independence and live on their own because of the risk that they doze off without wearing the ventilation mask or that, during the night, they do not hear the alarms and do not wake up.

A few studies have proposed the development of a system to wake up patients created specifically for this syndrome. Mayer et al. developed a mobile alarm system worn behind the ears that monitors the blood oxygen saturation level. If this drops below a pre-defined threshold, a loud acoustic signal is emitted to wake up the patient. However, the device has been tested only on one healthy subject; therefore, another study should be conducted to evaluate the usability of the prototype on people with CCHS [9]. Attali et al. tested on 20 healthy subjects and 20 patients with CCHS or Chronic Obstructive Pulmonary Disease (COPD) a device composed of a vibrating wristband and a phone application. In their study, they concluded that the use of vibrotactile stimulation alone is not able to awaken ventilator-dependent patients, including participants with CCHS. They suggest testing the efficacy of vibrotactile stimulation combined with an audio alarm [10]. In this context, our group developed an assistive device to improve assistance for patients with CCHS and help overcome the previously listed problem [6]. The device is coupled with a pulse-oximeter and carries out various multisensory stimulation strategies (acoustic, tactile, and proprioceptive stimuli) depending on the SpO_2 blood concentration level and duration of desaturation. The idea is to lead to a certain awakening of the patient in critical conditions. In fact, the most intense sensory stimulation is used in life-threatening situations. If the device is able to awaken patients, it will increase the everyday safety and independence of teenagers and adults with CCHS. The device has been tested in two previous studies. In the first one, through the involvement of eight healthy subjects, it was demonstrated that the device works correctly, guarantees rapid awakenings, and does not affect the user's sleep [11]. In the other one, the device was tested on a group of five individuals with CCHS, and it was found to be relatively effective in inducing wakefulness without impacting sleep quality. However, the results are considered preliminary due to the small sample size, which limited the ability to extensively test each actuator on all participants [12].

Another aspect that was reported in [12] was the efficacy of the device in inducing arousals, defined as a rapid shift in the electroencephalography (EEG) frequency lasting at least 3 s but no more than 15 s [13]. This phenomenon has been studied in adult patients with breathing disorders, showing the importance of arousal for recovery after desaturations. Indeed, the arousal is thought to be a protective reflex against hypoxemia. However, the effect of arousals in children and adolescents is still debated [14–17], and there is very limited knowledge about arousals events and their effects on subjects affected by CCHS.

This manuscript describes the first attempt to clinically validate the device previously developed by our group [11], thus paving the way to its applicability as an assistive device for CCHS patients.

Specifically, this manuscript describes the results of a multicenter clinical trial aimed at testing the device on 15 patients with CCHS of different ages. Particularly, we aimed to (1) analyze its efficacy in waking them up, in reducing the duration of desaturation, and assess if multisensory stimulation affects patients' sleep efficiency in comparison with typical night setup; (2) investigate if the presence of arousals on the EEG traces enables a faster recovery of the saturation level; (3) verify whether a stimulation device is generally superior to others in waking patients.

2. Materials and Methods

2.1. Participants

The study population comprised 15 patients with CCHS: 4 children (2 boys and 2 girls; age = 8 ± 4 years) and 11 young adults (3 boys and 8 girls; age = 22 ± 7 years). The patients were a subgroup of the cohort constituting the A.I.S.I.C.C. (Italian Association for Central Congenital Hypoventilation Syndrome) association. All patients breathed spontaneously without assistance during the daytime while needing invasive or non-invasive ventilator support during the night. Everyone has a genetically confirmed diagnosis of CCHS; the PHOX2B mutations include 14 cases with polyalanine repeat mutations (PARMs) and one with nonPARM (NPARM) frameshift mutations. The demographical and clinical characteristics of our cohort are summarized in Table 1.

Table 1. Participants' characteristics and site of the testing procedure. NIV: non-invasive ventilation. Tracheo: tracheostomy. PPPCS: Pediatric Pain and Palliative Care Service of the University of Padua.

Subject	Gender	Age (Years)	Gene Mutation	Type of Ventilation	Testing Location
S_001	F	18	PHOX2B 20/27 PARM	NIV	IRCCS E. Medea
S_002	M	5	PHOX2B 20/27 PARM	Tracheo	IRCCS E. Medea
S_003	M	5	PHOX2B 20/26 PARM	NIV	IRCCS E. Medea
S_004	F	18	PHOX2B frameshift NPARM	NIV	IRCCS E. Medea
S_005	F	19	PHOX2B 20/26 PARM	NIV	IRCCS E. Medea
S_006	F	16	PHOX2B 20/27 PARM	Tracheo	IRCCS E. Medea
S_007	M	17	PHOX2B 20/26 PARM	NIV	IRCCS E. Medea
S_008	F	11	PHOX2B 20/29 PARM	Tracheo	PPPCS
S_009	M	28	PHOX2B 20/26 PARM	NIV	Meyer Hospital

Table 1. *Cont.*

Subject	Gender	Age (Years)	Gene Mutation	Type of Ventilation	Testing Location
S_010	F	26	PHOX2B 20/25 PARM	Pacing	Meyer Hospital
S_011	M	22	PHOX2B 20/26 PARM	NIV/pacing	Meyer Hospital
S_012	F	12	PHOX2B 20/32 PARM	Tracheo	PPPCS
S_013	F	25	PHOX2B 20/26 PARM	Pacing	IRCCS E. Medea
S_014	F	39	PHOX2B 20/25 PARM	NIV	Meyer Hospital
S_015	F	23	PHOX2B 20/25 PARM	NIV	Meyer Hospital

Recruitment and testing were completed in three different Italian centers with expertise in the management of patients with CCHS: IRCCS E. Medea, Meyer Hospital, and the Pediatric Pain and Palliative Care Service of the University of Padua. The study was approved by the Ethic Committee of IRCCS Medea (PROT. NO 199/13-CE; date 9 April 2013) and conducted according to the guidelines of the Declaration of Helsinki. All participants were informed about the methodology and duration of the study, and written informed consent to participate was obtained from them or from their parents prior to inclusion in the protocol.

2.2. Device Description

The assistive awakening device used in this trial is coupled with a pulse-oximeter and carries out various multisensory stimulation strategies, depending on the SpO_2 level and the duration of the desaturation. The device has an Android tablet that dynamically monitors the SpO_2 level as measured using a pulse-oximeter and activates, according to an ad hoc developed software, different actuators such as a piezoelectric buzzer (acoustic stimuli), a small air fan (tactile stimulation), a vibrating pillow (tactile/proprioceptive stimulation), and a fire alarm (strong acoustic stimulation) (Figure 1) [6]. All the actuators are commercial devices with the following characteristics:

- Air fan (Blower—Squirrel Cage, Sparkfun Electronics, Niwot, CO, USA): outlet diameter of 33 mm, rated airflow 16 cubic feet per minute (CFM) and a fan speed of 3000–3500 revolutions per minute (rpm).
- Vibrating massage pillow (Pillow-massager E.R. Rovera, Lissone, Italy): dimensions $30 \times 16.5 \times 13$ cm.
- Piezoelectric buzzer (CET12A3.5, Sparkfun Electronics, Niwot, CO, USA): minimum Sound Pressure Level (SPL) of 85 dB.
- Fire alarm (ROSHNI LP (ROLP/SV, Fulleon, Cwmbran, UK)): acoustic stimulation of 100 dB.

To configure the device, four distinct severity levels (SLs) must be defined for each patient. These levels are determined by two key parameters: the maximum allowable time a patient can remain within a specific SpO_2 range and the corresponding SpO_2 value range. This dual approach enables the device to address both acute hypoxic episodes and prolonged mild hypoxia, which could pose a significant risk too. For each SL, one or more actuators can be configured, with adjustable stimulation intensity. This ensures complete customization of both the type and intensity of stimuli activated under various conditions. Additionally, the device records SpO_2 levels, heart rate, timestamps, and alarm triggers at a sampling rate of 1 Hz. It also includes a user interface that facilitates real-time SpO_2 monitoring and the efficient management of alarms [11,12].

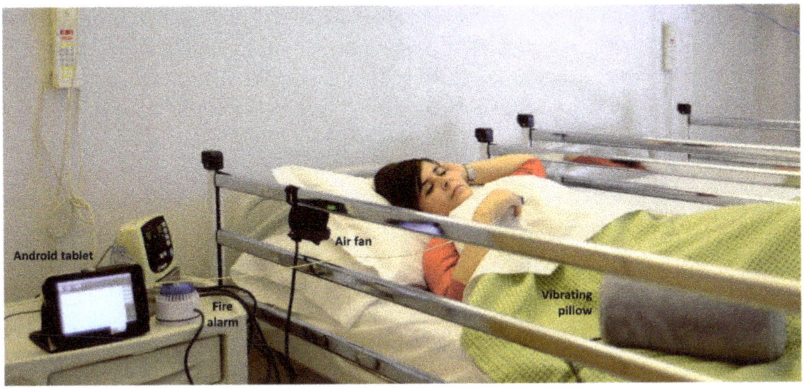

Figure 1. Assistive device with its actuators.

The device was developed by using a co-design process involving patients, their families, and doctors from the Italian Association for Congenital Central Hypoventilation Syndrome (AISICC) to ensure compliance and ease of use.

2.3. Study Design

The study protocol included 3 nights of testing per subject (Figure 2). During the first night (baseline night, B_N), the standard monitoring system of each participant was used (i.e., proper assistive ventilation device and pulse-oximeter), and polysomnographic data were acquired. This night was used to perform a baseline evaluation of patient sleep and desaturation events. During the test nights (T_{N1} and T_{N2}), the awakening device was connected to a pulse oximeter (Nonin Avant 9600, Nonin Medical, Plymouth, MN, USA) and desaturation events were recorded. The test nights were presented in a randomized way. T_{N1} differs from T_{N2} in that the subject also wears polysomnography sensors (Natus Embla N7000 or Natus Embletta X10 System, Natus Medical Incorporated, Middleton, WI, USA) to monitor electroencephalogram, respiratory flows, SpO_2, heart rate, and to evaluate sleep efficiency. Since, during this night, the patient is in a controlled sleep laboratory setting, the clinician changes the ventilator parameter to induce at least one desaturation. Using this method, we could assess device activation in borderline situations.

	Reference night	Test night 1	Test night 2
Devices used	• PSG	• **Awakening device** • PSG	• **Awakening device**
Evalueted events	• Spontaneous desaturations	• Spontaneous desaturations • Induced desaturations	• Spontaneous desaturations

Randomized order

Figure 2. Study design and setting for each night. PSG: polysomnography.

In the two test nights, the SpO_2 and time values associated with each SL were individually defined for each participant in agreement with his/her doctor. Only one actuator was activated for each SL. The fire alarm was always associated with SL4, which represents the most critical situation, while the other three actuators were randomly associated with each SL on each test night.

Each patient performed all acquisitions in the same center during three consecutive nights. One patient (S_008) completed only the reference night due to health problems not related to the clinical trial, while another (S_001) decided not to perform the reference data acquisition.

2.4. Data Acquisition

During the test nights, the different actuators were tested, thus providing us the parameters for identifying the efficacy of the device in waking up the participants, the effect of the stimulations on the participant's sleep efficiency, and the effect of arousals on the recovery of the saturation level.

The awakening device was acquired, along with a sample rate of 1 Hz, SpO_2 and beat-per-minute values, the time and type of actuators triggered, and the time the alarm remained active. The polysomnography sensors monitored the electroencephalogram, respiratory flow, SpO_2, and heart rate. SpO_2 values were also acquired through a standard pulse oximeter worn by each participant during all the nights.

2.5. Data Processing

Combining the information coming from the awakening device and the PSG, the following parameters were computed for each night and each actuator:

- number of spontaneous and induced desaturations that triggered the actuator;
- number of awakenings, time required for awakening, and time necessary for recovering the basal level of SpO_2;
- number of arousals and time required for the saturation level to recover after the arousal (evaluated only during the nights with the PSG sensors);
- time required for SpO_2 levels to return to baseline when no awakenings or arousals occurred;
- sleep efficiency.

Desaturation events were identified from the value of SpO_2 detected by the pulse oximeter and recorded by the awakening device. These events were categorized as either spontaneous or induced, depending on their cause: events triggered by a clinician modifying ventilator parameters were classified as induced, while all others were considered spontaneous. For each participant, the total number of events, categorized as either spontaneous or induced, was calculated. It was decided not to subdivide the desaturations on the basis of severity level in order for the results to have statistical consistency. Additionally, SpO_2 values were used to determine the recovery time following a desaturation for both types of events.

The offline analysis of the PSG recording, which was made by an expert clinician with several years of expertise, led to the identification of sleep stages, wake phases, and the presence of arousals during both spontaneous and induced desaturations. PSG data were analyzed with Somnologica Studio software (REM LOGIC 3 version 3.4.4.2413) by Embla N7000 and Embletta X10 System, and a scoring of the PSG tracks was performed using the age-appropriate criteria of the American Academy of Sleep Medicine [18]. Arousals were defined as a return to alpha or fast frequency EEG activity, well differentiated from the background, lasting at least 3 s but no more than 15 s [13]. The percentage of arousals was defined as the number of arousals over the number of non-awakenings events, calculated only for the nights for which these data (i.e., B_N and T_{N1}) were available. An analysis of the PSG data was also carried out to calculate sleep efficiency (i.e., sleep/wake ratio based on the number of movements measured). Furthermore, combining the SpO_2 data from the pulse oximeter and the EEG signal, the arousal effect was evaluated through a comparison between the time to recover basal SpO_2 after arousal and the time to recover basal SpO_2 if no arousal occurs.

To determine whether the patient was awake or asleep during the three nights, various types of data were analyzed. For B_N and T_{N1}, EEG data collected from the polysomnography sensor were utilized. During the remaining night, the participant's movements were visually assessed, and the moments when the patient manually silenced the alarm were taken as clear indications of wakefulness.

Then, we computed the device efficacy, defined as its ability to awaken the patient, as the number of awakenings over the total number of desaturation events (both induced and spontaneous), expressed as a percentage. By dividing the events based on the triggered actuator, the effectiveness of each actuator was likewise calculated.

Ultimately, we calculated the risk time, defined as the total time for which the patient's life is in danger due to spontaneous desaturations. This parameter accounts for two scenarios: the time before awakening if the patient wakes up, or the time required to return to normal SpO_2 levels if no awakening occurs, distinguishing between cases with arousal and those without. This time was computed when the device was available as well as without it (reference night).

2.6. Statistical Analysis

The data analysis included clustering the population into two subgroups: young adults and children (defined in the Section 2.1).

Concerning the statistical analysis, the normality of data distribution was computed using the one-sample Kolmogorov–Smirnov test. Since all the data were found to be not normally distributed, non-parametric statistical tests were used. A p-value < 0.05 was considered significant in all the tests.

First, the median and interquartile ranges (IQRs) of the percentages of awakenings were analyzed, comparing the values recorded during the test nights (T_{Ns}, i.e., both T_{N1} and T_{N2}) with those of the baseline night (B_N). The same analysis was performed for the percentage of arousals. For both parameters, differences between the test nights and the baseline night were evaluated using the Wilcoxon signed-rank test. In the second step, the data on the percentage of awakenings and arousals were clustered based on the triggered actuator, and the differences in efficacy among actuators were assessed using the non-parametric Friedman test.

Furthermore, we compared the risk time with and without the device and the recovery time in relation to the presence/absence of the arousal effect. For these temporal parameters, only spontaneous desaturations were considered, as induced desaturations represent non-physiological and highly critical situations that do not reflect typical conditions. Medians and interquartile ranges (IQRs) were calculated for each temporal parameter in T_{Ns} and B_N; differences between T_{Ns} and B_N were analyzed using the Mann–Whitney U test.

In the end, a comparison of sleep efficiency between T_{N1} and B_N was conducted using a Wilcoxon signed-rank test.

3. Results

Table 2 shows the total number of desaturation events (both induced and spontaneous) that occurred in the three nights, broken down by the type of actuator that is activated during the test nights.

Table 2. Number of total desaturations during the baseline night and the test nights (divided by the actuators that were elicited).

	Total Number of Desaturations				
	Baseline Night	Test Nights			
		Air Fan	*Buzzer*	*Vibrating Pillow*	*Fire Alarm*
Young adults (11)	768	207	158	170	17
Children (4)	256	191	66	92	12

3.1. Device Effectiveness: Awakenings, Risk Time, and Sleep Efficiency

Table 3 shows the percentage of awakening, the sleep efficiency, and the risk time during the test nights (with the device) and the baseline night (with the standard setting) on young adults and children. Interestingly, the percentage of awakenings on the test nights in young adults was statistically higher than on the night with the standard setting, with 25% (IQR = 21%) and 6% (IQR = 9%) of awakenings, respectively ($p = 0.018$). On the other hand, the device seems to have a reduced effect on children (N = 4, age = 8 ± 4), with 11% (IQR = 7%) of awakenings with the device and 3% (IQR = 5%) in the standard setting.

Table 3. Effects of the device on young adults and children in the test nights versus the baseline night [Median (IQR)].

	Young Adults		
	Test Nights (T_{Ns})	**Baseline Night (B_N)**	*p*
% awakenings	24.5 (21)%	5.6 (9.4)%	**0.018**
Sleep efficiency	71.3 (7.2)%	79.3 (10.8)%	0.153
% arousals	23 (23.4)%	0 (1.3)%	0.180
Risk time (s)	4 (7)	9 (31)	**<0.001**
	Children		
	Test Nights (T_{Ns})	**Baseline Night (B_N)**	*p*
% awakenings	10.7 (7.4)%	3.3 (5.4)%	0.180
Sleep efficiency	88.2 (9)%	88.2 (11)%	0.593
% arousals	29 (15.1)%	0 (1.3)%	0.109
Risk time (s)	6 (11)	3 (8)	**<0.001**

Sleep efficiency both in children and young adults was comparable in the nights with or without the use of the device. In fact, in young adults, the sleep efficiency was 71.3% (IQR = 7.2%) in T_{N1} and 79.3% (IQR =10.8%) in B_N. In children, the sleep efficiency was equal to 88.2% in both nights, with IQR = 9% in T_{N1} and IQR = 11% in B_N. Thus, the device does not affect the patient's sleep more than the standard setting used by the patient. In general, children have higher sleep efficiency with respect to adults.

Considering the risk time, young adults exhibited a shorter risk time in T_{Ns} compared to B_N ($p < 0.001$), with most of the risk time values on test nights concentrating below 100 s, while spreading over 300 s on the baseline night (Figure 3a). This result was opposite for children (Figure 3b), who showed higher median values of risk time during the test night. Nevertheless, Figure 3b shows that most of the risk time values on test nights concentrated below 100 s, reaching 300 s in a few cases and 1900 s during B_N. Furthermore, from a qualitative perspective, the children had a lower risk time in B_N with respect to young adults.

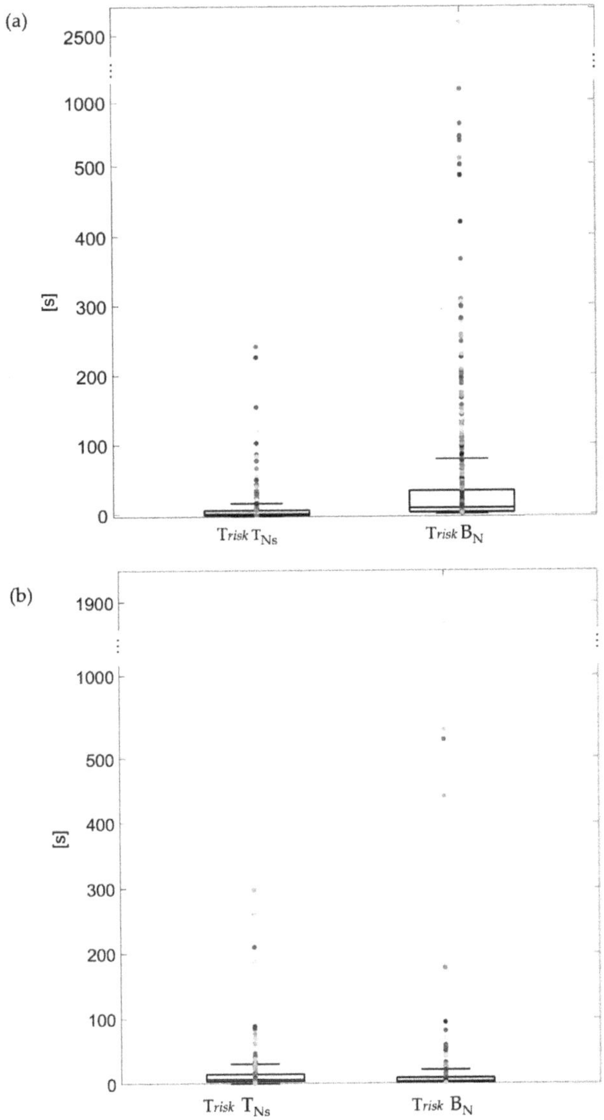

Figure 3. Risk time in young adults (**a**) and children (**b**). Each risk time is represented by a dot.

3.2. Arousal Effect

Table 3 shows that the percentage of arousals in young adults was higher in T_{Ns} with respect to B_N: 23% (IQR = 23%) and 0% (IQR = 1%), respectively. These results were also confirmed in children with 29% (IQR = 15%) of arousals in T_{Ns} with respect to 0% (IQR = 1%) in B_N. However, these differences were not statistically significant. Furthermore, young adults recovered significantly faster after an arousal (median = 4 s IQR = 6 s) caused by the activation of one of the stimulations performed by the device with respect to desaturations, during which the device did not cause arousals (median = 6 s, IQR = 25.5 s, $p < 0.001$). In contrast, in the children, an opposite trend was reported: the recovery time was 10 s (IQR = 19 s) and 3 s (IQR = 9 s), respectively ($p = 0.004$).

3.3. Differences Among Actuators

Table 4 shows the effects of the device on young adults and children divided by the type of actuators. The percentage of awakenings in young adults (N = 11, age = 22 ± 7) was 100% (IQR = 57%) for the fire alarm, while the vibrating pillow and the air fan showed lower and comparable efficacy. The worst results were obtained with the buzzer, with a percentage of awakenings of 23% (IQR = 67%). However, no significant difference was found among the stimulations. Unlike adults, in children, the most effective device was the vibrating pillow. The air fan had a slightly lower performance, while the buzzer and the fire alarm were not effective in waking them up.

Table 4. Effects of the device on young adults and children broken down by the type of triggered actuator [Median (IQR)].

			Young Adults		
	Air Fan	**Buzzer**	**Vibrating Pillow**	**Fire Alarm**	p
% awakenings	36.7 (65.5)%	23.3 (67)%	38.9 (51.5)%	100 (57)%	0.664
% arousals	19.2 (21)%	12.5 (46.1)%	0 (6.8)%	66.7 (50)%	0.482
Risk time (s)	4 (4.5)	6.5 (7)	4.5 (7)	1.5 (13.5)	0.366
			Children		
	Air Fan	**Buzzer**	**Vibrating Pillow**	**Fire Alarm**	p
% awakenings	13.6 (16.7)%	0 (3.7)%	18.8 (16.7)%	0 (0)%	0.223
% arousals	39.2 (21)%	2 (4.5)%	4.1 (15.4)%	66.7 (25)%	0.117
Risk time (s)	6 (11)	7 (20.25)	6 (11)	33 (0)	0.420

Concerning the percentage of arousal in young adults, the fire alarm is the device that caused the highest number of arousal with respect to the number of non-awakenings equal to 66.7% (IQR = 50%). In contrast, the vibrating pillow was not effective in causing arousals even if no significant difference was observed.

Finally, in young adults, the fire alarm was the device associated with the shortest risk time, while, in children, the air fan and the vibrating pillow were the actuators that most effectively reduced it. However, no statistical difference emerged when comparing the risk time among actuators in both groups.

4. Discussion

Concerning the aim of the project, the device is efficient in waking up young adults with CCHS; however, it is not effective on children. In fact, in young adults, our device has a higher percentage of awakenings with respect to the standard setting.

In young adults, the device is efficient in cases of dangerous situations, since the fire alarm, which is the alarm set in situations with higher risk for the patient, usually wakes them. Also, the fire alarm seems to be the device with the shortest risk time. The other devices are less efficient as the percentage of awakening is below 50%. A previous study tested the efficacy of a vibrotactile device for CCHS or COPD patients (aged between 19 and 24 years old). They concluded that the vibrating stimuli itself is not efficient [10].

This is confirmed by our project since the vibrating pillow itself awakens young adults only in 39% of cases. However, in our study, the difference between the four actuators was not statistically significant; this could suggest that everyone is more responsive to a different type of stimuli, confirming the importance of the modularity of the proposed device, namely, that each patient can choose which device to associate with each SL based on his/her sensitivity. Moreover, the percentage of awakenings on the test nights was statistically much higher than on the night with the standard setting in young adults. These results confirm that our device improves the patients' condition at night with respect to the common alarm integrated into the pulse oximeter. This is further confirmed by the significantly lower risk time when using the device with respect to the standard setting.

On the other hand, in children, the effectiveness in terms of both the number of awakenings and risk time is not confirmed. The percentage of awakening is not reduced with the device with respect to the standard setting, and it is possible to qualitatively appreciate the lower efficacy of all the actuators with respect to young adults. Also, the risk time is not lowered by the use of the device. However, risk time values were mainly concentrated under 100 s in both conditions. The fact that children do not react the same way as young adults to stimuli during sleep could be caused by a difference in sleep pattern that is characterized by important amounts of Slow Wave Sleep (SWS) that decrease sometime during puberty. Children have more periods of deep sleep, and it is, therefore, more difficult to wake them up [19,20], suggesting that the proposed device is not appropriate for this age group. Nevertheless, children do not live alone and do not need complete independence; therefore, the device could be a useful means to wake up their caregivers, reducing the habituation effect.

Regarding the effect of the device on arousals, the percentage of arousals corresponding to a desaturation and a stimulation activation is higher with respect to the same parameter when the standard setting is used both in young adults and children. However, the results of the statistical analysis show that the percentage of arousals in both groups does not depend on the used device. The importance of arousal for recovery after desaturation is thought to be a protective reflex against life-threatening hypoxemia in adults, while it is still debated in children and adolescents [14]. It is commonly stated in the literature that children with CCHS do not have arousal in response to endogenous hypoxemia and hypercapnia [17]. However, two studies contradict this conclusion. The first one tested the hypercapneic arousal responses of CCHS children (5.8 $\pm$ 1.2) during sleep while their home ventilators were used. During the night, a rapid increase in the inspired carbon dioxide tension was induced, and it has been shown that most CCHS children have arousal responses to hypercapnia [16]. Huang et al. studied the arousal associated with gas exchange abnormalities in CCHS patients (aged 13 $\pm$ 7 years). The study was performed by disconnecting the ventilator from the patients and evaluating the presence of arousal through overnight polysomnography. They concluded that children/youth with CCHS have frequent arousals associated with gas exchange abnormalities during sleep and that they occurred during active but not quiet sleep [15].

Another study conducted by McNamara et al. found that, in children (aged 1–14 years) with Obstructive Sleep Apnea (OSA), respiratory events were often terminated spontaneously, and that the duration of apnoea associated with arousal was longer compared with self-terminating apnoea [21]. This conclusion is supported by our findings in the children's sample, where recovery time is extended when arousals occur compared to when they do not. Conversely, in young adults, recovery time is shorter with arousal than without. This may be due to an effect observed in some studies, where an improvement in ventilation during sleep has been seen in patients who actively move during rapid eye movement sleep or even when they are passively moved [22]. In our study, arousal is not the primary mechanism for recovery from desaturation, as only 23% of non-awakenings in children and 29% in young adults are associated with arousal. Nevertheless, this may have a protective effect in young adults.

Significantly, sleep efficiency was not affected by the presence of the device in both groups. In general, in healthy school-aged children, sleep efficiency is usually around 90% [23], while in healthy adolescents and adults, sleep efficiency is considered 'good' if it is higher than 85%. Therefore, in our population, this parameter is slightly below average during all the nights.

This study presents some limitations. The first one is related to the sample size, as the study was conducted only on 15 subjects, and the number of activations for certain actuators was relatively low. Particularly, the results obtained for the children's group should be interpreted with caution, as they are based on tests conducted with only four subjects. Nevertheless, the target population for the device consists of adolescents and young adults. In the case of children, we anticipate that the device's stimulations could be directed toward the caregiver, thereby supporting their assistive role. Additionally, the limited number of recorded desaturation events restricted the ability to discern differences across varying severity levels of desaturation. Moreover, a limitation of the device stems from the use of commercially available actuators for which not all the stimulation characteristics (e.g., frequency and amplitude of the vibrations) are known. Future studies should better characterize the effect of stimuli manipulation on the device's effectiveness. Future developments of the device could leverage AI-based pattern recognition to improve its responsiveness to desaturation events, thereby enhancing its ability to dynamically adjust to individual responses. Moreover, the next step of validation will include the testing of the device at patients' homes to see how it works in their familiar environment over an extended period. Furthermore, testing on the caregivers of children with CCHS will be performed to see if the device also elicits improvements in parents' quality of life.

In conclusion, the awakening device is efficient on adolescents/youth affected by CCHS; however, it is less effective on children. Therefore, the device could be useful to wake up caregivers in response to child desaturation. The results suggest that the device proposed is effective in improving domiciliary care and the quality of life of young people who want more independence, even if it would be useful to collect more data since the patient sample size is quite small.

Author Contributions: Conceptualization, E.B., C.P., A.C. and F.M.; methodology, E.B., C.P. and S.R.; formal analysis, F.F., C.A. and S.R.; investigation, E.B., C.P., F.M., F.F., N.N., I.C. and C.A.; data curation, E.B., C.P. and S.R.; writing—original draft preparation, S.R.; writing—review and editing, E.B., C.P. and S.R.; supervision, E.B. and C.P.; project administration, E.B.; funding acquisition, E.B. and A.C. All authors have read and agreed to the published version of the manuscript.

Funding: This research was supported by the Italian Ministry of Health (RC 2012/2013 and RC 2024/2025 to E. Biffi). This work was also partially supported by Associazione Italiana per la Sindrome da Ipoventilazione Centrale Congenita Sindrome di Ondine (AISICC).

Institutional Review Board Statement: The study was conducted in accordance with the Declaration of Helsinki and approved by the Ethic Committee of IRCCS Medea (PROT. NO 199/13-CE; date 9 April 2013).

Informed Consent Statement: Informed consent was obtained from all subjects involved in the study.

Data Availability Statement: The data presented in this study are available upon request from the corresponding author.

Acknowledgments: Authors thank all of the participants and their families for their support and involvement.

Conflicts of Interest: The authors declare no conflicts of interest.

References

1. Trang, H.; Samuels, M.; Ceccherini, I.; Frerick, M.; Garcia-Teresa, M.A.; Peters, J.; Schoeber, J.; Migdal, M.; Markstrom, A.; Ottonello, G.; et al. Guidelines for diagnosis and management of congenital central hypoventilation syndrome. *Orphanet J. Rare Dis.* **2020**, *15*, 252. [CrossRef] [PubMed]
2. Kasi, A.S.; Li, H.; Jurgensen, T.J.; Guglani, L.; Keens, T.G.; Perez, I.A. Variable phenotypes in congenital central hypoventilation syndrome with PHOX2B nonpolyalanine repeat mutations. *J. Clin. Sleep Med.* **2021**, *17*, 2049–2055. [CrossRef] [PubMed]
3. O'Brien, L.M.; Holbrook, C.R.; Vanderlaan, M.; Amiel, J.; Gozal, D. Autonomic function in children with congenital central hypoventilation syndrome and their families. *Chest* **2005**, *128*, 2478–2484. [CrossRef] [PubMed]
4. Di Lascio, S.; Benfante, R.; Cardani, S.; Fornasari, D. Research Advances on Therapeutic Approaches to Congenital Central Hypoventilation Syndrome (CCHS). *Front. Neurosci.* **2021**, *14*, 615666. [CrossRef] [PubMed]
5. Leppänen, T.; Kainulainen, S.; Korkalainen, H.; Sillanmäki, S.; Kulkas, A.; Töyräs, J.; Nikkonen, S. Pulse Oximetry: The Working Principle, Signal Formation, and Applications. In *Advances in the Diagnosis and Treatment of Sleep Apnea*; Advances in Experimental Medicine and Biology; Springer: Cham, Switzerland, 2022; Volume 1384, pp. 373–385. [CrossRef]
6. Cavalleri, M.; Carcano, A.; Morandi, F.; Piazza, C.; Maggioni, E.; Reni, G. A new device for the care of Congenital Central Hypoventilation Syndrome patients during sleep. In Proceedings of the 2013 35th Annual International Conference of the IEEE Engineering in Medicine and Biology Society (EMBC), Osaka, Japan, 3–7 July 2013; pp. 2445–2448. [CrossRef]
7. Mathur, S.; Laifman, E.; Keens, T.G.; Kun, S.; Ward, S.L.D.; Perez, I.A. Children with Congenital Central Hypoventilation Syndrome Do Not Wake up to Ventilator Alarms. *Sleep Breath.* **2022**, *26*, 1277–1280. [CrossRef] [PubMed]
8. Vanderlaan, M.; Holbrook, C.R.; Wang, M.; Tuell, A.; Gozal, D. Epidemiologic Survey of 196 Patients with Congenital Central Hypoventilation Syndrome. *Pediatr. Pulmonol.* **2004**, *37*, 217–229. [CrossRef] [PubMed]
9. Mayer, J.; Junger, P.; Hokenmaier, L.; Pott, P.P. Wearable wake-up system for CCHS patients. *Curr. Dir. Biomed. Eng.* **2022**, *8*, 245–248. [CrossRef]
10. Attali, V.; Lavault, S.; Guerder, A.; Al-Youssef, S.; Dudoignon, B.; Taytard, J.; Arnulf, I.; Faure, M.; Straus, C.; Similowski, T.; et al. Awakening efficacy of a vibrotactile device in patients on home nocturnal ventilatory assistance and healthy subjects as family caregiver proxies. *Chronic Respir. Dis.* **2020**, *17*, 1479973120983331. [CrossRef] [PubMed]
11. Biffi, E.; Piazza, C.; Cavalleri, M.; Taddeo, P.; Carcano, A.; Morandi, F.; Reni, G. An assistive device for congenital cen-tral hypoventilation syndrome outpatients during sleep. *Ann. Biomed. Eng.* **2014**, *42*, 2106–2116. [CrossRef] [PubMed]
12. Biffi, E.; Piazza, C.; Morandi, F.; Avantaggiato, P.; Formica, F.; Carcano, A.; Borgatti, R.; Reni, G. Preliminary data on the usability and efficacy of an assistive device for the Congenital Central Hypoventilation Syn-drome: An observational study. In Proceedings of the XIV Mediterranean Conference on Medical and Biological Engineering and Computing 2016, Paphos, Cyprus, 31 March–2 April 2016.
13. Togo, F.; Cherniack, N.S.; Natelson, B.H. Electroencephalogram characteristics of autonomic arousals during sleep in healthy men. *Clin. Neurophysiol.* **2006**, *117*, 2597–2603. [CrossRef] [PubMed]
14. Remmers, J.E.; Degroot, W.J.; Sauerland, E.K.; Anch, A.M. Pathogenesis of upper airway occlusion during sleep. *J. Appl. Physiol.* **1978**, *44*, 931–938. [CrossRef] [PubMed]
15. Huang, J.; Colrain, I.M.; Panitch, H.B.; Tapia, I.E.; Schwartz, M.S.; Samuel, J.; Pepe, M.; Bandla, P.; Bradford, R.; Mosse, Y.P.; et al. Effect of sleep stage on breathing in children with central hypoventilation. *J. Appl. Physiol.* **2008**, *105*, 44–53. [CrossRef] [PubMed]
16. Marcus, C.L.; Bautista, D.B.; Amihyia, A.; Ward, S.L.D.; Keens, T.G. Hypercapneic arousal responses in children with congenital central hypoventilation syndrome. *Pediatrics* **1991**, *88*, 993–998. [PubMed]
17. Weese Mayer, D.E.; Shannon, D.C.; Keens, T.G.; Silvestri, J.M. Idiopathic Congenital Central Hypoventilation Syndrome. *Am. J. Resp. Crit. Care Med.* **1999**, *60*, 368–373.
18. Berry, R.B.; Brooks, R.; Gamaldo, C.E.; Harding, S.M.; Lloyd, R.M.; Quan, S.F.; Troester, M.M.; Vaughn, B.V. AASM Scoring Manual Updates for 2017 (Version 2.4). *J. Clin. Sleep Med.* **2017**, *13*, 665–666. [CrossRef] [PubMed]
19. Gaudreau, H.; Carrier, J.; Montplaisir, J. Age-related modifications of NREM sleep EEG: From childhood to middle age. *J. Sleep Res.* **2001**, *10*, 165–172. [CrossRef] [PubMed]
20. Bes, F.; Schulz, H.; Navelet, Y.; Salzarulo, P. The distribution of slow-wave sleep across the night: A comparison for infants. *Sleep* **1991**, *14*, 5–12. [CrossRef] [PubMed]
21. McNamara, F.; Issa, F.G.; Sullivan, C.E. Arousal pattern following central and obstructive breathing abnormalities in infants and children. *J. Appl. Physiol.* **1996**, *81*, 2651–2657. [CrossRef] [PubMed]

22. Hager, A.; Koch, W.; Stenzel, H.; Hess, J.; Schöber, J. Effects of movement and work load in patients with congenital centra hypoventilation syndrome. *Eur. J. Prev. Cardiol.* **2007**, *14*, 294–298. [CrossRef] [PubMed]
23. Montgomery-Downs, H.E.; O'brien, L.M.; Gulliver, T.E.; Gozal, D. Polysomnographic characteristics in normal pre-school an early school-aged children. *Pediatrics* **2006**, *117*, 741–753. [CrossRef] [PubMed]

sensors

MDPI

rticle

Exploring the Link Between Motor Functions and the Relative Use of the More Affected Arm in Adults with Cerebral Palsy

sabelle Poitras [1,2], Jade Clouâtre [1,3], Alexandre Campeau-Lecours [1,3] and Catherine Mercier [1,2,*]

1 Centre for Interdisciplinary Research in Rehabilitation and Social Integration, CIUSSS de la Capitale-Nationale, Quebec City, QC G1M 2S8, Canada; isabelle.poitras@ucalgary.ca (I.P.); jade.clouatre.1@ulaval.ca (J.C.); alexandre.campeau-lecours@gmc.ulaval.ca (A.C.-L.)
2 School of Rehabilitation Sciences, Laval University, Quebec City, QC G1V 0A6, Canada
3 Department of Mechanical Engineering, Laval University, Quebec City, QC G1V 0A6, Canada
* Correspondence: catherine.mercier@rea.ulaval.ca

Abstract: Individuals with hemiparetic cerebral palsy (CP) exhibit reduced use of their more affected (MA) arm, yet the factors that influence its use during activities of daily living remain elusive. The objectives of this study were to describe the relative use of the MA arm during an ecological task, examine its relationship with the level of impairment, and investigate its association with performance in various unilateral and bilateral tasks. Methods: Participants took part in two sessions comprising robotic assessments and clinical assessments of motor functions, as well as accelerometry measurement during kitchen tasks. Four variables were derived from accelerometry data. Stepwise regression analyses were used to identify the best contributors to the accelerometry variables among robotic and clinical assessments. Results: Nineteen adults with CP (34.3 years old ± 11.5; MACS I = 7, II = 6, III = 6) were included. The *Use Ratio* measured during the kitchen tasks ranged between 0.10 and 0.63. The best predictors of all accelerometry metrics were two bilateral assessments (r^2 = 0.23–0.64). Conclusions: The importance of assessing bilateral tasks was reaffirmed by the key role played by two bilateral tasks in determining the relative use of the MA arm. The results support the use of intensity-based accelerometry metrics to measure MA arm use.

Keywords: accelerometry; activities of daily living; motor function; cerebral palsy; bimanual coordination; upper extremity

1. Introduction

Individuals who have hemiparetic cerebral palsy (CP) exhibit more pronounced motor impairments in one hand than the other [1]. The arm displaying more impairments is referred to as the more affected (MA) arm, while the other arm is referred to as the less affected (LA) arm. This disparity in motor function between the two arms leads to increased attention given to the MA arm, for both assessments and interventions [2]. Indeed, most assessments that are used to characterize upper extremity motor functions are either unilateral—extrapolating impairments observed in the MA arm to bilateral motor functions —or subjective—relying on self-reported questionnaires (e.g., ABILHAND-Kids [3]) or clinicians' observations (i.e., Assisting Hand Assessment [4]). While these assessments provide valuable insights into the performance of the MA arm, they are subject to certain biases (e.g., underestimation of bilateral impairment, recall bias, reliance on the clinician's experience, etc.) [5–7]. Furthermore, bilateral upper extremity motor functions have been underexplored in adults with CP [8,9], leading to even fewer validated options for quantitative clinical assessments in this population, while the assessments that are available do not offer normative data [7,10]. This is an important concern, as most activities of daily living require the use of both arms in a coordinated manner.

Interestingly, the use of robotic devices for quantifying upper extremity impairment has extended to various neurologically impaired populations, including individuals who have experienced stroke [11], people living with multiple sclerosis [12], children with CP [13] and, more recently, adults with CP [14]. This technology enables quantitative assessment of both bilateral and unilateral upper extremity functions, providing normative values that allow for comparison with age- and sex-matched healthy controls [15]. This quantitative approach allows for the use of standardized tasks to tackle the mechanisms that underlie the observed decrease in motor performance. This system has been used to assess performance in different types of bilateral tasks, which can be classified according to a model [16] in children [17] and adults [14,18] with CP. This model classifies bilateral tasks according to two characteristics: (1) the symmetry of arm movements (asymmetric or symmetric task); and (2) the conceptualization of the task goal (independent goals or common goal). Children with CP used different motor strategies compared with their peers when performing symmetric and asymmetric tasks while also demonstrating worse overall motor performance. This suggests that the type of task has a significant impact on their motor performance [19,20]. However, little is known about the bilateral performance of adults with cerebral palsy during symmetric and asymmetric tasks. Indeed, only three studies have addressed this question: one identified worse performance during an asymmetric task [14], while the other two showed that adults with CP tend to slow down their less affected arm to match the capabilities of their more affected arm [8,9]. The use of robotic devices gives interesting insights on potential reasons explaining bilateral impairments. However, a primary limitation of robotic devices is that they are not ecological because they restrict the number of degrees of freedom and the influence of gravity. This potentially limits the ability to generalize conclusions to a broader context.

Recently, the use of accelerometers has been proposed to address this limitation and offer a more ecologically valid assessment of upper extremity use during daily activities. These systems are portable, small, easy to use, and capable of providing valid results across various populations [21–23], including in adults with CP [24,25]. Accelerometers generally quantify either the intensity of arm use [21,26] or the amount of time of arm use [27,28]. Measuring arm use in the context of daily activities is particularly important given a phenomenon known as "developmental disregard" in individuals with CP. Developmental disregard is defined as the underuse of the MA arm during activities of daily living, despite assessments of the upper extremity's actual capacity indicating that the person should be capable of performing the task with their MA arm or both arms [29–32]. This underuse could lead to a decrease in motor capacity in the unused hand, resulting in further disabilities [29,32]. However, accelerometry data do not provide information on the reason why the MA arm is not used to a greater extent. As a result, measuring developmental disregard and understanding which factor contributes to it remains a challenge.

Given the fact that each assessment method has strengths and limitations, a multimodal assessment approach was used, combining clinical, robotic, and accelerometry assessments as the potential to provide insights on the relationship between upper extremity capacities and upper extremity use in real-world contexts. Therefore, the first objective of this study was to describe the relative use of the MA arm during an ecological task and to assess the difference of relative use of the MA across different levels of motor impairments (Manual Ability Classification System (MACS) I, II, and III) in adults with CP. The second objective was to assess the relationship between the relative use of their MA arm during an ecological task and their motor functions, measured using either clinical or robotic assessment tools.

To attain these two objectives, we assessed MA arm use using accelerometers worn on each wrist during kitchen tasks. The kitchen task was chosen as it is a common everyday activity requiring numerous bilateral movements. Four metrics were derived, focusing either on the intensity or duration of arm use, as well as on either the global relative use of each limb or specifically on periods of time where both arms were used in combination one with the other. We also employed a set of clinical and robotic assessments to measure both bilateral and unilateral motor functions. Because clinical and robotic assessments have very different requirements (primarily given that clinical assessments have a strong focus on manual functions while robotic ones focus on proximal motor control), both types of metrics were tested in separate regression models.

2. Materials and Methods

2.1. Participants

Participants were recruited from various sources, including through health records at the Centre Intégré Universitaire de Santé et de Services Sociaux de la Capitale-Nationale (CIUSSS-CN), through patient organizations, and through the Université Laval mailing list. Eligible participants met specific criteria, including being aged 18 to 65 years old, having a diagnosis of hemiparetic CP, being capable of performing a transfer with minor assistance to sit in the robotic device, and having a level of I, II, or III (mild to moderate impairments) on the MACS scale. Exclusion criteria included cognitive impairments or uncorrected visual problems that could interfere with the assessment tasks. Ethical approval for the study was obtained from the local ethics committee (Ethics #2018-609, CIUSSS-CN), and all participants provided written informed consent before participation.

The MACS level is a clinical assessment used to characterize participants' ability to manipulate objects during everyday activities. Level I indicates mild, barely visible impairments, while level III indicates significant difficulties in manipulating objects, requiring task adaptation.

2.2. Experimental Setup

Participants engaged in two assessment sessions, each lasting approximately three hours. The procedure for each session is described in Table 1. The session duration allowed time for participants to take a break between each assessment, reducing the potential impact of fatigue on motor performance. These sessions included various robotic tasks and clinical assessments. The first session involved performing robotic tasks using a bilateral Kinarm Exoskeleton Lab (Kinarm, Kingston, ON, Canada) (see Figure 1 for a visual representation of the experimental setup), along with four of the clinical assessments. The second session involved performing an Observation-based assessment of the involvement of the MA arm as well as a set of kitchen tasks. Each participant chose the recipe of their choice (the choices were baking a cake, baking cookies, or making marshmallow treats). To complete the session, participants were required to gather ingredients from the pantry and bring them to the kitchen, prepare the recipe, clean up, set the table, prepare tea or coffee, eat the dessert, drink the tea or coffee, clear the table, and wash the dishes (duration of the task between 1 h 30 min and 2 h 30 min). The duration of the task varied across participants, as the more impaired individuals generally took longer to complete the task compared with those with milder impairments. However, all participants completed the task, and the analyses were selected to minimize the impact of this difference on the accelerometry results (i.e., relative metrics). The kitchen tasks required participants to move around the kitchen, either by walking or by using a wheelchair. They wore an ActiGraph GT9X Link (sampling rate of 100 Hz, internal memory of 4 GB, accelerometer dynamic range of ±8 g, ActiGraph LLC, Pensacola, FL, USA) on each wrist while performing the task (i.e., accelerometry metrics were calculated from this task; see Figure 2 for the experimental setup for the accelerometry assessment). The two sessions were scheduled less than two weeks apart for most participants, except for one participant who experienced a four-week gap due to being affected by COVID during this period. The robotic tasks included three motor tasks, one bilateral asymmetric independent goal task (Object Hit), one bilateral symmetric common goal task (Ball on Bar), and one unilateral task (Visually Guided Reaching). The clinical assessments included five motor tasks, one bilateral asymmetric independent goal task (Observation-based assessment of the involvement of the MA arm), one bilateral symmetric common goal task (Two-Arm Coordination Test), two unilateral tasks (Jebsen–Taylor Hand Function Test and Box and Block test), and one measurement of grip strength (Jamar hand-grip dynamometer). The tasks were selected to complement each other in terms of type (i.e., there was a combination of bilateral and unilateral tasks).

Table 1. Assessment details for each session.

Session 1 (<3 h)	**Session 2 (~3 h)**
1. Informed consent and initial clinical history interview (~30 min) 2. Object Hit (~7 min) 3. Ball on Bar (~8 min) 4. Visually Guided Reaching of the MA and LA arm (~10 min) 5. Two-Arm Coordination (~15 min) 6. Jebsen–Taylor Hand Function Test of the MA and LA arm (~20 min) 7. Box and Block test (~10 min) 8. Grip strength (~8 min)	1. Observation-based assessment of the involvement of the MA arm (~30 min) 2. Kitchen task (~1 h 30 min to 2 h 30 min)

Legend: Robotic assessments are in blue, clinical assessments are in green, and accelerometry assessment is in red. Three hours was the maximum duration of the session for people having more impairments and having more fatigue (i.e., they required more frequent and longer breaks).

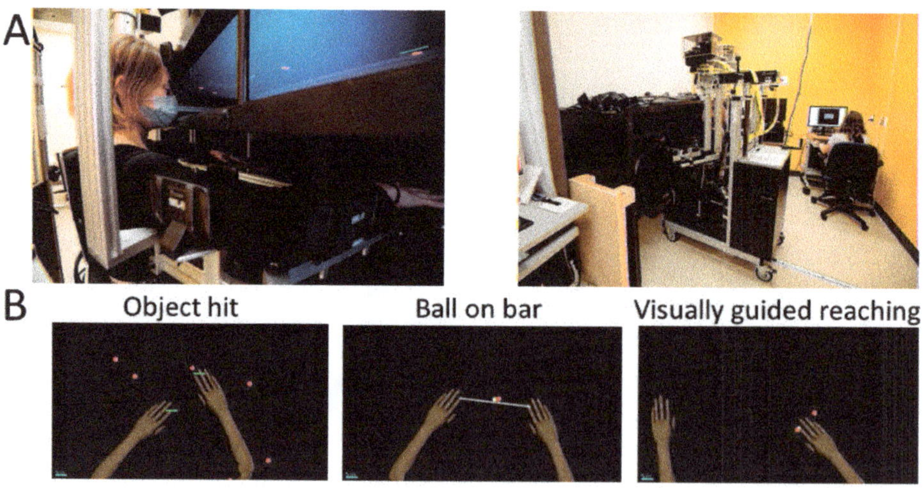

Figure 1. (**A**) Experimental setup for the Kinarm Exoskeleton Lab and (**B**) workspace representation of the Object Hit, Ball on Bar, and Visually Guided Reaching tasks.

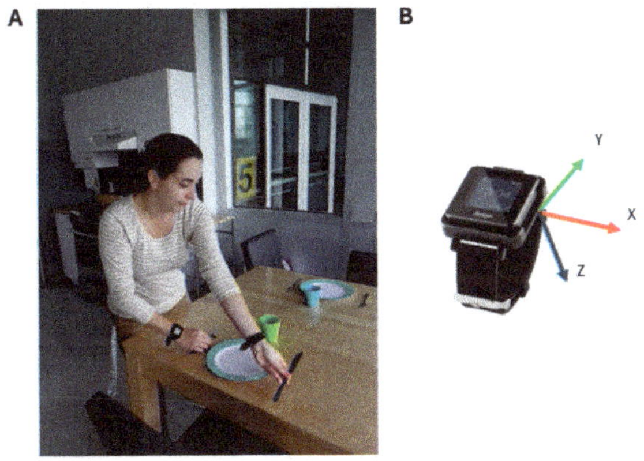

Figure 2. Experimental setup for the accelerometry assessment. (**A**). Participant wearing one accelerometer at each wrist while setting the table. (**B**). Accelerometer used for the assessment including a representation of the *x*-, *y*-, and *z*-axes.

2.3. Accelerometry Processing

The extraction of raw accelerometry data was conducted using ActiLife 6 software (ActiGraph LLC, Pensacola, FL, USA, sampling rate of 100 Hz). The offline pre-processing of data was performed using a custom MATLAB program (MATLAB version 9.6.0 (R2022b), MathWorks Inc., Natick, MA, USA) as detailed in [33], resulting in the calculation of activity counts (ACs). ACs were computed using the vector magnitude ($AC = \sqrt{{s_{xi}}^2 + {s_{yi}}^2 + {s_{zi}}^2}$), representing the norm of the AC on the *x*-, *y*-, and *z*-axes (s_{xi}, s_{yi}, and s_{zi} denote the sum of AC for a 1 s epoch). The data were then separated into epochs of 1 s, as demonstrated as optimal in adults with CP [25]. Accelerometry data were only gathered during the kitchen task.

2.4. Metrics Calculations

Four metrics (detailed below) were computed to measure the relative use of each limb: 1—*Magnitude Ratio*; 2—*Use Ratio*; 3—*Percentage of Bilateral Use*; 4—*Bilateral Arm Use Index* (*BAUI*). For the *Use Ratio* and the *Percentage of Bilateral Use*, an AC threshold of 100 was employed as these are time-based measurements, and this method has been validated by [24]. These four accelerometry metrics made it possible to test the combination of two factors: 1—focusing either on the intensity (i.e., *Magnitude Ratio* and *BAUI*) or duration (i.e., *Use Ratio* and *Percentage of Bilateral Use)* of arm use; and 2—focusing either on the global relative use of each limb (i.e., *Magnitude Ratio* and *Use Ratio*) or specifically on periods of time when both arms are used in combination with one another (i.e., *BAUI* and *Percentage of Bilateral Use*).

A fifth metric, *Bilateral Magnitude*, was extracted to provide visual presentation of the data, but it was not used for analyses.

2.4.1. *Magnitude Ratio* (Metric Focusing on Intensity + Global Relative Use)

The *Magnitude Ratio* represents the contribution of each upper extremity in a specific activity [26]. A vector of *Magnitude Ratio* was calculated for each epoch of 1 s, allowing us to visualize data for the whole task. The formula used was as follows:

$$Magnitude\ Ratio\ = \log\frac{AC\ of\ the\ MA\ arm}{AC\ of\ the\ LA\ arm} \tag{1}$$

where the AC of the MA arm represents the total AC of the MA arm, while the AC of the LA arm represents the total AC of the LA arm.

This yielded a value between −7 and 7 for each epoch of 1 s. A value of −7 represented more use of the LA arm, while a value of 7 represented more use of the MA arm. Movements that were only unilateral (e.g., where the LA arm was moving while the MA arm was still) were given an artificial value of −7 for the LA arm and 7 for the MA arm, as presented in [26]. A value of 0 indicated equal use of both arms. To gain an overview of the overall use of the upper extremities, the median value of the vector was calculated.

2.4.2. *BAUI* (Metric Focusing on Intensity + Bilateral Use)

The *BAUI* represents the ratio of the intensity of bilateral use [21]. (*BAUI* > 1 represents a higher intensity of use of the MA arm, *BAUI* < 1 represents higher intensity of use of the LA arm, *BAUI* = 1 represents equal intensity of u of both arms). The formula used was as follows:

$$BAUI = \frac{\sum(AC_{MA}\ when\ AC_{MA} \neq 0\ and\ AC_{LA} \neq 0)}{\sum(AC_{LA}\ when\ AC_{MA} \neq 0\ and\ AC_{LA} \neq 0} \quad (2)$$

where $\sum(AC_{MA} \neq 0\ AND\ AC_{LA} \neq 0)$ represents the summation of AC where both arms (MA and LA) are moving simultaneously.

2.4.3. *Use Ratio* (Metric Focusing on Duration + Global Relative Use)

The *Use Ratio* represents the proportion of time one arm was used in relation to the other (*Use Ratio* > 1 represents more use of the MA arm, *Use Ratio* < 1 represents more use of the LA arm, *Use Ratio* = 1 represents equal use of both arms). The formula used was as follows:

$$Use\ Ratio = \frac{movement\ duration\ LA\ arm\ (AC_{LA} \geq 100)}{movement\ duration\ MA\ arm\ (AC_{MA} \geq 100)} \quad (3)$$

where the $AC_{LA} \geq 100$ represents the AC of the LA arm exceeding the threshold of 100, and $AC_{MA} \geq 100$ represents the AC of the MA arm exceeding the threshold of 100.

2.4.4. *Percentage of Bilateral Use* (Metric Focusing on Duration + Bilateral Use)

The *Percentage of Bilateral Use* represents the percentage of time the two arms moved simultaneously. The formula used was as follows:

$$Percentage\ of\ Bilateral\ Use = \frac{\sum(AC_{MA} \geq 100\ AND\ AC_{LA} \geq 100)}{\sum AC_{total}} \quad (4)$$

where $AC_{MA} \geq 100\ AND\ AC_{LA} \geq 100$ represents the number of epochs where the AC of the MA arm and the AC of the LA arm exceeded the threshold of 100, and the AC_{total} represents the number of epochs where at least one arm was moving.

2.4.5. *Bilateral Magnitude*

As mentioned above, the *Bilateral Magnitude* was extracted solely for descriptive purposes. In combination with the *Magnitude Ratio*, it makes it possible to provide a visual representation of the intensity of the use of upper extremities use by means of density plots [26].

A vector of *Bilateral Magnitude* was calculated for each epoch, allowing us to visualize data for the whole task. The formula used was as follows:

$$Bilateral\ Magnitude = AC\ of\ the\ MA\ arm + AC\ of\ the\ LA\ arm \quad (5)$$

where the AC of the MA arm represents the total AC of the MA arm, while the AC of the LA arm represents the total AC of the LA arm.

2.5. Robotic Assessments

For all robotic assessments, the raw values of the *Task Score* were converted to a z-score by the system based on a methodology presented here: https://kinarm.com/kinarm-products/kinarm-standard-tests (accessed on 20 January 2025).

2.5.1. Object Hit

In the Object Hit task, the participant used both hands to hit balls that appeared at the far end of the screen and moved towards them, spanning different positions from the middle to the sides [34]. Participants encountered a total of 300 balls, and the speed of the balls increased progressively. The task was performed twice, but the analysis concentrated on the second attempt only to reduce any potential learning effect [35].

2.5.2. Ball on Bar

In the Ball on Bar task, the participant was given a virtual bar to hold between their hands with a virtual ball positioned on it [36]. The goal was to successively reach four targets by positioning the virtual ball accurately on each target. The task includes three levels of difficulty, where the first level was the easiest and the third level was the most challenging, characterized by increased movement of the ball and a higher risk of it falling off the bar. The task was completed twice, with the analysis focusing on the second attempt to minimize learning effects [35].

2.5.3. Visually Guided Reaching

In the Visually Guided Reaching task, the participant had to reach four targets that were distributed at a 10 cm radius from the initial target [11]. The targets were presented in a pseudorandom order. The aim was to reach the targets as quickly and precisely as possible. This task was performed with the LA arm first, and then with the MA arm.

2.6. Clinical Assessments

2.6.1. Observation-Based Assessment of the Involvement of the MA Arm

In the Observation-based assessment of the involvement of the MA arm, the participant had to perform 7 different tasks (1—cleaning up the table; 2—making coffee; 3—setting the table for two; 4—pouring a glass of water from a pitcher; 5—cutting a piece of mastic; 6—folding two towels; 7—putting toothpaste on a toothbrush) while being video-recorded. The main goal of this assessment is to evaluate the integration of the MA arm during various bimanual tasks by scoring different aspects of the assisting hand's performance, such as grasping and releasing (see [7] for the detailed list of criteria). Two clinicians have rated the relative involvement of the MA arm offline, as presented in [7], which has been shown to have a good reliability ($\tau b = 0.84$).

2.6.2. Two-Arm Coordination Test

In the Two-Arm Coordination Test, the participants had to move an apparatus on a traced star as quickly and precisely as possible [37]. The task required bimanual coordination as both hands had to work together to successfully complete the task. Pushing or pulling on two handles allowed participants to perform up–down and right–left displacements. Participants performed the task four times in each direction (i.e., in a clockwise or counterclockwise direction), and the starting direction was randomized across participants. A one-minute practice session was conducted at the beginning of the testing to ensure that participants would be assessed on their motor performance and not their understanding of the task. The main variable for this test was the performance index, representing the multiplication of the time and the number of errors (i.e., number of times the stylus fell outside the drawing line) +1. Based on [10], an average of the third and fourth trials were used, as a learning plateau was demonstrated after the third trial. The average score for the clockwise and counterclockwise trials was calculated, as a Wilcoxon signed-rank test did not show a significant difference between the two directions. The Two-Arm Coordination Test was shown as a valid assessment to evaluate bimanual coordination in children having cerebral palsy [10].

2.6.3. Jebsen–Taylor Hand Function Test

The Jebsen–Taylor Hand Function Test includes seven unilateral tasks (1—writing a sentence; 2—turning cards over; 3—picking up small objects; 4—simulating feeding; 5—stacking checkers; 6—lifting light objects, 7—lifting heavy objects) that were performed by the participants with their LA arm first and then their MA arm after [38]. The main variable was the total time required to complete all the tasks. The total time was converted into a z-score based on normative values provided in [38]. The Jebsen–Taylor Hand Function Test was shown as a reliable assessment to assess unilateral capacity in children having cerebral palsy [39].

2.6.4. Box and Block Test

The Box and Block test required the participant to move blocks from one side of a wooden box to the other for 1 min. Participants were not allowed to throw blocks to the other side or to grab more than one block at a time. Participants had a 30 s practice period before starting the test to make sure they understood the instructions. The main variable was the number of blocks successfully sent to the other side of the box. The number of blocks was converted into a z-score based on the normative data provided in [40]. They performed the test twice, with the analysis focusing on the second attempt only as the Wilcoxon signed-rank test showed a significant difference between the first and the second attempt ($p = 0.01$). The Box and Block test was shown as a reliable assessment to assess unilateral capacity in children having cerebral palsy [41].

2.6.5. Grip Strength

To measure the grip strength, a hand grip dynamometer was used (Jamar, Performance Health, Mississauga, ON, Canada). Participants were asked to grip the handle of the dynamometer as hard as they could, and the peak value of the attempt was recorded. Three attempts were conducted for each hand, and the mean value of these trials was used for analysis. The testing was performed in a random order between hands, with a 1 min break between each trial to avoid fatigue. In cases where there was a high discrepancy across trials, a fourth trial was conducted, and the two most similar values were then averaged. The mean of the peak values obtained was then converted to a z-score based on the normative values provided in the hand grip dynamometer user's guide [42]. Reliability of the Jamar hand dynamometer was shown for the assessment of grip strength in individuals having cerebral palsy [43].

2.7. *Statistical Analysis*

Descriptive statistics (comprising mean and standard deviation (SD)) were calculated for sociodemographic variables and accelerometry metrics. One participant was excluded from the *Use Ratio* analyses as they were an outlier and the inclusion of their results would have led to an abnormal distribution of data. After this exclusion, normality testing showed that all data were normally distributed (see Figure S1 in the Supplementary Materials). Kruskal–

Wallis tests were performed on accelerometry metrics (i.e., *Magnitude Ratio, BAUI, Use Ratio, Percentage of Bilateral Use*) to assess the difference in upper extremity use across levels of impairments (MACS). Stepwise, forward, and backward regression analyses were performed for accelerometry metrics according to two regression models: 1—the Robotic Assessment Model (comprising the following tasks: Object Hit, Ball on Bar, and Visually Guided Reaching); and 2—the Clinical Assessments Model (comprising the following assessments: Observation-based assessment of the involvement of the MA arm, Two-Arm Coordination Test, Jebsen–Taylor Hand Function Test, Box and Block test, and grip strength). The adjusted r-squared value (r^2) for each model and accelerometry metric was reported to account for differences in the number of values entered in each model. Two models were employed to account for the important differences between robotic and clinical assessments (notably, the fact that clinical assessments have a strong focus on manual function while robotic assessments focus on proximal motor control). Our objective was to identify the most significant contributor for each assessment method. For all statistical analyses, the alpha threshold was set to 0.05.

3. Results

3.1. Sample Description

Nineteen participants were recruited for this study (see Table 2 for information on sociodemographic and clinical characteristics). Eighteen of the participants were able to complete all planned assessments, while one participant was unable to complete the Two-Arm Coordination Test due to poor grasping capacities (i.e., the participant was unable to hold the handles). One participant performed only one attempt for the Object Hit and the Ball on Bar tasks due to muscle fatigue and an increase in spasticity. The results of the first attempt were used for this participant as the Wilcoxon signed-rank test showed no effect of trial at the group level (a comparison between first and second attempts resulted in a p-value > 0.05). Table 3 and Figure 3 show the distribution of the results of motor assessments.

Table 2. Sociodemographic and clinical characteristics of the participants.

Total Number of Participants	19
Age (years)	34.3 ± 11.5
Sex (female (F), male (M))	F = 58% M = 42%
More affected side (right (R), left (L)) *	R = 63% L = 37%
Handedness (right (R), left (L)) *	R= 42% L = 58%
Percentage of participants for each level of the Manual Ability Classification System	I = 37% II = 31.5% III = 31.5%

* Note that one participant was right-handed but their more affected arm was their right arm.

Table 3. Mean and 95% confidence interval (z-score) by motor assessment.

		Mean [95%—Confidence Interval]
Robotic Assessments	Object Hit	3.1 [2.37–3.76]
	Ball on Bar	1.7 [1.66–3.9]
	Visually Guided Reaching	2.9 [1.9–3.9]

Table 3. *Cont.*

		Mean [95%—Confidence Interval]
Clinical Assessments	Observation-based assessment of the involvement of the MA arm	59.3 [52.1–66.4]
	Two-Arm Coordination	155.5 [90.6–220.4]
	Jebsen–Taylor Hand Function Test	25.9 [7.0–44.9]
	Box and Block test	−6.1 [−10.8–−2.9]
	Grip strength	−2.6 [−3.3–−1.96]

Legend: Grey cells represent robotic assessments.

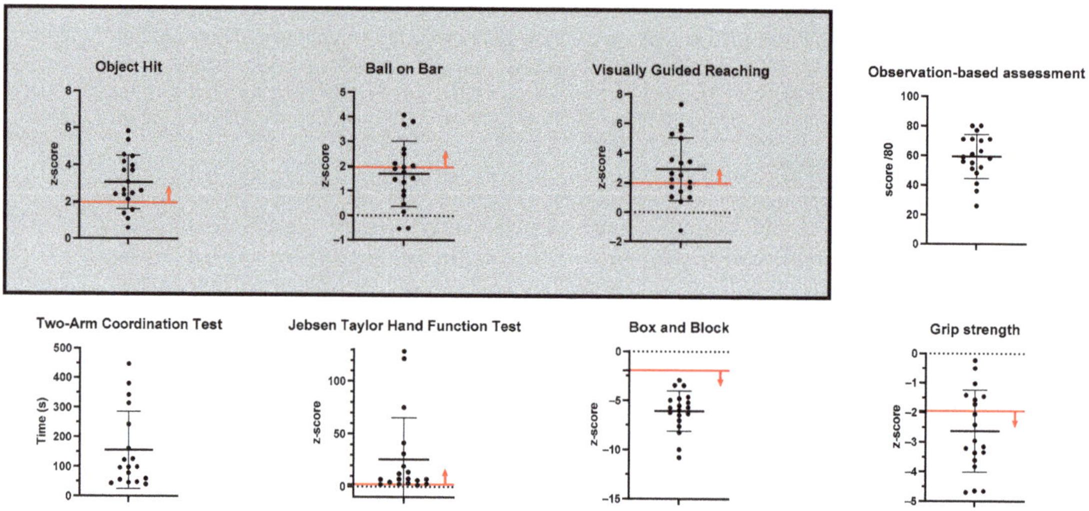

Figure 3. Histograms showing the distribution of results for each assessment. Robotic assessments are displayed within a grey square. The red line indicates the cutoff for normative data when available, with the direction of the arrow pointing toward the presence of impairments.

3.2. Description of Upper Extremity Use Using Accelerometry During Kitchen Tasks

Figure 4 displays density plots that illustrate the distribution of the intensity of upper limb use intensity in three representative subjects, one for each of the MACS levels (see Figure S2 in the Supplementary Materials for the density plot for each of the 19 subjects). The *Bilateral Magnitude* (y-axis on the density plots) was similar across MACS levels ((mean ± SD), MACS I: 140.4 ± 29.7; MACS II: 147.9, ± 31.6; MACS III: 118.8 ± 65.4) which shows that the intensity of the combination of MA and LA arm movements did not change based on the severity of participants' impairments, with the LA arm compensating any lack of MA use. The shift of the density plot toward the left (i.e., negative *Magnitude Ratio*) shows that the participants used their LA arm with a greater intensity during both bilateral and unilateral movements and that this asymmetry was more important among more severely impaired individuals. The column of data seen at a *Magnitude Ratio* of 7 showed that adults with a MACS level of III displayed almost no unilateral movements with their MA arm, while less impaired individuals still used their MA arm unilaterally, although to a lesser extent (i.e., the column at 7 is smaller than the column at −7).

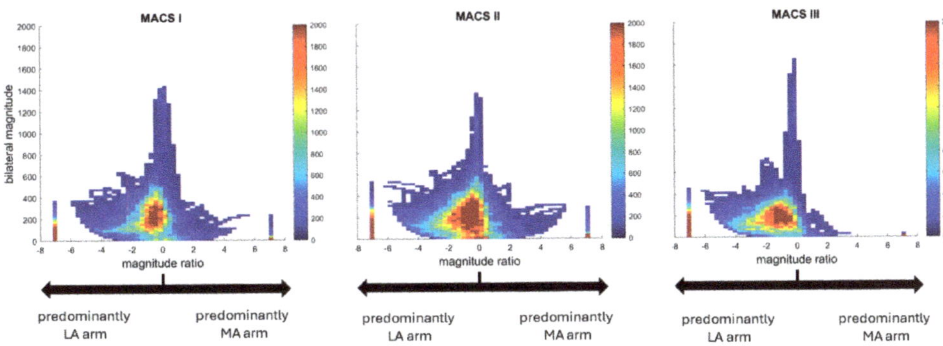

Figure 4. Distribution of upper limb use intensity for representative subjects across levels of impairment. The x-axis represents the *Magnitude Ratio*, i.e., the relative contribution of each upper extremity in terms of intensity. A negative value represents a larger use of the MA arm while a positive value represents a larger use of the LA arm. A value of 0 means that both arms are used equally. The column of data at -7 represents unilateral movement of the LA arm, and the column of data at 7 represents unilateral movements of the MA arm. The y-axis represents the intensity of bilateral use (*Bilateral Magnitude*). The color scale represents the frequency at which each combination happened, ranging from blue (less frequently) to red (more frequently). MACS = Manual Ability Classification Scale.

Table 4 reports descriptive data for each accelerometry metric of interest and compares these metrics across MACS levels. The results show that the two metrics that focus on intensity (i.e., *Magnitude Ratio* and *BAUI*) are distinguished across MACS levels, but this is not the case for metrics that focus on duration of use, although a trend was observed for the *Use Ratio*, showing that participants with worse motor capacities tend to use their MA arm less.

Table 4. Mean ($\pm$standard deviation) of each accelerometry metric and their comparison across levels of impairment.

		MACS I	MACS II	MACS III	Total	p-Value
Intensity	*Magnitude Ratio*	**-0.69 ± 0.46**	**-1.02 ± 0.28**	**-1.63 ± 0.75**	**-1.09 ± 0.64**	**0.047**
	Bilateral Arm Use Index	**0.71 ± 0.18**	**0.52 ± 0.10**	**0.47 ± 0.14**	**0.58 ± 0.18**	**0.03**
Duration	*Use Ratio*	0.47 ± 0.09	0.37 ± 0.10	0.30 ± 0.16	0.38 ± 0.13	0.15
	Percentage of Bilateral Use	26.1 ± 13.5	24.2 ± 6.9	16.2 ± 14.0	22.4 ± 12.1	0.42

Legend: The left column indicates whether the metric focused on intensity or duration of use. Cells in grey correspond to metrics that focus on global use, while white cells correspond to metrics that focus on bilateral use. The significance level for the Kruskal–Wallis tests was set at $p \leq 0.05$. Significant results appear in bold; MACS = Manual Ability Classification Scale.

3.3. *Relationship Between Robotic and Clinical Assessments and Upper Limb Use in Real-Life Activities*

Table 5 shows the results of the stepwise and forward regression analyses as they provided identical results. The results for the backward models are not presented for clarity but yielded identical results for the intensity-based metrics and similar results for the duration-based metrics. The presented models were chosen based on the results of the previous section (i.e., intensity-based metrics allowed us to distinguish across MACS levels). For the Robotic Assessment Model, the only variable entered in the model was the

Ball on Bar test (a bilateral symmetric common goal task). For the Clinical Assessments Model, for most of the metrics (except for the *Magnitude Ratio*), the variable integrated in the model was the Observation-based assessment of the involvement of the MA arm (bilateral independent goal task). Interestingly, most of the assessments integrated in the models were bilateral tasks, regardless of whether the accelerometry metrics focused on global relative use or specifically on bilateral use.

Table 5. Results of the stepwise and forward regression analysis for each accelerometry metric, using either the Robotic Assessment Model or the Clinical Assessment Model.

		Robotic Assessment Model	Clinical Assessment Model
Intensity	*Magnitude Ratio*	Ball on Bar ($r^2 = 0.43$, $p = 0.001$)	1- Box and Block test ($r^2 = 0.72$, $p < 0.001$) 2- Box and Block test and Jebsen–Taylor Hand and Function ($r^2 = 0.82$, $p < 0.001$)
	Bilateral Arm Use Index	Ball on Bar ($r^2 = 0.23$, $p = 0.02$)	Observation-based assessment of the involvement of the MA arm ($r^2 = 0.60$, $p < 0.001$)
Duration	*Use Ratio*	Ball on Bar ($r^2 = 0.27$, $p = 0.02$)	Observation-based assessment of the involvement of the MA arm ($r^2 = 0.64$, $p < 0.001$)
	Percentage of Bilateral Use	Ball on Bar ($r^2 = 0.25$, $p = 0.02$)	Observation-based assessment of the involvement of the MA arm ($r^2 = 0.43$, $p = 0.002$)

Legend: The Robotic Assessment Model comprised the following tasks: Object Hit, Ball on Bar, and Visually Guided Reaching. The Clinical Assessment Model comprised the following tests: Observation-based assessment of the involvement of the MA arm, Two-Arm Coordination Test, Jebsen–Taylor Hand Function Test, Box and Block test, and the grip strength test. Grey cells represent the metric focusing on the relative use of the upper extremity.

4. Discussion

The first objective of this study was to describe relative MA arm use during an ecological task and test whether it differed across different levels of motor impairments (MACS I, II, and III) in adults with CP. The results indicate that metrics focusing on intensity, as opposed to duration of use of each arm, have a better capacity to discriminate across the different levels of manual impairment, as assessed using MACS. The second objective was to assess the relationship between relative use of the MA arm and motor functions, assessed with either robotic or clinical assessments. Among the metrics focusing on intensity, the *Magnitude Ratio* was the one being predicted by both robotic and clinical assessments (r^2 of 0.43 and 0.82, respectively). However, the same robotic assessment, the Ball on Bar task, was identified as the best predictor of accelerometry metrics. For the clinical assessments, most of the accelerometry metrics were predicted by the Observation-based assessment of the involvement of the MA arm, while the *Magnitude Ratio* was predicted by the Box and Block test and the Jebsen–Taylor Hand Function Test. These results reaffirm the importance of assessing the use of both arms during ecological tasks. Indeed, it is well established that the majority of activities of daily living require the coordinated use of both arms [16,23,44,45], a concept known as bimanual coordination. The term "bilateral use", as used in this article, refers to the use of the upper extremities regardless of whether they are used simultaneously or sequentially. This term was preferred to enhance clarity and encompasses both the coordination and use of the upper extremities as assessed in this study.

Magnitude Ratio and *Use Ratio* have been studied in various populations, allowing for a comparison with data from the literature. The range of the *Magnitude Ratio* (−0.69 to −1.63) observed in the present study clearly reveals asymmetry of the arm used compared with the one reported in healthy subjects (−0.06 to −0.16) [26,44,46] (a value of 0 indicated equal use of both arms). These assessments are quite well aligned, although they suggest a bit less asymmetry in our sample, with results being reported in the individual with stroke (i.e., −1.3 to −2.2) [26,47] and children with CP (i.e., −1.7) [48]. The same observations are seen in the *Use Ratio*, showing a clear asymmetry, even among participants classified as MACS I (i.e., 0.3 to 0.47) compared with reference values in healthy subjects (i.e., 0.71 to 1.00) [21,46,49,50] (*Use Ratio* = 1 represents equal use of both arms). Our results contribute additional insights into the bilateral use of upper extremities, encompassing both the time spent moving both arms simultaneously and the relative intensity of movements when this occurs. Specifically, our findings reveal that asymmetry of intensity between both arms during simultaneous movements (referred to as *BAUI*) also make it possible to discriminate across levels of manual impairments. Overall, the fact that only metrics that focused on intensity of use (*Magnitude Ratio* and *BAUI*) were able to discriminate between levels of manual impairments suggests that these metrics should be favored over those that focus on duration of arm use.

Despite the different ability of accelerometry metrics to discriminate across levels of manual impairments, they all showed a similar pattern of results for the regression models, in which Ball on Bar and the Observation-based assessment of the involvement of the MA arm were almost systematically identified as the best predictors. It is interesting to note that these two assessments focus on bimanual function, suggesting that impairments in bimanual function specifically interfere with the successful integration of the MA arm in an ecological task. Among the robotic assessments, two bilateral tasks were tested: a symmetric common goal task (Ball on Bar) and an asymmetric independent goals task (Object Hit). Although several components of these two tasks have been shown to be impaired in adults with CP [14], our results align with those of Decraene et al. [17], who demonstrated that the Ball on Bar task offers a more discriminative assessment than the Object Hit task when evaluating different aspects of bilateral functioning (i.e., spatiotemporal coupling and interlimb differences) in children with CP. On the one hand, the fact that the Observation-based assessment of the involvement of the MA arm was the best predictor of accelerometry is not surprising, as this assessment focuses specifically on the integration of the MA arm into bimanual activities, which is what is measured with accelerometry. On the other hand, this tool relies on observation, while many other clinical assessments offer a more quantitative approach and normative data. This finding is in line with the findings of a study reporting that the frequency of wrist movements measured with accelerometry was correlated to the observer's report during the Assisting Hand Assessment test in children with CP (i.e., our Observation-based assessment of the involvement of the MA arm was developed based on the Assisting Hand Assessment test) [51]. Notably, the tasks that were assessed were mainly asymmetric with independent goals. While this might appear to contradict the results of the Robotic Assessment Model, important differences between the tasks need to be kept in mind. For example, the Object Hit task has much higher requirements for quick visuomotor processing compared with the everyday tasks (e.g., cooking or folding towels) performed in the corresponding clinical assessment. Another important difference is that, in the Observation-based assessment of the involvement of the MA arm, participants were instructed to use their arm as they typically would at home, allowing them to employ their preferred strategies. In contrast, the other clinical assessments provided specific instructions on how to perform the tasks, minimizing compensatory movements (e.g., during the Jebsen–Taylor Hand Function Test, participants were required to use a cylindrical grasp when lifting the can). This could explain the strong relationship between the Observation-based assessment of the involvement of the MA arm and the accelerometry metrics as they assess closely related concepts. When looking at the two common goal tasks, the Two-Arm Coordination Test requires the ability to correctly hold the handles of the apparatus, which was sometimes a limiting factor, while the Ball on Bar test required only movements of shoulders and elbows. Nevertheless, the results of both models support the importance of performing assessments that specifically focus on bimanual functions in individuals with CP.

4.1. Clinical Relavance

The accelerometry metrics indicate that, even among less severely impaired participants, adults with CP tend to underuse their MA arm despite having the capacity to use it. This tendency is even more pronounced in individuals with greater impairments. This is a significant observation, as most adults with CP do not receive treatment for their upper extremity impairments [52], further reinforcing the phenomenon of developmental disregard. This underscores the critical need for targeted interventions for adults with CP, who are often left on their own upon reaching adulthood. Our findings demonstrate the necessity of interventions focusing on arm use and particularly on the intensity of use. The small *Magnitude Ratio* and *BAUI* not only indicate that adults with CP use their MA hand less frequently but also reveal that it is primarily used to support the movement of their LA arm. These results highlight the need for a paradigm shift in CP care for adults. The fact that CP is considered a non-progressive disorder does not mean that nothing can be done to improve their functional abilities.

4.2. Study Limitations

This study has several limitations that should be acknowledged. First, the small number of participants included in the study reduced the generalizability of results. However, recruiting an evenly distributed sample across the three MACS levels helped mitigate the risk of bias. The small number of participants did not allow for analyses based on age and sex. This would have been an interesting consideration, as it is well established that motor capacity declines with age [53,54] and that there is a difference between the motor function of men and women [55]. Second, the lack of normative data for two of the clinical assessments used (i.e., the Observation-based assessment of the involvement of the MA arm and the Two-Arm Coordination Test) may have influenced the relationship with the accelerometry metrics. This issue reflects a longstanding challenge for adults with CP, as many assessments were originally developed for different populations or for children, leading to a scarcity of objective assessments of bilateral coordination tailored specifically to adults with CP. The robotic system used in this study did not provide an ecological environment to assess upper extremity functions as it is not representative of everyday life. Moreover, the position of the arm in the robotic device did not allow for measuring the pronation/ supination, which is important when performing activities of daily living. These limitations may have contributed to the weaker relationship found in the Robotic Assessment Model as the robotic device did not assess hand dexterity or postural control and removed the impact of gravity on upper extremities, limiting the impact of weakness. Fourthly, we collected accelerometry data for a specific set of tasks, including cooking, setting the table, eating, and drinking, which is not fully representative of the integration of the MA arm across the broader spectrum of activities of daily living. Our laboratory-based study allowed us to assess unilateral and bilateral functions in a controlled environment, serving as an essential first step. Further studies are needed to explore upper limb integration across a broader range of activities. Finally, we used a clinical measurement for grip strength that only considers the peak value of muscle contraction. This approach does not allow for an analysis of the dynamics of muscle contraction. Investigating this aspect would be an interesting avenue for future studies, as it is known that children with CP exhibit a different pattern of muscle activation compared with a control group [56].

5. Conclusions

In conclusion, the integration of robotic, clinical, and accelerometry assessments offers valuable insights into the factors contributing to upper extremity use in adults with CP. Our results support the use of intensity-based accelerometry metrics to measure MA arm use during daily activities and robotic or clinical assessments that focus on bimanual function to predict MA arm integration during ecological tasks, such as cooking or eating. More studies targeting the difference of bilateral task demands are required to better understand the mechanisms that explain developmental disregard as it leads to long-term disabilities [57]. Moreover, to address the limitations of the current study, further research should include a larger sample size, examine the impact of age on bilateral use, and gather accelerometry data outside of the laboratory.

Supplementary Materials: The following supporting information can be downloaded at: https://www.mdpi.com/article/10.3390/s25030660/s1, Figure S1: Distribution of data for the four accelerometry metrics. Mean and standard deviation values are displayed; Figure S2: Distribution of upper limb use intensity for each subject.

Author Contributions: I.P.: Conceptualization, data curation, formal analysis, investigation, methodology, software, project administration, writing—original draft; J.C.: software, writing—review and editing; A.C.-L.: supervision, software, writing—review and editing; C.M.: supervision, project administration, methodology, conceptualization, writing—review and editing. All authors have read and agreed to the published version of the manuscript.

Funding: This research was funded by grants from the Université Laval Research Chair in Cerebral Palsy (Fondation de l'Université Laval, #0021; C.M. is the chairholder) and the Fonds de recherche du Québec—Santé (FRQ-S; #251649). I.P. was supported by a fellowship from the Canadian Institutes of Health Research. C.M. also holds the Canada Research Chair in Pain and Sensorimotor Rehabilitation. A.C.-L. is supported by Research Scholar Awards from FRQ-S (J2).

Institutional Review Board Statement: Ethical approval for the study was obtained from the local ethics committee (Ethics #2018-609, CIUSSS-CN).

Informed Consent Statement: All participants provided written informed consent before participation.

Data Availability Statement: The raw data supporting the conclusions of this article will be made available by the authors without undue reservation.

Conflicts of Interest: The authors declare that the research was conducted in the absence of any commercial or financial relationships that could be construed as potential conflicts of interest.

References

1. Basu, A.P.; Pearse, J.E.; Baggaley, J.; Watson, R.M.; Rapley, T. Participatory design in the development of an early therapy intervention for perinatal stroke. *BMC Pediatr.* **2017**, *17*, 33. [CrossRef]
2. Rich, T.L.; Menk, J.S.; Rudser, K.D.; Feyma, T.; Gillick, B.T. Less-Affected Hand Function in Children with Hemiparetic Unilateral Cerebral Palsy: A Comparison Study with Typically Developing Peers. *Neurorehabilit. Neural Repair* **2017**, *31*, 965–976. [CrossRef] [PubMed]
3. Arnould, C.; Penta, M.; Renders, A.; Thonnard, J.L. ABILHAND-Kids: A measure of manual ability in children with cerebral palsy. *Neurology* **2004**, *63*, 1045–1052. [CrossRef] [PubMed]
4. Krumlinde-Sundholm, L.; Holmefur, M.; Kottorp, A.; Eliasson, A.-C. The Assisting Hand Assessment: Current evidence of validity, reliability, and responsiveness to change. *Dev. Med. Child. Neurol.* **2007**, *49*, 259–264. [CrossRef]
5. Choi, B.C.; Pak, A.W. A catalog of biases in questionnaires. *Prev. Chronic Dis.* **2005**, *2*, A13. [PubMed]
6. Mahtani, K.; Spencer, E.A.; Brassey, J.; Heneghan, C. Catalogue of bias: Observer bias. *BMJ Evid.-Based Med.* **2018**, *23*, 23. [CrossRef] [PubMed]
7. Gagné-Pelletier, L.; Poitras, I.; Flamand, V.H.; Mercier, C. Reliability of an observation-based scoring grid to assess bimanual performance during unstandardized tasks in adults living with cerebral palsy. *Disabil. Rehabil.* **2023**, *46*, 3733–3738. [CrossRef]
8. Langan, J.; Doyle, S.T.; Hurvitz, E.A.; Brown, S.H. Influence of Task on Interlimb Coordination in Adults with Cerebral Palsy. *Arch. Phys. Med. Rehabil.* **2010**, *91*, 1571–1576. [CrossRef] [PubMed]
9. Lott, C.; Johnson, M.J. Upper limb kinematics of adults with cerebral palsy on bilateral functional tasks. In Proceedings of the 2016 38th Annual International Conference of the IEEE Engineering in Medicine and Biology Society, Orlando, FL, USA, 16–20 August 2016; IEEE Engineering in Medicine and Biology Society. Annual International Conference. Volume 2016, pp. 5676–5679.
10. Riquelme, I.; Arnould, C.; Hatem, S.M.; Bleyenheuft, Y. The Two-Arm Coordination Test: Maturation of Bimanual Coordination in Typically Developing Children and Deficits in Children with Unilateral Cerebral Palsy. *Dev. Neurorehabil* **2019**, *22*, 312–320. [CrossRef]
11. Coderre, A.M.; Amr Abou, Z.; Dukelow, S.P.; Demmer, M.J.; Moore, K.D.; Demers, M.J.; Bretzke, H.; Herter, T.M.; Glasgow, J.I.; Norman, K.E.; et al. Assessment of Upper-Limb Sensorimotor Function of Subacute Stroke Patients Using Visually Guided Reaching. *Neurorehabilit. Neural Repair* **2010**, *24*, 528–541. [CrossRef] [PubMed]
12. Simmatis, L.E.; Jin, A.Y.; Taylor, S.W.; Bisson, E.J.; Scott, S.H.; Baharnoori, M. The feasibility of assessing cognitive and motor function in multiple sclerosis patients using robotics. *Mult. Scler. J.-Exp. Transl. Clin.* **2020**, *6*, 2055217320964940. [CrossRef] [PubMed]
13. Kuczynski, A.M.; Semrau, J.A.; Kirton, A.; Dukelow, S.P. Kinesthetic deficits after perinatal stroke: Robotic measurement in hemiparetic children. *J. Neuroeng. Rehabil.* **2017**, *14*, 13. [CrossRef] [PubMed]
14. Poitras, I.; Dukelow, S.P.; Campeau-Lecours, A.; Mercier, C. Robotic assessment of bilateral and unilateral upper limb functions in adults living with cerebral palsy. *J. Neuroeng. Rehabil.* **2024**, *21*, 144. [CrossRef]
15. Scott, S.H.; Lowrey, C.R.; Brown, I.E.; Dukelow, S.P. Assessment of Neurological Impairment and Recovery Using Statistical Models of Neurologically Healthy Behavior. *Neurorehabil Neural Repair* **2022**, *37*, 394–408. [CrossRef] [PubMed]
16. Kantak, S.; Jax, S.; Wittenberg, G. Bimanual coordination: A missing piece of arm rehabilitation after stroke. *Restor. Neurol. Neurosci.* **2017**, *35*, 347–364. [CrossRef] [PubMed]
17. Decraene, L.; Orban de Xivry, J.-J.; Kleeren, L.; Crotti, M.; Verheyden, G.; Ortibus, E.; Feys, H.; Mailleux, L.; Klingels, K. In-depth quantification of bimanual coordination using the Kinarm exoskeleton robot in children with unilateral cerebral palsy. *J. Neuroeng. Rehabil.* **2023**, *20*, 154. [CrossRef] [PubMed]
18. Poitras, I.; Campeau-Lecours, A.; Mercier, C. Relationship between somatosensory and visuo-perceptual impairments and motor functions in adults with hemiparetic cerebral palsy. *Neurorehabilit. Neural Repair* **2024**, *15*, 1425124. [CrossRef] [PubMed]
19. Rudisch, J.; Butler, J.; Izadi, H.; Zielinski, I.M.; Aarts, P.; Birtles, D.; Green, D. Kinematic parameters of hand movement during a disparate bimanual movement task in children with unilateral Cerebral Palsy. *Hum. Mov. Sci.* **2016**, *46*, 239–250. [CrossRef]
20. Volman, M.J. Spatial coupling in children with hemiplegic cerebral palsy during bimanual circle and line drawing. *Mot. Control* **2005**, *9*, 395–416. [CrossRef]
21. Hoyt, C.R.; Van, A.N.; Ortega, M.; Koller, J.M.; Everett, E.A.; Nguyen, A.L.; Lang, C.E.; Schlaggar, B.L.; Dosenbach, N.U.F. Detection of Pediatric Upper Extremity Motor Activity and Deficits with Accelerometry. *JAMA Netw. Open* **2019**, *2*, e192970. [CrossRef]
22. Lang, C.E.; Wagner, J.M.; Edwards, D.F.; Dromerick, A.W. Upper extremity use in people with hemiparesis in the first few weeks after stroke. *J. Neurol. Phys. Ther.* **2007**, *31*, 56–63. [CrossRef] [PubMed]
23. Bailey, R. Assessment of Real-World Upper Limb Activity in Adults with Chronic Stroke. Ph.D. Thesis, Washington University, Washington, DC, USA, 2015; 148p.

4. Poitras, I.; Clouâtre, J.; Campeau-Lecours, A.; Mercier, C. Accelerometry-Based Metrics to Evaluate the Relative Use of the More Affected Arm during Daily Activities in Adults Living with Cerebral Palsy. *Sensors* **2022**, *22*, 1022. [CrossRef]
5. Poitras, I.; Gagné-Pelletier, L.; Clouâtre, J.; Flamand, V.H.; Campeau-Lecours, A.; Mercier, C. Optimizing Epoch Length and Activity Count Threshold Parameters in Accelerometry: Enhancing Upper Extremity Use Quantification in Cerebral Palsy. *Sensors* **2024**, *24*, 1100. [CrossRef] [PubMed]
6. Bailey, R.R.; Klaesner, J.W.; Lang, C.E. Quantifying Real-World Upper-Limb Activity in Nondisabled Adults and Adults with Chronic Stroke. *Neurorehabil Neural Repair* **2015**, *29*, 969–978. [CrossRef] [PubMed]
7. Uswatte, G.; Giuliani, C.; Winstein, C.; Zeringue, A.; Hobbs, L.; Wolf, S.L. Validity of Accelerometry for Monitoring Real-World Arm Activity in Patients with Subacute Stroke: Evidence from the Extremity Constraint-Induced Therapy Evaluation Trial. *Arch. Phys. Med. Rehabil.* **2006**, *87*, 1340–1345. [CrossRef] [PubMed]
8. Heye, A.-L.; Kersting, C.; Kneer, M.; Barzel, A. Suitability of accelerometry as an objective measure for upper extremity use in stroke patients. *BMC Neurol.* **2022**, *22*, 220. [CrossRef]
9. Zielinski, I.M.; Jongsma, M.L.; Baas, C.; Aarts, P.B.; Steenbergen, B. Unravelling developmental disregard in children with unilateral cerebral palsy by measuring event-related potentials during a simple and complex task. *BMC Neurol.* **2014**, *14*, 6. [CrossRef]
0. Zielinski, I.M.; Steenbergen, B.; Aarts, P.B.M.; Green, D.; Jongsma, M.L.A. Developmental disregard in children with unilateral cerebral palsy is accompanied by a lack of movement related mu-suppression. *Dev. Med. Child. Neurol.* **2016**, *58* (Suppl. S6), 34.
1. Houwink, A.; Geerdink, Y.A.; Steenbergen, B.; Geurts, A.C.; Aarts, P.B. Assessment of upper-limb capacity, performance, and developmental disregard in children with cerebral palsy: Validity and reliability of the revised Video-Observation Aarts and Aarts module: Determine Developmental Disregard (VOAA-DDD-R). *Dev. Med. Child. Neurol.* **2013**, *55*, 76–82. [CrossRef] [PubMed]
2. Zielinski, I.M.; Steenbergen, B.; Baas, C.; Aarts, P.B.; Jongsma, M.L. Neglect-like characteristics of developmental disregard in children with cerebral palsy revealed by event related potentials. *BMC Neurol.* **2014**, *14*, 221. [CrossRef]
3. Poitras, I.; Clouâtre, J.; Bouyer, L.J.; Routhier, F.; Mercier, C.; Campeau-Lecours, A. Development and Validation of Open-Source Activity Intensity Count and Activity Intensity Classification Algorithms from Raw Acceleration Signals of Wearable Sensors. *Sensors* **2020**, *20*, 6767. [CrossRef] [PubMed]
4. Tyryshkin, K.; Coderre, A.M.; Glasgow, J.I.; Herter, T.M.; Bagg, S.D.; Dukelow, S.P.; Scott, S.H. A robotic object hitting task to quantify sensorimotor impairments in participants with stroke. *J. Neuroeng. Rehabil.* **2014**, *11*, 47. [CrossRef]
35. Mang, C.S.; Whitten, T.A.; Cosh, M.S.; Scott, S.H.; Wiley, J.P.; Debert, C.T.; Dukelow, S.P.; Benson, B.W. Test-retest reliability of the KINARM end-point robot for assessment of sensory, motor and neurocognitive function in young adult athletes. *PLoS ONE* **2018**, *13*, e0196205. [CrossRef] [PubMed]
36. Lowrey, C.; Jackson, C.; Bagg, S.; Dukelow, S.; Scott, S. A Novel Robotic Task for Assessing Impairments in Bimanual Coordination Post-Stroke. *Int. J. Phys. Med. Rehabil.* **2014**, *S3*, 002. [CrossRef]
37. Lafayette Instrument. *Two-Hand Coordination Test—User Instructions*, 2nd ed.; Lafayette Instrument: Lafayette, IN, USA, 2016. Available online: https://lafayetteevaluation.com/products/two-arm-coordination/ (accessed on 20 January 2025).
38. Jebsen, R.H.; Taylor, N.; Trieschmann, R.B.; Trotter, M.J.; Howard, L.A. An objective and standardized test of hand function. *Arch. Phys. Med. Rehabil.* **1969**, *50*, 311–319. [PubMed]
39. Araneda, R.; Ebner-Karestinos, D.; Paradis, J.; Saussez, G.; Friel, K.M.; Gordon, A.M.; Bleyenheuft, Y. Reliability and responsiveness of the Jebsen-Taylor Test of Hand Function and the Box and Block Test for children with cerebral palsy. *Dev. Med. Child. Neurol.* **2019**, *61*, 1182–1188. [CrossRef] [PubMed]
40. Mathiowetz, V.; Volland, G.; Kashman, N.; Weber, K. Adult norms for the Box and Block Test of manual dexterity. *Am. J. Occup. Ther.* **1985**, *39*, 386–391. [CrossRef] [PubMed]
41. Liang, K.-J.; Chen, H.-L.; Shieh, J.-Y.; Wang, T.-N. Measurement properties of the box and block test in children with unilateral cerebral palsy. *Sci. Rep.* **2021**, *11*, 20955. [CrossRef]
42. AbilityOne, H. *Hydraulic Hand Dynamometer Owner's Manual*; Sammons Preston Rolyan: Bolingbrook, IL, USA, 2003.
43. Sugiyama, T.; Whitney, D.G.; Schmidt, M.; Haapala, H.; Bowman, A.; Peterson, M.D.; Hurvitz, E.A. Measuring grip strength in adolescents and adults with cerebral palsy in a clinic setting: Feasibility, reliability, and clinical associations. *Dev. Med. Child. Neurol.* **2024**, *66*, 87–94. [CrossRef]
44. Bailey, R.R.; Klaesner, J.W.; Lang, C.E. An Accelerometry-Based Methodology for Assessment of Real-World Bilateral Upper Extremity Activity. *PLoS ONE* **2014**, *9*, e103135. [CrossRef]
45. Bailey, R.R.; Birkenmeier, R.L.; Lang, C.E. Real-world affected upper limb activity in chronic stroke: An examination of potential modifying factors. *Top. Stroke Rehabil.* **2015**, *22*, 26–33. [CrossRef]

46. Bailey, R.R.; Lang, C.E. Upper-limb activity in adults: Referent values using accelerometry. *J. Rehabil. Res. Dev.* **2013**, *50*, 1213–1222. [CrossRef] [PubMed]
47. Essers, B.; Biering Lundquist, C.; Verheyden, G.; Brunner, I.C. Determinants of Different Aspects of Upper-Limb Activity after Stroke. *Sensors* **2022**, *22*, 2273. [CrossRef]
48. Goodwin, B.M.; Sabelhaus, E.K.; Pan, Y.C.; Bjornson, K.F.; Pham, K.L.D.; Walker, W.O.; Steele, K.M. Accelerometer Measurements Indicate That Arm Movements of Children with Cerebral Palsy Do Not Increase After Constraint-Induced Movement Therapy (CIMT). *Am. J. Occup. Ther.* **2020**, *74*, 7405205100p1–7405205100p9. [CrossRef] [PubMed]
49. Porta, M.; Leban, B.; Orrù, P.F.; Pau, M. Use of bilateral wrist-worn accelerometers to characterize upper limb activity time, intensity and asymmetry of use in physically demanding and sedentary working task. *Int. J. Ind. Ergon.* **2022**, *92*, 103359. [CrossRef]
50. Dawe, J.; Yang, J.F.; Fehlings, D.; Likitlersuang, J.; Rumney, P.; Zariffa, J.; Musselman, K.E. Validating Accelerometry as a Measure of Arm Movement for Children with Hemiplegic Cerebral Palsy. *Phys. Ther.* **2019**, *99*, 721–729. [CrossRef] [PubMed]
51. Howcroft, J.; Fehlings, D.; Zabjek, K.; Fay, L.; Liang, J.; Biddiss, E. Wearable wrist activity monitor as an indicator of functional hand use in children with cerebral palsy. *Dev. Med. Child. Neurol.* **2011**, *53*, 1024–1029. [CrossRef]
52. Hurvitz, E.A.; Whitney, D.G.; Waldron-Perrine, B.; Ryan, D.; Haapala, H.J.; Schmidt, M.; Gray, C.; Peterson, M.D. Navigating the Pathway to Care in Adults with Cerebral Palsy. *Front. Neurol.* **2021**, *12*, 734139. [CrossRef] [PubMed]
53. Swinnen, S.P.; Heuninckx, S.; Van Impe, A.; Goble, D.J.; Coxon, J.P.; Wenderoth, N. Aging and Movement ControlThe Neural Basis of Age-related Compensatory Recruitment. In *Motor Control: Theories, Experiments, and Applications*; Danion, P.F., Latash, P.M., Eds.; Oxford University Press: Oxford, UK, 2010.
54. Yan, J.H.; Thomas, J.R.; Stelmach, G.E. Aging and rapid aiming arm movement control. *Exp. Aging Res.* **1998**, *24*, 155–168.
55. Liutsko, L.; Muiños, R.; Tous Ral, J.M.; Contreras, M.J. Fine Motor Precision Tasks: Sex Differences in Performance with and without Visual Guidance across Different Age Groups. *Behav. Sci.* **2020**, *10*, 36. [CrossRef]
56. Charles, J. Upper extremity muscle activation in children with unilateral cerebral palsy during an auditory cued repetitive task: Effects on bimanual coordination. *J. Pediatr. Rehabil. Med.* **2017**, *10*, 19–26. [CrossRef]
57. Basu, A.P.; Pearse, J.; Kelly, S.; Wisher, V.; Kisler, J. Early Intervention to Improve Hand Function in Hemiplegic Cerebral Palsy. *Front. Neurol.* **2015**, *5*, 281. [CrossRef] [PubMed]

sensors

MDPI

Review

Electromyography Signal Acquisition, Filtering, and Data Analysis for Exoskeleton Development

Jung-Hoon Sul [1,*], Lasitha Piyathilaka [1], Diluka Moratuwage [1], Sanura Dunu Arachchige [1], Amal Jayawardena [2], Gayan Kahandawa [2] and D. M. G. Preethichandra [1]

1 School of Engineering and Technology, Central Queensland University, Rockhampton, QLD 4701, Australia; l.piyathilaka@cqu.edu.au (L.P.); d.moratuwage@cqu.edu.au (D.M.); s.dunuarachchige@cqu.edu.au (S.D.A.); d.preethichandra@cqu.edu.au (D.M.G.P.)

2 Institute of Innovation, Science and Sustainability, Federation University Australia, Churchill, VIC 3842, Australia; a.jayawardena@federation.edu.au (A.J.); g.appuhamillage@federation.edu.au (G.K.)

* Correspondence: j.sul@cqu.edu.au

Abstract: Electromyography (EMG) has emerged as a vital tool in the development of wearable robotic exoskeletons, enabling intuitive and responsive control by capturing neuromuscular signals. This review presents a comprehensive analysis of the EMG signal processing pipeline tailored to exoskeleton applications, spanning signal acquisition, noise mitigation, data preprocessing, feature extraction, and control strategies. Various EMG acquisition methods, including surface, intramuscular, and high-density surface EMG, are evaluated for their applicability in real-time control. The review addresses prevalent signal quality challenges, such as motion artifacts, power-line interference, and crosstalk. It also highlights both traditional filtering techniques and advanced methods, such as wavelet transforms, empirical mode decomposition, and adaptive filtering. Feature extraction techniques are explored to support pattern recognition and motion classification. Machine learning approaches are examined for their roles in pattern recognition-based and hybrid control architectures. This article emphasizes muscle synergy analysis and adaptive control algorithms to enhance personalization and fatigue compensation, followed by the benefits of multimodal sensing and edge computing in addressing the limitations of EMG-only systems. By focusing on EMG-driven strategies through signal processing, machine learning, and sensor fusion innovations, this review bridges gaps in human–machine interaction, offering insights into improving the precision, adaptability, and robustness of next generation exoskeletons.

Keywords: electromyography (EMG); exoskeleton; EMG signal processing; human-machine interface

1. Introduction

Wearable robotics, both powered (active) and non-powered (passive) exoskeletons, have advanced rapidly over the past two decades with their applications ranging from physical rehabilitation and mobility assistance to industrial support and military augmentation [1]. Exoskeletons are designed to assist or augment human motion functions by replicating and/or enhancing the movements of limbs [2]. To achieve seamless human–robot interactions, various sensors and technologies have been developed to anticipate and respond to a user's movement intentions in real-time. These techniques include electromyography (EMG), mechanomyography, electrical impedance myography, ultrasound, force myography, and near-infrared spectroscopy. Among the key technological components, the most prevalent device is EMG [3], whose signals provide a direct window into neuromuscular activation patterns [4]. EMGs have become instrumental in developing intuitive and human-in-the-loop interfaces for exoskeleton systems [5], offering a direct correlation between the neural command signals and the resulting movements.

Despite its potential, the application of EMG in exoskeleton development presents a range of technical challenges. These include issues related to signal acquisition such as difficulties in real-time signal processing [6], including noise filtering and feature extraction, and complexities in data analysis and interpretation for control algorithms. Moreover, variations in skin impedance, movement artifacts [7], and individual anatomical differences can significantly affect the quality and reliability of EMG signals. These challenges underscore the necessity for a thorough understanding of the end-to-end EMG processing pipeline, from acquisition to analysis, to develop reliable and adaptive exoskeletons.

This review aims to provide a comprehensive analysis of EMG signal processing techniques in the context of exoskeleton development. While numerous studies have addressed EMG signal processing in general biomedical or rehabilitation contexts, relatively few studies have focused exclusively on the unique demands and applications of EMG in exoskeletons. Moreover, this paper evaluates the role of emerging multimodal frameworks that integrate EMG with inertial, visual, and neuroelectric signals to enhance system adaptability and robustness. The integration of edge computing further supports real-time processing and personalized control strategies, enabling home-based and outpatient rehabilitation scenarios. By narrowing the scope to this specific application, the present review offers a detailed synthesis that bridges the gap with an emphasis on EMG signal acquisition, processing (filtering and post-processing), methods of EMG signal analysis, and the application of EMG in exoskeleton developments.

2. EMG Signal Acquisition for Exoskeletons

Accurate acquisition of EMG signals is a critical first step in developing effective control strategies for assistive and rehabilitative exoskeletons. In contrast to general biomedical applications, where post hoc analysis or offline classification may be acceptable, EMG acquisition in exoskeletons must enable real-time interpretation of user intent with high temporal fidelity and robustness [8]. These signals serve as the primary interface between human motor intent and machine response, enabling real-time control and adaptive assistance. The EMG system must reliably extract neuromuscular signals under dynamic, noisy, and mobile conditions—ensuring that the exoskeleton responds intuitively and safely to user intent [8]. The choice of the EMG acquisition method directly impacts the system's responsiveness, reliability, and user comfort. To support various control requirements and application contexts, several types of EMG signals are utilized, each offering distinct advantages and limitations. These EMG signal types and their suitability for exoskeleton development are explored, and their key characteristics are compared in Table 1.

2.1. Types of EMG Signals

Different types of EMG signals provide varying levels of detail, invasiveness, and applicability. The main EMG signal types utilized in exoskeleton applications include the following:

- Surface Electromyography (sEMG)
- Intramuscular Electromyography (iEMG)
- High-Density Surface Electromyography (HD-sEMG)
- Electroneurography (ENG)

Table 1. Comparison of EMG signal types for exoskeleton applications.

Type	Advantages	Limitations	Applicability
sEMG	- Non-invasive, easy to use - Comfortable for extended use - Real-time control feasible	- Sensitive to noise and motion artifacts - Limited to superficial muscles	Widely used in commercial exoskeletons
iEMG	- High signal specificity - Accessible to deep	- Invasive and uncomfortable - Clinical expertise required	Research and diagnostic studies
HD-sEMG	- High spatial resolution - Improved pattern recognition accuracy	- Bulky and expensive - High computational cost	Research and experimental control
ENG	- Motor intent detected before muscle activation	- Highly invasive - Limited to experimental studies	Emerging research technology

2.1.1. Surface EMG (sEMG)

sEMG captures muscle activation signals non-invasively through electrodes placed on the skin over target muscles. It is the most used method for real-time control of exoskeletons, especially for detecting user intentions and providing assistive torque or motion commands. Crucially, sEMG enables inference of user intent before observable movement, which is vital for responsive and intuitive exoskeleton behavior [8]. Although sEMG is sensitive to motion artifacts and variations in electrode placement, its ease of use and comfort make it ideal for wearable devices [7,9]. However, in dynamic exoskeleton applications, challenges such as signal drift, motion-induced impedance shifts, and real-time noise must be overcome to ensure continuous and reliable control [9].

2.1.2. Intramuscular EMG (iEMG)

iEMG involves inserting fine-wire or needle electrodes directly into the muscle tissue to record signals from individual motor units or deep muscles. This method provides high signal specificity and minimal crosstalk, making it suitable for detailed biomechanical analysis and research-grade exoskeleton systems. However, due to its invasive nature and the requirement for clinical expertise, it is impractical for daily assistive use [10,11].

2.1.3. High-Density Surface EMG (HD-sEMG)

HD-sEMG utilizes a grid of closely spaced surface electrodes to capture high-resolution spatial and temporal muscle activity patterns. This technology enhances the accuracy of pattern recognition algorithms, enabling better differentiation between muscle activations. Its fine spatial resolution makes it promising for high-DOF exoskeletons and precise movement classification. Although HD-sEMG offers improved control strategies, it requires complex signal processing and is currently more prevalent in research environments [12,13]. However, its hardware bulk and computational requirements currently limit field deployment in wearable systems.

2.1.4. Electroneurography

Electroneurography (ENG) records electrical signals from peripheral nerves rather than muscle tissue. This method allows for the early detection of motor commands before muscle activation, offering the potential for highly responsive exoskeleton control. However, current ENG systems are invasive and primarily experimental, with limited application in commercial exoskeletons [14].

2.2. EMG Sensor Technologies for Exoskeleton Control

Accurate and reliable EMG signal acquisition is essential for enabling intuitive and responsive exoskeleton control systems. Unlike static clinical environments, exoskeletons operate under dynamic conditions where the user and device are constantly in motion. As such, EMG sensors must remain robust against motion artifacts, electrode displacement, and variable skin impedance [8]. The effectiveness of these systems largely depends on the selection of appropriate sensor technologies, which must balance signal quality, user comfort, integration complexity, and real-time processing requirements [15]. In the context of exoskeleton development, EMG sensors are employed not only to capture muscle activation patterns but also to ensure seamless human–machine interaction in both assistive and rehabilitative applications [16,17]. EMG sensors can be broadly classified into surface electrodes, intramuscular electrodes, wearable and flexible EMG devices, and hybrid sensor systems, each offering distinct advantages and limitations for exoskeleton control.

2.2.1. Surface Electrode Technologies

Surface electrodes are the most widely used non-invasive method for EMG signal acquisition in exoskeleton systems [18]. Dry electrodes offer ease of application and reusability, making them suitable for short-term use in controlled environments. However, their susceptibility to motion artifacts and high skin-electrode impedance can compromise signal quality during dynamic exoskeleton-assisted movements [19]. The skin-electrode impedance is influenced by several factors, including the electrical resistance of the outer layer of the skin, moisture levels (dryness), the type of electrode used, the pressure applied to the electrode, and presence of contaminants such as sweat or body hair [20–22].

On the other hand, wet electrodes provide higher signal fidelity, which is beneficial for precise control tasks in exoskeletons requiring accurate muscle activation detection. Nonetheless, their long-term use is limited by discomfort, gel drying, and the risk of skin irritation [23]. These wet electrodes usually use an Ag/AgCl-based piece and a gel combination as the electrode. They are specifically used in laboratory experiments and medical examinations due to their dependability [21]. However, once the gel begins to dry, the same issues that arise with impedance are also present in wet electrodes. Due to the time-consuming nature and discomfort associated with their use, wet electrodes are not preferred by wearers.

Textile-based electrodes integrated into wearable garments offer improved user comfort and mobility, making them ideal for long-term exoskeleton-assisted rehabilitation and monitoring [24]. Moreover, according to [22], textile-based electrodes are comparable to wet electrodes and much better for non-laboratory long-term use. However, challenges remain in maintaining signal fidelity and reducing susceptibility to motion-induced noise by impedance [25].

The most common method for minimizing the effects of the skin-electrode impedance is skin preparation [20–22]. Usually, before attaching an electrode, the skin area is shaved, abrased, and cleaned again with alcohol [20]. Moreover, according to [26], there are frontiers where researchers have developed novel textile-based electrodes to overcome the drawbacks of the existing electrodes. Also, there are instances where novel sensors, specifically textile-based electrodes, were tested to overcome the disadvantages of the existing EMG electrodes [20–22,26–28]. However, a proper solution for mitigating the adverse effects of skin impedance has yet to be found as the skin-electrode interface is yet to be understood [21].

Lastly, capacitive (non-contact) electrodes are highly desirable for shared exoskeleton systems and hygienic applications, as they avoid direct skin contact [29]. However, they are highly sensitive to electrode placement and body movement, often requiring advanced signal processing to ensure reliable control performance. Therefore, selecting a suitable surface EMG sensor involves a trade-off between robustness, wearability, signal integrity, and system complexity [8].

2.2.2. Intramuscular (Invasive) Electrodes

Intramuscular electrodes provide highly localized and precise EMG signal acquisition, offering accurate detection of deep muscle activations required for high-degree-of-freedom exoskeleton control [30]. Despite their superior signal quality, the invasive nature of these electrodes, along with user discomfort and clinical risks, limits their use to specialized medical exoskeleton applications and research environments. These electrodes provide unmatched precision for detailed muscle activation but are confined to niche or clinical applications due to their invasiveness [30].

2.2.3. Wearable and Flexible EMG Devices

Wearable EMG devices, such as the Myo armband, simplify the integration of EMG sensing into exoskeleton control frameworks for gesture recognition and basic control tasks [31]. However, their fixed electrode configurations and limited adaptability often restrict their performance in complex, high-precision exoskeleton applications. Flexible and stretchable EMG sensors made from advanced materials such as graphene and conductive polymers provide improved comfort and conformability, which is highly beneficial for long-term monitoring in wearable exoskeleton systems [32]. These technologies are particularly promising for soft exoskeletons and rehabilitation devices, although challenges related to long-term durability and signal stability remain. Textile electrodes, in particular, face performance degradation over time due to sweat absorption and wear-induced pressure variability. These issues can be mitigated through adaptive impedance tracking and automatic recalibration strategies during idle periods. While these emerging devices show promise for lightweight integration, their susceptibility to signal drift under extended use must be addressed for practical deployment.

2.2.4. Hybrid EMG Sensors

Hybrid EMG sensor systems combine EMG with complementary sensing modalities, such as inertial measurement units (IMUs) and electroencephalography (EEG), to enhance motion intent detection and improve control accuracy in exoskeletons [33]. Emerging multimodal frameworks also incorporate thermal sensing and bioimpedance feedback, providing richer physiological state information that can be leveraged to assess fatigue or muscle readiness [34]. Such integration supports robust intent inference in outpatient or unsupervised settings, where EMG alone may be insufficient. These multimodal architectures are particularly well-suited to real-world exoskeleton scenarios, where robustness to noise, delay, and misclassification is critical [8]. By leveraging data fusion, hybrid systems offer enhanced control robustness and adaptability beyond what standalone EMG systems can provide [33].

In summary, each EMG sensor modality presents unique advantages and trade-offs when applied to exoskeleton systems (see Table 2). While sEMG and HD-sEMG are preferred for real-time applications due to their non-invasiveness and rich signal content, they remain vulnerable to motion artifacts and electrode shifts. Intramuscular EMG provides precision but lacks wearability. Hybrid and flexible sensors offer a promising compromise, particularly when enhanced with multimodal fusion and adaptive signal processing strategies. Consequently, no single sensor type fully satisfies all exoskeleton-specific requirements; sensor selection must therefore consider application-specific trade-offs between robustness, comfort, and integration complexity [35].

Table 2. Comparison of EMG sensor types for exoskeleton applications, evaluating signal fidelity, wearability and comfort, robustness to noise, and integration complexity.

Sensor Type	Signal Fidelity	Wearability and Comfort	Robustness to Noise	Integration Complexity
Surface EMG	Moderate	High	Low to moderate	Low
Intramuscular EMG	High	Low	High	High
High-Density sEMG	Very High	Low to Moderate	Moderate	High
Textile-based EMG	Moderate	Very High	Low to Moderate	Moderate
Capacitive EMG	Low to Moderate	Very High	Low	High
Hybrid EMG	High	Moderate	High	Very High

2.3. *Noise and Artifacts in EMG Signals*

EMG signals are inherently weak and highly susceptible to various types of noise and artifacts, which can significantly degrade data quality and compromise the reliability of control strategies [36]. In exoskeleton applications, where precise and timely muscle activation detection is essential for seamless human–machine interaction, the impact of such interferences becomes even more critical. Effective identification and mitigation of noise sources are therefore fundamental to ensuring accurate signal acquisition, robust filtering, and reliable data analysis. This section focuses on the three most prevalent sources of noise and artifacts encountered in EMG-based exoskeleton control systems—motion artifacts, power-line interference (PLI), and crosstalk from adjacent muscles.

2.3.1. Motion Artifacts

Motion artifacts primarily result from mechanical disturbances at the skin-electrode interface, which are common during dynamic movements associated with exoskeleton-assisted tasks. These disturbances occur due to electrode displacement, cable motion, or changes in skin tension as the user performs physical activities. Consequently, low-frequency noise components—typically in the range of 0 to 20 Hz—are introduced into the EMG signal, potentially masking critical muscle activation cues. This is particularly problematic in exoskeleton control systems, where timely and accurate detection of user intent is essential for generating appropriate assistive responses. Mitigating motion artifacts through optimized electrode placement, secure fastening methods, and effective signal preprocessing is therefore crucial for ensuring reliable exoskeleton performance in real-world environments [36].

2.3.2. Power-Line Interference (PLI)

PLI is a pervasive source of electromagnetic noise, typically cantered at 50 Hz or 60 Hz depending on power supply frequencies. In the context of exoskeleton systems, which often operate in electrically noisy environments such as industrial settings or rehabilitation clinics, this interference can be coupled into the EMG acquisition system through poorly shielded electrodes, cables, and acquisition hardware. The resulting strong sinusoidal component can overwhelm true muscle activity signals, degrading the control system's ability to interpret user intent accurately. Employing robust hardware designs with proper shielding and high common-mode rejection, along with advanced filtering techniques, is essential to minimize the impact of power-line interference in exoskeleton applications [37].

2.3.3. Crosstalk from Adjacent Muscles

Crosstalk occurs when EMG electrodes inadvertently capture electrical activity from muscles adjacent to the intended target muscle. In exoskeleton control, this phenomenon can lead to ambiguous or misleading interpretations of muscle activation patterns, negatively affecting motion intent detection and control precision. This challenge is particularly significant when using sEMG in regions with densely packed muscles, such as the forearm, shoulder, or lower limb, which are commonly involved in exoskeleton-assisted movements [38]. Key factors contributing to crosstalk include electrode size, placement accuracy, inter-electrode distance, and the anatomical proximity of surrounding muscles. To address this, it is critical to implement optimized electrode configurations and advanced signal processing techniques that effectively isolate true muscle activation signals from interfering sources. Approaches such as high-density EMG arrays, blind source separation, and spatial filtering are increasingly being explored to enhance signal fidelity and improve control accuracy in wearable systems for exoskeleton-related applications [39,40].

Therefore, effective management of these noise sources is essential to improve the robustness, responsiveness, and user comfort of EMG-based exoskeleton control systems, ultimately enabling more natural and intuitive human–machine interactions.

3. EMG Signal Processing: Filtering and Preprocessing

EMG signals are typically of low magnitude, often in the microvolt range before amplification, and are therefore highly prone to contamination from various noise sources. Common interferences include power-line interference, baseline wandering, white Gaussian noise, motion artifacts, and high-frequency electronic noise. These noise components can cause significant distortion, resulting in erroneous signal representations in the time domain and overlapping spectra in the frequency domain. Such distortions hinder the accurate extraction of physiological information from raw EMG data. Consequently, effective preprocessing is essential to isolate the true EMG signal and ensure reliable analysis in both clinical and research applications.

3.1. *Traditional Filtering Methods*

One of the foundational techniques in EMG signal preprocessing is band-pass filtering, typically configured within the frequency range of 20–500 Hz. This filtering strategy serves a dual purpose: it preserves the spectral components that are physiologically relevant to muscle activity, while simultaneously eliminating extraneous noise that may obscure or distort the signal. The lower cutoff frequency, usually set at 20 Hz, is particularly effective in mitigating baseline drift, which can arise from sweat accumulation, slow movement of the electrode-skin interface, or respiration-induced body movements. It also attenuates motion artifacts, which are typically low-frequency oscillations caused by mechanical disturbances or poor electrode adhesion. Conversely, the upper cutoff, generally fixed at 500 Hz, is aimed at suppressing high-frequency noise originating from external electromagnetic sources, such as laboratory equipment, nearby electronic devices, or cable resonance phenomena.

This 20–500 Hz range is not arbitrary; it has been empirically validated to encompass the bulk of the electrophysiological energy generated by skeletal muscles during voluntary contractions. Notably, the dominant energy content of EMG signals is concentrated between 20 and 150 Hz, where the most diagnostically informative motor unit action potentials occur [41]. A widely recommended implementation of band-pass filtering is through the Butterworth filter, which is favored for its maximally flat frequency response in the passband and minimal phase distortion. When configured with an appropriate slope (e.g., 12 dB/octave), the Butterworth filter effectively balances noise reduction and signal fidelity, making it a staple in both clinical and experimental EMG applications.

In addition to these broadband noise sources, power-line interference (PLI) remains a pervasive and recurring issue in EMG recordings. This interference manifests as a narrow-band sinusoidal component at 50 Hz or 60 Hz, corresponding to the local power supply frequency. It originates from the coupling between the EMG electrodes and the surrounding electrical infrastructure and can significantly degrade signal quality, particularly when the SNR is already low [42]. To mitigate this, researchers often employ notch filters—narrow-band rejection filters specifically tuned to the PLI frequency. These filters are designed to remove the unwanted sinusoidal component while preserving adjacent signal frequencies. However, care must be taken in their design; overly aggressive notch filters can introduce spectral leakage or distort signal morphology.

Multiple studies have evaluated the effectiveness of notch filtering and have demonstrated its utility in a variety of settings. For instance, Ladrova et al. [42] compared several filtering techniques, including notch filters, wavelet transforms, and adaptive noise cancelers, and found that properly configured notch filters provided an efficient and low-complexity solution for suppressing PLI without introducing significant signal distortion [42]. Nonetheless, in environments where PLI varies over time or coexists with other noise sources, hybrid approaches or advanced spectral estimation methods may offer better performance.

3.2. *Advanced Noise Reduction Techniques*

Modern EMG recordings often face challenges beyond what traditional linear filters can handle. These include non-stationary noise, overlapping spectral interference, and the need for real-time adaptability in wearable and prosthetic systems. In response to these challenges, advanced signal denoising techniques have evolved, providing improved time–frequency resolution, adaptivity, and resilience to artifacts. Among the most widely adopted are the Wavelet Transform (WT), Empirical Mode Decomposition (EMD), and Kalman-based adaptive filtering methods.

3.2.1. Wavelet Transform (WT)

WT is particularly advantageous in EMG preprocessing due to its ability to represent signals across multiple scales, making it ideal for capturing transient and time-varying features common in biosignals. Unlike Fourier analysis, which assumes stationarity, wavelet analysis allows localized filtering, isolating both short-duration spikes and sustained low-frequency components.

Wavelet-based denoising typically involves decomposing the EMG signal into multiple levels of detail and approximation coefficients, applying a thresholding algorithm (e.g., soft or hard thresholding), and reconstructing the signal using only the coefficients presumed to contain muscle activity. Recent studies show that wavelet thresholding significantly improves signal-to-noise ratio (SNR) while retaining physiologically meaningful features [43].

Hybrid models, which combine multiple signal processing techniques, have gained increasing attention for their ability to enhance noise suppression while preserving important signal features in biomedical applications. The wavelet hybrid model proposed by Abbaspour et al. [44] presents a robust two-stage approach for eliminating electrocardiogram

(ECG) interference from sEMG signals by combining an Adaptive Neuro-Fuzzy Inference System (ANFIS) with wavelet transform [44]. In the first step, ANFIS is employed to model and suppress the nonlinear and time-varying ECG artifacts present in the contaminated EMG signal. However, low-frequency noise components in the range of 0–15 Hz often remain after ANFIS processing. Given that surface EMG signals primarily occupy the 5–500 Hz frequency range, this residual low-frequency noise can significantly degrade signal quality. To further enhance the denoising process, the second stage uses wavelet transform with nonlinear thresholding as a post-processing technique. The wavelet transform enables signal decomposition across multiple time scales, allowing for the precise identification and removal of remaining low-frequency interference without distorting the underlying EMG signal. By integrating the adaptive learning capabilities of ANFIS with the time–frequency localization strengths of wavelet analysis, the wavelet hybrid model effectively suppresses ECG noise while preserving the essential features of the EMG signal.

3.2.2. Empirical Mode Decomposition (EMD)

EMD is a nonlinear, data-driven technique that decomposes a signal into intrinsic oscillatory modes, known as Intrinsic Mode Functions (IMFs). Unlike wavelet transforms, EMD does not require the selection of basic functions, making it highly adaptive and capable of handling signals with complex time-varying behavior. In EMG processing, EMD has proven effective in isolating signal components corresponding to motion artifacts, power-line interference, and baseline drift. Andrade et al. [45] applied EMD to real and synthetic EMG signals, showing improved noise attenuation compared to wavelet-based filtering, particularly in signals with overlapping frequency bands.

Advanced versions of EMD techniques include combining a median filter (MF) to effectively remove impulsive noise from IMFs [46]. These filtered IMFs are then recombined to form a new signal, which undergoes a second EMD process to generate improved IMFs under the IEMD framework. The results indicate that the proposed IEMD method enhances the discriminative capability of these features compared to the conventional EMD.

3.2.3. Kalman Filtering and Adaptive Filtering

Kalman filtering is a recursive Bayesian estimation technique widely used for dynamic signal estimation in noisy environments. It models the EMG signal as a state-space process, where the observed measurements are considered noisy observations of the true underlying signal. The Kalman filter iteratively estimates the signal state by minimizing the mean square error between the predicted and observed measurements. This approach adapts to time-varying signal characteristics, making it suitable for real-time EMG signal enhancement [47]. Its ability to optimally combine prior information and current measurements results in effective noise suppression, particularly for Gaussian noise and slow-varying disturbances. However, the performance of Kalman filtering depends heavily on accurate modeling of signal and noise statistics, which can be challenging due to the complex nature of EMG signals.

Adaptive filtering, on the other hand, involves algorithms that dynamically adjust filter parameters based on the incoming signal characteristics, without requiring a priori knowledge of signal statistics. Common adaptive algorithms applied to EMG signal filtering include the Least Mean Squares (LMS) [48] and Recursive Least Squares (RLS) [49], filters. These methods iteratively minimize the error between the filter output and a desired response, effectively tracking changes in noise characteristics such as motion artifacts and electrode shifts. Adaptive filters are particularly valuable in scenarios with non-stationary noise, as they can continuously update their parameters to maintain optimal filtering performance. These filtering techniques have emerged as effective solutions for mitigating ECG artifacts in sEMG recordings, particularly when monitoring muscles near the heart [36]. These methods dynamically adjust filter parameters to minimize the influence of ECG interference without significantly distorting the underlying muscle signals. Nonetheless, adaptive filtering may suffer from convergence issues or require careful tuning of step-size parameters to balance adaptation speed and stability.

3.3. Noise Reduction Challenges in Exoskeleton-Based EMG Systems

Exoskeleton applications present unique challenges for EMG signal denoising that distinguish them from other EMG-based systems such as prosthetic limbs or stationary rehabilitation devices. These challenges stem from the inherently dynamic human–exoskeleton interaction, the tight physical integration of EMG sensors with mechanical components, and the strict real-time constraints required for closed-loop control. Overcoming these issues is essential for preserving signal integrity and ensuring safe, responsive actuation in assistive technologies [50].

A primary concern is the prevalence of non-stationary and movement-induced artifacts. During exoskeleton use, muscle activation typically coincides with substantial limb movement, generating artifacts such as motion-induced signal distortions, fluctuating skin-electrode impedance, and crosstalk between adjacent muscles [36]. Unlike prosthetic systems, which often operate under more constrained movement patterns, exoskeletons are used for complex, multi-joint, and often load-bearing activities. These factors increase the variability and noise content of the EMG signals, complicating effective extraction of the underlying motor intent.

Another critical challenge is sensor–mechanism interference. EMG electrodes are frequently placed in close proximity to rigid or semi-rigid exoskeleton components, resulting in exposure to mechanical vibrations [51] and electromagnetic interference (EMI) from actuators, motors, and joint encoders [52]. These interferences commonly overlap with the frequency range of EMG signals, making it difficult for conventional linear filters to effectively separate noise from the signal without introducing distortion or latency.

Real-time processing constraints further complicate signal denoising in exoskeleton applications. Because these systems require rapid interpretation of user intent to drive timely and safe actuation, EMG signals must be processed with minimal latency. Therefore, denoising techniques must not only be robust but also computationally efficient. Filtering algorithms must strike a careful balance between suppressing noise and preserving relevant signal features critical for downstream classification or control tasks [50].

Subject- and task-specific variability introduces additional complexity. Users differ in their physiology, movement strategies, and sensor attachment conditions, and the tasks performed with the exoskeleton may involve variable levels of intensity, duration, and muscle group engagement. These factors result in highly individualized signal characteristics, making fixed or non-adaptive filtering approaches less effective. Consequently, noise reduction strategies for exoskeleton-based EMG systems must often incorporate adaptive or personalized filtering schemes to maintain performance across users and conditions.

In addition to controlled laboratory settings, wearable and rehabilitation exoskeletons are increasingly being deployed in outpatient environments and real-world daily living scenarios, which are characterized by unpredictable movements and variable environmental conditions. These movement-rich contexts exacerbate noise-related challenges by introducing frequent posture changes, abrupt limb motions, and fluctuating ambient interference [53]. As such, the robustness of EMG filtering methods becomes even more critical. Filters that rely on stationarity assumptions or fixed-frequency band rejection often perform inadequately under these dynamic and nonlinear conditions. In contrast, adaptive methods such as wavelet-based thresholding, empirical mode decomposition (EMD), and Kalman filters have demonstrated superior robustness due to their ability to adjust to evolving signal characteristics in real time.

Wavelet-based thresholding is particularly effective in handling non-stationary EMG signals commonly encountered in dynamic tasks. Adaptive thresholding techniques, such as soft or level-dependent thresholding [54], can then suppress transient artifacts while preserving motor-relevant signal features. This approach is especially useful in outpatient and rehabilitation settings, where sudden movements or external impacts can cause unpredictable signal fluctuations.

EMD offers another powerful strategy for adaptive EMG denoising. EMD decomposes a complex signal into IMFs based on local extrema without assuming any prior basis functions [55]. Since it is inherently data-driven and nonlinear, EMD is well-suited for non-stationary and subject-specific EMG signals. In exoskeleton systems, low-frequency IMFs often capture motion artifacts and baseline drift, which can be selectively removed while retaining higher-frequency components associated with muscle activity. Moreover, EMD's flexibility enables it to adapt to a wide range of task dynamics and muscle recruitment patterns, enhancing its utility across diverse outpatient rehabilitation activities.

Kalman filtering and its extended or unscented variants provide an optimal framework for estimating the true EMG signal in the presence of dynamic and noisy measurements [56]. These filters use a probabilistic model of system dynamics and noise characteristics to recursively estimate the signal state. In exoskeleton applications, Kalman filters can be integrated into control loops to simultaneously denoise and interpret EMG signals in real time. Their robustness stems from their predictive and adaptive nature—by continuously updating their internal model based on incoming observations, they can track gradual or abrupt changes in signal statistics caused by user motion, fatigue, or electrode displacement. Moreover, Kalman filters can incorporate biomechanical constraints or musculoskeletal models to further enhance their estimation accuracy under real-world movement conditions.

Collectively, these adaptive denoising methods offer significant advantages for rehabilitation and outpatient exoskeleton use. Their ability to respond to variable noise sources, individual differences in physiology, and contextual changes in task execution makes them more robust than traditional linear filters. Nonetheless, ensuring their practical deployment requires careful consideration of computational efficiency, parameter tuning, and real-time implementation constraints, especially for embedded systems. Continued research into lightweight, hybrid, and learning-enhanced variants of these methods could further improve their robustness and applicability in wearable neuroprosthetic and assistive technologies.

4. EMG Signal Analysis Methods for Exoskeleton Control

EMG analysis has been established for quite some time. In the past, the signals obtained from EMGs had limited applications due to the absence of effective signal processing methods. However, with advancements in computational technologies, EMG-based applications have become much more prevalent at present [57]. Once the EMG data have been processed, the subsequent step involves analyzing these data to extract meaningful information. Several techniques can be employed to achieve this. These techniques can primarily be categorized into two groups. First, there are traditional methods where basic statistical and mathematical principles are applied to the EMG signals. Second, relatively novel approaches, such as machine learning, are utilized to capture significant information, including motion and gesture recognition.

4.1. Feature Extraction Techniques

One of the primary applications of the EMG feature extraction is in developing and controlling exoskeletons. Since humans directly utilize exoskeletons as assistive devices, the effects on the user can be directly monitored through muscle signals captured by EMG sensors. Additionally, when it comes to active exoskeleton control, employing EMG sensors enables the exoskeleton to operate harmoniously with the human, creating a human–machine symbiosis. To achieve these tasks, it is crucial to process and analyze EMG signals. After preprocessing the EMG signals as outlined in the previous chapter, the next step is to proceed with their analysis. This analysis is divided into three primary areas, as shown in Figure 1, namely feature extraction, pattern recognition, and muscle synergy analysis. The following subsections explore each of these areas in detail.

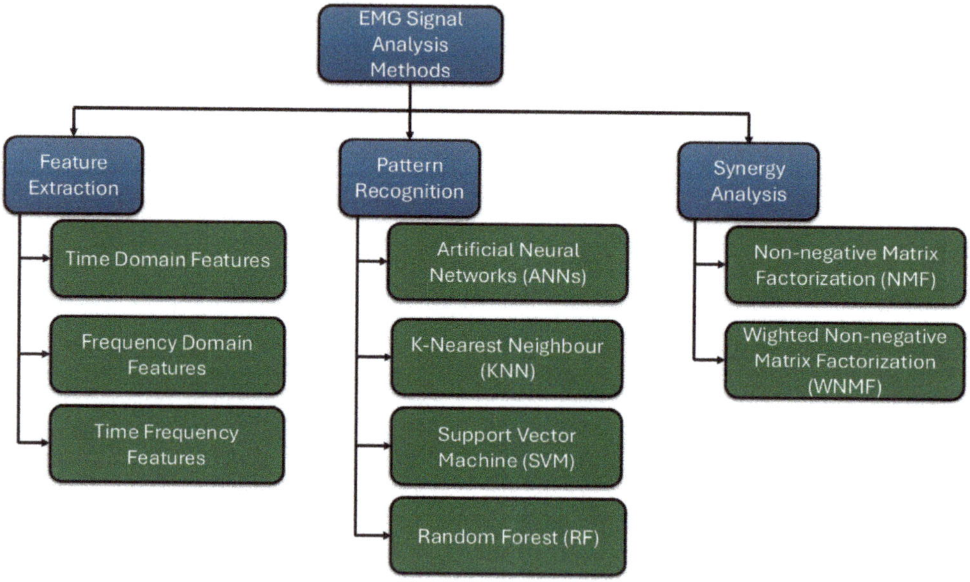

Figure 1. Classification of EMG signal analysis methods (main classifications in blue and their sub-classifications in green).

4.1.1. Time-Domain Features

As the name implies, time domain features are characteristics derived from a signal within the time domain. These features can provide valuable real-time insights into the signals. In the context of EMGs, such features specifically serve to capture the muscle activity of various muscles during different movements [58].

Commonly used time-domain features in the EMG field include Mean Absolute Value (MAV) and Root Mean Square (RMS) [59]. These two features offer crucial insights in engineering applications where the muscle force generated is of significant value [60]. However, upon closer examination, these metrics also provide specific insights. The Mean Absolute Value (MAV) serves as a more direct representation of muscle contractions or activity. In contrast, the Root Mean Square (RMS) offers insights into muscle effort and energy expenditure during a particular motion [61]. When evaluating computational costs, MAV is relatively less expensive than RMS [62]. Another time-domain feature utilized in the analysis of electromyography (EMG) data is the Zero Crossing Rate (ZCR). As the name indicates, ZCR represents the count of instances in which the EMG signal crosses the zero level within a specified time unit. This measurement serves as an indication of the frequency of muscle activation and the timing of muscular contractions [60].

4.1.2. Frequency-Domain Features

When considering frequency domain features relevant to exoskeleton applications, Power Spectral Density (PSD) can be identified as a significant metric. PSD in EMG signal analysis is primarily utilized to evaluate the strength of the EMG signal across its frequency content. In other words, this feature is instrumental in assessing muscle activity, as commonly noted in scientific literature. Two key metrics derived from PSD are Median Frequency (MDF) and Mean Frequency (MNF) [63]. Both of these parameters serve as reliable indicators of muscle fatigue, particularly during isometric tasks [64]. Although both parameters are useful for assessing muscle fatigue, the MDF is preferred due to its reduced sensitivity to outliers [63,64]. However, the calculation of MDF may incur slightly higher computational costs compared to MNF due to the specific methodology employed in its computation [64]. Regarding exoskeletons, both parameters serve as significant features in determining the amount of power required by the wearer over a given duration, especially as the wearer's fatigue increases the power required by the wearer over a given duration, especially as the wearer's fatigue increases.

4.1.3. Time-Frequency Features

The analysis of time-frequency features in EMG is essential for comprehending the time-varying motions and dynamic characteristics associated with particular movements. This is especially critical in applications such as exoskeletons, where the identification of movements and movement patterns is paramount; hence, the importance of time-frequency features cannot be overstated. The Short-Time Fourier Transform (STFT) is one of the most commonly used time-frequency features in EMG analysis. In STFT, dynamic signals are divided into short-time segments, and as the name suggests, those parts are then subjected to the Fourier Transform. Each signal segment is subjected to this process. According to scientific literature, this method is applicable when the muscle contraction patterns change over time [65]. On the other hand, WT decomposes an EMG signal into components at various scales [66]. In simpler terms, this method is capable of providing insights into the transient features of EMG signals, making it ideal for tasks such as gesture detection based on EMG signals [66,67].

4.2. EMG Pattern Recognition for Motion Control

Processing signals, as mentioned in the previous section, has apparent limitations with respect to exoskeleton-related applications. Specifically, those EMG signals illustrate the changes in a muscle under a particular scenario. Thus, in applications where human and machine symbiosis is important, EMG pattern recognition plays a significant role. In a contemporary era marked by the increasing prominence of Machine Learning, EMG pattern recognition emerges as a viable technique for the control of exoskeletons, harnessing these machine learning methodologies.

As illustrated in Figure 1, four primary machine techniques are used to analyze EMG signals [68]. The first is supervised learning, where human intervention is required to label and sort data during the algorithm training [68,69]. The second category is unsupervised learning, in which no explicit training is provided; instead, the machine learning algorithm identifies patterns within the data [69]. Supervised learning, on the other hand, utilizes labeled data and employs algorithms that learn a mapping from inputs to known outputs. In contrast, unsupervised learning analyzes unlabeled data to discover hidden patterns or groupings without prior training labels [70]. In scientific literature, there are only a few instances where unsupervised machine learning algorithms have been utilized to recognize patterns in EMG signals [68,71,72]. However, in most cases, these algorithms are employed as a technique to address new EMG data with anomalies after supervised learning has already been applied. Therefore, this review will not focus on unsupervised learning.

Supervised learning has emerged as a prominent area of research in the analysis of EMG data. Numerous studies conducted in recent years have successfully implemented methods for motion pattern recognition. According to scientific literature, it can be identified that Artificial Neural Networks (ANNs) have been commonly utilized in EMG-based motion recognition [68,73–77]. The human brain's structure inspires these ANNs and has a high potential for accurate motion recognition due to its excellent performance in developing nonlinear connections [75]. Nonetheless, researchers have identified several drawbacks associated with this technique. The inherent "black box" characteristic of neural networks, which hinders the understanding or alteration of their internal operations, raises concerns regarding their performance under unfamiliar future conditions [78]. Moreover, the necessity for a substantial volume of training data represents another issue that must be addressed [78]. Also, in instances of training with backpropagation—a widely utilized method for training neural networks—this network-related error may become trapped in a local minimum error instead of the global minimum error, leading the networks to produce erroneous outputs [79]. However, it is worth noting that backpropagation allows for the construction of Convolutional Neural Networks (CNNs) and Recurrent Neural Networks (RNNs), which are derived from multi-layered ANNs. These models serve as powerful tools in the classification and recognition of EMG motion data [80]. Furthermore, according to the authors of [81], neural network-based EMG analysis methods are capable of analyzing and classifying EMG signals in real-time with greater accuracy. This characteristic renders this approach significantly more suitable for exoskeleton control.

Instead of ANNs, there are quite a few other machine learning-based techniques that have been successfully utilized in EMG pattern recognition. K-Nearest Neighbor (KNN) is one of the simplest algorithms used to classify or recognize patterns in EMG signals. In this method, new data is classified based on the nearest data point [82]. However, this method incurs significant computational costs during the prediction phase, as it necessitates comparing the latest data point with all training data points. Moreover, the capability to make correct decisions in the presence of multiple scenarios (classes) is troublesome in this method [82]. More accurate Support Vector Machine (SVM) and Random Forest (RF) methods have also been used in EMG motion classification. Theoretically, the RF algorithm, a derivation of the decision tree method, has high accuracy and is capable of handling large amounts of data [83]. This method is inherently resistant to outliers, which is crucial for EMG analysis, given the noisy signals that persist even after signal filtering [83]. However, RF becomes extremely computationally expensive once the dataset becomes larger and requires careful tuning of the algorithm [84]. On the other hand, Support Vector Machines (SVMs) serve as a robust classifier for noisy data and demonstrate superior generalization capabilities compared to other methodologies [85]. However, increased computational requirements arise when the number of data points increases, and the manual selection method for the kernel and parameters is observed as a disadvantage of this approach for EMG classification [86].

4.3. Muscle Synergy Analysis for Exoskeleton Control

Muscle synergy analysis is recognized as a crucial aspect of the symbiotic relationship between humans and exoskeletons. Human movement is governed by the central nervous system (CNS). Additionally, it is well-established that the human musculoskeletal system consists of redundant degrees of freedom when performing various movements. Consequently, it has been theorized that the CNS simplifies human motor functions by employing linear combinations of synergies, which are motor commands sent to different groups of muscles that activate them simultaneously [87,88]. These synergies serve as an efficient and parsimonious method for controlling and simplifying spatiotemporal patterns of muscle activation, thereby reducing the degrees of freedom that need to be coordinated within the human body [87,88]. Identifying these synergies can enhance the detection of human motion and gestures, which would be particularly advantageous in contexts where exoskeleton control is necessary. These synergies are typically identified through EMG signals and have been employed in many applications, including the control of exoskeletons [87–93].

According to a recent scientific review on synergy analysis, several primary algorithms have been utilized in this field, as illustrated in Figure 1. The review [87] indicates that 85% of the scientific literature employs non-negative Matrix Factorization (NMF) for synergy analysis. In academic terms, non-negative NMF is a methodology utilized for decomposing and simplifying EMG signals into simple components. NMF can be explained in the following equation [87,94,95].

$$D = CS \tag{1}$$

where D is given non-negative matrix, and C and S are reduced rank non-negative matrices. In an EMG application, D is a matrix representing EMG readings from different muscles over a specific timeframe [94,95]. C is the synergy matrix, which indicates which muscles are activated together, while S is the activation pattern, illustrating when the synergy is active [94,95]. Optimizing the synergy and activation matrices can facilitate accurately identifying motions and gestures for exoskeleton control. Furthermore, this technique holds significant value in developing rehabilitation exoskeletons for paralyzed patients, as their motor functions are compromised and synergies may not be clearly defined [90,93,94]. However, with pre-existing data on synergy, it becomes feasible for the exoskeleton to deliver the necessary support for the intended motions [90,93,94]. Except for NMF, weighted NMF (WNMF), a derivation of NMF, is the second most used algorithm for synergy analysis [87]. All other methods, which include Principal Component Analysis (PCA) [96], Independent Component Analysis (ICA) [97], Factor Analysis (FA) [98], and Autoencoders (Neural Networks) [99], have only been utilized in less than 3% of existing literature, indicating their limitations [87]. In conclusion, recognizing complex motion patterns is critically important for delivering essential support through exoskeletons to meet the user's specific requirements and ensure optimal comfort during their use.

5. Application of EMG in Exoskeleton Development

Wearable robotic exoskeletons emerge as a transformative class of assistive technology that bridges the interface between human intention and robotic actuation. These devices are designed to enhance, support, or restore voluntary movement in users across a broad spectrum of contexts, from individuals with mobility impairments to industrial workers facing repetitive strain. A major challenge in realizing intuitive and efficient human–robot interaction lies in decoding user intent with precision. As shown in Figure 2, EMG, which captures the electrical activity of muscles during contraction, offers a compelling bio signal for driving exoskeleton control systems due to its ability to provide real-time feedback about neuromuscular activity [35,100].

EMG signals can be collected non-invasively using sEMG or invasively through intramuscular techniques. While sEMG is more widely adopted in wearable robotics due to its practicality, it is more susceptible to noise, crosstalk, and skin impedance variations [101]. Intramuscular EMG provides greater spatial resolution but is limited in long-term applications due to its invasive nature. Regardless of the recording technique, the raw EMG signal must be carefully processed through a series of steps, including band pass filtering, full wave rectification, smoothing, and normalization to make it suitable for control [102,103].

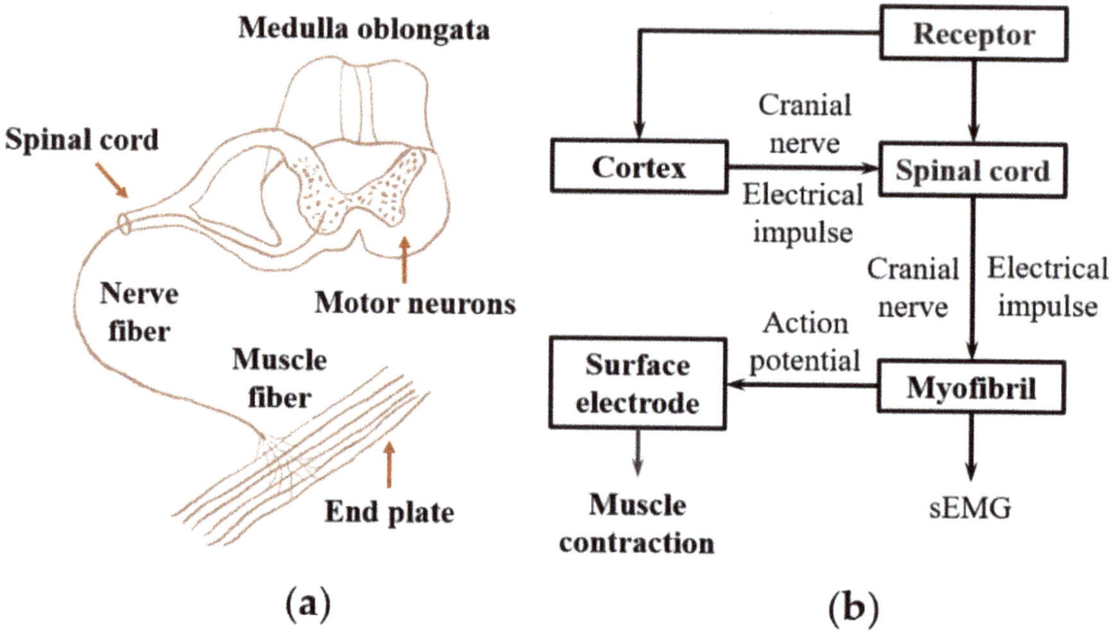

Figure 2. The principle of generation of the EMG signal. (**a**) The structure of the neuromuscular system. (**b**) The schematic of the EMG signal transduction in the nerve and muscle system. Adapted from Fang et al. [100], licensed under CC BY 4.0.

5.1. EMG-Based Control Strategies

The utility of EMG for exoskeletons depends not only on the fidelity of the signal but also on the robustness of the control algorithm that interprets it. Broadly, EMG-based control strategies fall into the following three categories: threshold-based control, pattern recognition (PR) based control, and hybrid systems that combine EMG with other sensory inputs.

5.1.1. Threshold-Based Control

Threshold-based control is a foundational approach where actuation is triggered when the EMG signal exceeds a user-defined amplitude, as depicted in Figure 3. This method assumes a direct correlation between muscle activation strength and intended motion [104–106]. For example, when the EMG signal from the forearm flexors exceeds a threshold, a robotic hand might be commanded to close. While simple and computationally efficient, this method lacks finesse in differentiating graded force levels or distinguishing between multiple movement classes [35,107].

Despite its limitations, threshold-based control remains relevant in scenarios demanding rapid, binary actuation, such as hand open/close tasks or gait initiation. It is especially useful in early rehabilitation phases where gross motor activation is the primary goal. However, its reliance on fixed thresholds poses issues related to fatigue, electrode displacement, and signal variability over time. Such factors can render the system unreliable without frequent recalibration [108].

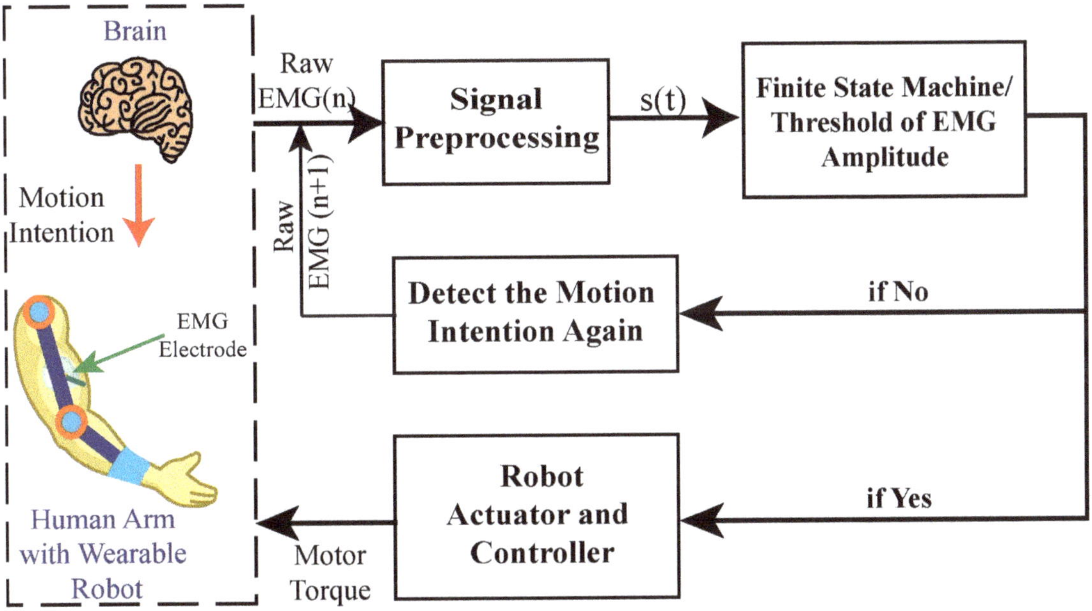

Figure 3. The conceptual block diagram for threshold-based (On–Off/Finite State Machine) myoelectric control system. Adapted from Fu et al. [106], licensed under CC BY 4.0.

5.1.2. Pattern Recognition-Based Control

To achieve more refined control, pattern recognition (PR) techniques are employed. PR based systems involve the extraction of discriminative features from EMG signals (e.g., Mean Absolute Value, zero crossing, waveform length), followed by classification into predefined motion categories using machine learning algorithms [109]. Classifiers like Linear Discriminant Analysis (LDA), Support Vector Machines (SVM), and Artificial Neural Networks (ANNs) are commonly used [110,111]. The complete EMG pattern recognition pipeline is illustrated in Figure 4, starting from data acquisition and preprocessing, through feature extraction and dimensionality reduction, to final classification using machine learning algorithms. More recently, deep learning techniques such as Convolutional Neural Networks (CNNs) and Long Short-Term Memory (LSTM) networks have been adopted to exploit the temporal dependencies in EMG signals [112].

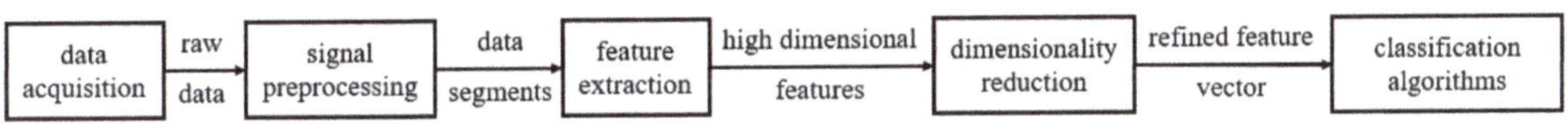

Figure 4. The pipeline of performing EMG pattern recognition. Adapted from Fang et al. [100], licensed under CC BY 4.0.

This paradigm is particularly suited for upper limb exoskeletons and myoelectric prostheses, where a range of gestures or tasks must be interpreted from EMG. PR allows for multi-DOF (degree of freedom) control, proportional force estimation, and even co-contraction detection. However, its effectiveness is tempered by the need for large training datasets, sensitivity to inter- and intra-subject variability, and degradation in performance due to factors like fatigue or environmental noise [113,114]. To address these issues, researchers have explored techniques such as domain adaptation, unsupervised learning, and transfer learning to improve generalizability. While effective in controlled environments, real-world applications still pose significant challenges in maintaining classifier robustness without extensive recalibration.

5.1.3. Hybrid Control Strategies

A growing body of work now focuses on hybrid control systems, which combine EMG with additional sensors such as IMUs, EEG, and pressure sensors [115]. These systems aim to mitigate the limitations of EMG-only strategies by integrating redundant or complementary information. For instance, while EMG indicates intention, IMUs can provide limb orientation and velocity, improving accuracy in classifying complex motions [116].

In populations with weak or unreliable muscle activation, EEG offers an alternative pathway for interpreting motor intent. Hybrid EEG–EMG systems have been used to facilitate control in users with spinal cord injuries or advanced neuromuscular disorders [117]. Additional sensors like force transducers help monitor user–device interaction forces, contributing to adaptive impedance control and safety assurance [6]. These multimodal approaches have proven to improve classification accuracy, robustness to sensor artifacts, and overall adaptability of exoskeleton systems. However, they also increase system complexity, power consumption, and computational demands, which leads to the next critical issue: real-time signal processing.

5.2. Real-Time Processing Challenges

Achieving high-performance EMG control in exoskeletons hinges on the ability to process signals with minimal delay. The end-to-end latency from muscle activation to actuation must typically fall below 100 ms to preserve natural responsiveness and avoid destabilizing the user [118].

5.2.1. Computational Latency and Hardware Constraints

EMG processing pipelines involve several stages: analog-to-digital conversion, filtering, segmentation, feature extraction, and classification. Each must be optimized for speed and accuracy. Embedded systems used in wearable robotics, such as microcontrollers or System-on-Chip (SoC) platforms, offer limited resources, thus demanding algorithmic efficiency [115]. Hardware accelerators, FPGAs, and lightweight machine learning models have been proposed to address these constraints. Moreover, communication delays, particularly in wireless setups, must be minimized using protocols like BLE or Wi-Fi Direct, which require tight synchronization between sensor nodes and processing units [119].

5.2.2. Adaptive Calibration for User-Specific Variations

Inter- and intra-subject variability is another major obstacle. Muscle fatigue, electrode drift, skin impedance, and posture shifts alter the EMG signal distribution, reducing the reliability of static classifiers. Solutions include real-time normalization of EMG amplitudes, adaptive filtering (e.g., RLS and Kalman filters), and models capable of online learning [115,120]. Recent approaches also include confidence-based prediction systems that trigger recalibration protocols when uncertainty exceeds predefined thresholds [121]. Semi-supervised and unsupervised learning are further explored to reduce the user burden during long-term operation. Together, these adaptations form the foundation for the next generation of systems: personalized and intelligent exoskeletons.

5.3. Personalized and Adaptive Exoskeleton Control

The ultimate goal of EMG-based exoskeletons is to provide tailored assistance that adapts in real-time to the needs, intentions, and physiological states of individual users. Personalization becomes particularly important in clinical settings, where no two patients share the same rehabilitation trajectory or muscular response profile.

5.3.1. AI-Driven Adaptive Controllers

AI-driven controllers, particularly those based on reinforcement learning (RL), have shown promise in personalizing exoskeleton behavior. These systems learn optimal control policies by interacting with the user and adapting to feedback such as muscle activation patterns, gait asymmetry, or energy consumption [122–124]. Figure 5 illustrates a reinforcement learning-based architecture for EMG hand gesture recognition, where raw EMG signals are processed and classified using either a Deep Q-Network (DQN) or a Double-DQN to determine the intended gesture.

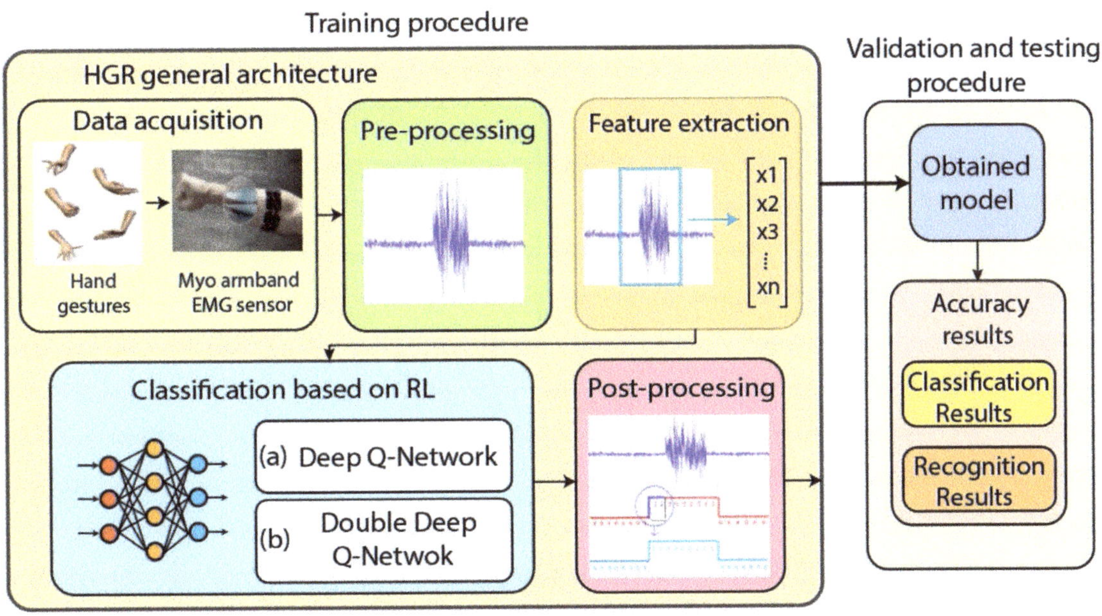

Figure 5. Hand gesture recognition architecture based on EMG signals and reinforcement learning (RL). The classification stage can employ either Deep Q-Network (DQN) or Double-DQN for motion intent decoding. Adapted from Caraguay et al. [124], licensed under CC BY 4.0.

Personalization is achieved through iterative learning: the controller adjusts joint torque, stiffness, or movement timing to minimize muscular effort or enhance movement symmetry [123,125]. Deep neural networks like LSTMs are used to capture temporal patterns and forecast future movement needs, allowing pre-emptive adjustments [112]. Multimodal sensors (e.g., EMG + IMU + force) further enhance the ability of these controllers to detect context changes (e.g., level walking vs. incline) and adapt assistance dynamically [126]. Bayesian optimization offers another route for tuning control parameters with minimal user feedback, especially useful in early-stage rehabilitation [127].

5.3.2. Muscle Fatigue Compensation Techniques

Fatigue presents a unique challenge for EMG control. It alters both the amplitude and frequency characteristics of EMG signals, potentially misleading classifiers trained under fresh conditions [120]. Spectral features such as Median Frequency (MF) and Mean Power Frequency (MPF) have been widely used to detect fatigue. As fatigue progresses, these values decline, signaling a need to modify assistance levels [128]. Changes in muscle synergy, which reflect how muscle groups coordinate, are also indicative of fatigue and can be leveraged for adaptive control using dimensionality reduction techniques like NNMF [129].

Fuzzy logic and neuro-fuzzy controllers excel in this context due to their tolerance for imprecision and their ability to incorporate heuristics into control schemes [130]. Adaptive filters, such as RLS or wavelet-based denoisers, offer real-time compensation for fatigue-induced signal degradation [107]. Finally, user-in-the-loop optimization frameworks allow users to provide subjective feedback, enabling the system to adjust torque or stiffness based on perceived exertion and comfort [9].

5.4. Limitations of EMG Only Control Compared to Multimodal Biosensing Approaches

EMG has been widely used as a control signal for robotic exoskeletons, prostheses, and human machine interfaces due to its ability to reflect voluntary muscle activation. However, relying on EMG signals alone presents several limitations, particularly in real world and rehabilitation settings. Multimodal biosensing approaches that integrate other physiological signals such as force sensing, electroencephalography, inertial motion data, or skin temperature can significantly improve the accuracy, robustness, and usability of these systems.

5.4.1. Signal Variability and Instability

One major limitation of EMG based systems is their sensitivity to changes in skin impedance, electrode positioning, sweating, and muscle fatigue. These factors lead to signal drift and unstable performance over time. Zheng et al. [131] found that EMG performance deteriorates significantly under sweat-related impedance changes, while force myography remained more stable under the same conditions. Similarly, Nazari and Zheng [132] noted that EMG-based interfaces often require frequent recalibration to address the variability stemming from electrode placement and user-specific muscle physiology. The study highlights that combining EMG with complementary modalities such as sonomyography or inertial sensors can improve signal robustness and reduce the burden of recalibration.

5.4.2. Lack of Contextual Awareness

EMG provides information about local muscle activity but does not capture external context, limb orientation, or movement intention at a higher level. As a result, EMG only systems may not perform well in complex tasks such as grasping different objects or adapting to changing environments. Zandigohar et al. [133] demonstrated that combining EMG signals with visual and gaze data significantly enhances grasp intent inference by integrating environmental context, improving accuracy compared to EMG-only approaches.

In another study, Al Quraishi and co-authors [134] demonstrated that integrating EEG with EMG improved robustness and intent recognition, especially during task transitions.

5.4.3. Decreased Performance Under Fatigue or Impairment

During extended use or in users with reduced muscular function, EMG signal strength and quality can diminish. This reduction makes control less reliable and may result in false or missed commands. Zheng et al. [131] noted that the combination of EMG with force signals improved classification accuracy even when fatigue was present. Meanwhile, Zeng et al. [135] demonstrated that ultrasound, when fused with EMG, enhances force estimation robustness during fatigue, outperforming EMG alone.

5.4.4. Susceptibility to Noise and Crosstalk

EMG signals are prone to motion artifacts, electrical interference, and signal mixing from neighboring muscles, which can confuse classification algorithms. Zandigohar et al. [133] found that EMG signals were affected by movement artifacts, and this issue was addressed by incorporating vision-based inputs. Al Quraishi et al. [134] showed that combining EEG with EMG improved signal quality and interpretation in noisy environments.

5.4.5. Limited Resolution and Low Intent Classification

EMG based control often lacks the ability to produce continuous or multi-level control, especially when using threshold methods or simple classifiers. This limits the range of motions and reduces natural interaction. Zheng et al. [131] reported that EMG alone resulted in gesture recognition accuracy of 81.5 percent, while combining it with force sensing improved accuracy to over 91 percent. Zandigohar et al. [133] similarly demonstrated that EMG plus vision improved grasp prediction accuracy from 81.6 percent to 95.3 percent.

5.5. Benefits of Integrating Edge Computing in Wearable EMG Systems for Home Monitoring

Wearable EMG systems are becoming increasingly important in home-based health monitoring and assistive applications. Their functionality and reliability can be significantly enhanced by integrating edge computing platforms that process data locally rather than transmitting it to remote cloud servers. This approach presents several key advantages for real-time EMG signal interpretation and control in wearable systems.

5.5.1. Minimization of Response Delays and Improvement of Real-Time Performance

Processing EMG signals directly on embedded platforms or nearby edge devices allows for rapid computation and decision making. This local computation ensures that movement intentions or physiological assessments can be interpreted within milliseconds, which is critical for closed-loop motor control, such as in prosthetics or exoskeletons. Studies such as those by Covi et al. [136] demonstrated that adaptive edge computing architectures, particularly those leveraging neuromorphic principles, significantly reduce latency and support timely actuation responses in wearable biomedical systems.

5.5.2. Enhancement of Data Privacy and Security

By confining data processing to local devices, edge computing significantly reduces the transmission of sensitive physiological data over networks. This localized data handling offers better control over user privacy and supports compliance with healthcare data protection regulations. Jeong et al. [137] demonstrated that their portable EMG and ECG monitoring system employs smartphone-based adaptive digital filtering to minimize interference without introducing latency, effectively preserving data privacy and delivering reliable real-time diagnostics in home environments.

5.5.3. Reduction in Power and Communication Overhead

Transmitting continuous streams of raw EMG data requires substantial bandwidth and power, particularly in battery-powered wearable devices. Edge platforms enable devices to transmit only essential summaries or alerts, thereby conserving energy and reducing wireless network demand. This capability extends the operational lifetime of wearable systems, which is vital for long-term use in home environments. For example, biomedical devices that transmit only essential processed summaries, instead of full resolution EMG signals, demonstrate notable energy savings over Bluetooth Low Energy (BLE) connections. For example, in a study on wireless biomedical sensors, the authors found that transmitting a single averaged value rather than raw 4 kHz signals reduced Bluetooth module power consumption from 3 mA (at 10 ms intervals) to just 0.9 mA above a 50 ms interval indicating that data reduction strategies can save substantial energy [138].

5.5.4. Capability for Adaptive Local Signal Processing

Edge-integrated systems can perform essential preprocessing steps such as noise filtering, signal rectification, feature extraction, and pattern recognition without external support. This allows the device to adjust processing parameters in response to changes in the user's condition, signal quality, or environmental factors. Such adaptability improves the robustness and usability of wearable EMG systems during prolonged or daily use. As demonstrated by Salkić et al. [139], implementing an edge computing framework on a compact platform (like Raspberry Pi) allowed real-time preprocessing and classification of wearable sensor data highlighting the feasibility of adaptive, on-device processing in practical applications.

5.5.5. Enabling Instantaneous Feedback and Personalized Assistance

With computation and decision making occurring locally, wearable EMG systems can provide immediate feedback to the user or activate actuators in real time. This is particularly beneficial for rehabilitation and therapeutic use, where timely feedback can improve motor learning and recovery outcomes. For example, a real-time hand-exoskeleton system incorporating local EMG classification coupled with a virtual reality feedback loop effectively synchronized user movement with visual feedback, enhancing user engagement and adherence to training protocols [140].

5.6. Enhancing Muscle Fatigue Compensation via Bioimpedance-Integrated EMG Systems

Muscle fatigue is a common challenge in prolonged use of wearable assistive technologies such as exoskeletons and prostheses. Traditional EMG-based systems detect fatigue through changes in signal amplitude, frequency content, or muscle activation patterns. However, these metrics alone often suffer from inter-subject variability and susceptibility to noise, sweat, and signal drift. An emerging solution is the integration of bioimpedance (BI) measurements alongside EMG to monitor the physiological state of muscles more comprehensively.

BI, especially through multifrequency or electrical impedance myography (EIM), measures muscle tissue resistance and reactance to alternating currents and is sensitive to changes in fluid distribution and cellular structure. Studies have shown that impedance magnitude and phase vary significantly under muscle fatigue conditions. Vescio et al. [141] reported statistically significant impedance changes during fatigue protocols, and Kusche and Ryschka (2019) demonstrated that combining BI with EMG improves contraction detection in noisy conditions [34].

Integrating EMG and BI enables a dual-modality approach that combines electrophysiological activity (EMG) with structural and fluidic muscle condition (BI). Kusche and Ryschka [34] demonstrated a wearable system combining both modalities for more robust contraction recognition in noisy environments. They found that BI signals remained stable under mechanical disturbances that affected EMG, allowing better segmentation of valid muscle activity. Similarly, Huang et al. [142] applied electrical impedance myography during dynamic contractions and observed impedance changes that correlated with fatigue progression, confirming that BI provides consistent indicators of muscle condition, even as EMG signal quality diminishes.

Furthermore, the fusion of the EMG–BI data can support machine learning models that are more resilient to transient fluctuations and can generalize better across sessions and users. By incorporating BI data into fatigue compensation algorithms, wearable systems can dynamically adjust assistance levels, rest intervals, or alert mechanisms, thereby minimizing risk of overuse injuries and improving user comfort. For instance, Jaiswal et al. [143] demonstrated that machine learning frameworks combining EMG and inertial data significantly enhanced fatigue state classification compared to using EMG alone, underscoring the benefit of multimodal integration for sustained wearable performance.

5.7. *Optimizing Adaptive Calibration Using Multimodal Biofeedback*

Traditional EMG-based control systems for exoskeletons often rely solely on signal amplitude or pattern recognition to infer user intent. However, this approach may struggle to maintain reliability across extended sessions due to factors like electrode displacement, skin impedance changes, or muscle fatigue. To improve robustness and personalization, recent research has emphasized the importance of adaptive calibration systems supported by multimodal biofeedback.

One effective approach is the use of human-in-the-loop learning paradigms, where the system continuously refines its control parameters based on real-time user feedback. Peternel et al. [144] demonstrated a system where EMG signals were integrated with adaptive impedance control to teach robotic movements through user demonstration. This allowed the exoskeleton to iteratively minimize EMG effort, adjusting torque outputs based on the user's physiological response in real time.

Beyond EMG alone, vibrotactile feedback has emerged as a powerful modality for enhancing motor learning and calibration. De Angelis et al. [145] conducted a systematic review and meta-analysis showing that vibrotactile feedback improves motor performance, especially in balance and gait training for neurological patients. These tactile cues act as external feedback mechanisms that help the user better align their intent with the exoskeleton's output. In rehabilitation contexts, this has proven particularly valuable in reducing the cognitive load required to learn and maintain proper control strategies.

Additionally, combining BI signals with EMG provides real-time insights into the structural and fluidic state of muscles. Kusche and Ryschka [34] developed a wearable system that used both EMG and BI for muscle activity detection, demonstrating that BI remained more stable in the presence of mechanical artifacts and sweating conditions where EMG would typically degrade. This fusion enabled more consistent calibration by filtering out invalid muscle activations and dynamically adjusting thresholds and gain factors.

These findings suggest that multimodal calibration, which leverages complementary biosignals like vibrotactile feedback and BI, not only enhances user safety but also minimizes the need for frequent manual recalibration. In future applications, machine learning algorithms may be integrated into this multimodal framework to autonomously learn user-specific signal signatures and adapt the control logic over time.

5.8. Inclusion of Additional Bioelectric Modalities to Improve Gesture Recognition Accuracy in Noisy Environments

EMG-based control systems are widely used for gesture recognition in wearable assistive technologies. However, their accuracy can be significantly compromised in noisy environments due to issues such as muscle fatigue, signal crosstalk, motion artifacts, and electrode displacement. To address these limitations, researchers have proposed integrating additional bioelectric modalities such as EEG and electrooculography (EOG) with EMG to enhance system robustness and classification performance.

Hybrid systems that combine EEG and EMG have been shown to improve gesture recognition accuracy by leveraging both central nervous system (cortical) signals and peripheral muscular activation. For example, Kawase et al. [146] developed a hybrid brain-machine interface (BMI) for controlling an upper limb exoskeleton in patients with paresis. In their system, EEG signals were used to detect the user's motor intention, while EMG was employed for fine tuning joint angle estimation. The combination significantly improved control accuracy, even in impaired users, highlighting the benefits of using multiple physiological channels.

Another area of active research involves the integration of EMG signals with gaze tracking and EOG to improve intention detection in assistive robotic systems. For instance, Zandigohar et al. [133] introduced a multimodal human–machine interface that combines EMG with visual input including gaze orientation and environmental context using a fusion model to infer user intent more accurately. Their findings showed that this approach significantly enhanced gesture recognition, especially under conditions of muscle fatigue or external noise. The inclusion of gaze data provided an additional contextual layer, helping to disambiguate overlapping EMG signal patterns and improving the overall reliability of the system.

The inclusion of additional bioelectric modalities also supports more flexible and adaptive machine learning architectures. Multimodal deep learning models can learn temporal and spatial correlations across signal types, enabling more nuanced interpretation of user intent. Furthermore, these systems may offer improved generalizability across sessions and users by reducing reliance on any single, noise-sensitive modality. For example, Wei and Ren [147] developed a multimodal generative model that augments EMG data with virtual IMU signals, resulting in a 2–13% accuracy improvement in gesture recognition compared to EMG-only models comparable to physical IMU fusion high-lighting the power of multimodal learning even without extra hardware

Overall, incorporating modalities such as EEG, EOG, or even skin conductance can significantly enhance the resilience and accuracy of gesture recognition systems in challenging operational contexts. As wearable technologies move toward home and clinical use, this multimodal approach represents a promising direction for robust human–machine interfacing.

6. Conclusions

This review has presented a comprehensive overview of the end-to-end electromyography (EMG) signal processing pipeline, ranging from acquisition and filtering to feature extraction and advanced machine learning algorithms and closing with its application in exoskeleton development. Surface EMG (sEMG) remains the most widely adopted type due to its non-invasive nature, ease of integration, and potential for real-time application.

However, the variability remains a challenge particularly in dynamics or ambulatory environments. Intramuscular EMG and emerging methods like High-Density (HD) sEMG and Electroneurography (ENG) offer improved specificity and fidelity while they are often limited by invasiveness or equipment complexity.

Robust signal acquisition must be complemented by effective noise mitigation strategies. Traditional band-pass and notch filters offer foundational denoising capabilities, while modern techniques provide real-time adaptive solutions. The combination of these approaches enables the preservation of biologically meaningful signal content necessary for reliable control inputs. Feature extraction methods offer critical insights into muscle activation and fatigue. They provide foundational data for pattern recognition algorithms, which are essential for interpreting motion intent in complex control systems. Despite these advancements, EMG-only control systems face challenges in robustness, especially in long-term, unsupervised, or fatigue prone situations. Multimodal biosensing approaches that integrate EMG with electroencephalography, bioimpedance, inertial sensing, and visual feedback offer significant improvements in accuracy, stability, and adaptability.

Machine learning has enabled high-accuracy classification of movement patterns. Furthermore, muscle synergy analysis plays a pivotal role in understanding neuromuscular coordination. This synergy centric approach reduces control complexity and allows for more nature and efficient interactions. Lastly, in the application domain, EMG-driven exoskeletons demonstrate promising utility across rehabilitation, industrial support, and mobility augmentation. Three main EMG-base control paradigms, namely threshold-based, pattern recognition-based, and hybrid systems, offer varying levels of complexity and adaptability. Real-time processing is a central hurdle in translating laboratory grade EMG control strategies into reliable field-deployable exoskeletons. Solutions are increasingly leaning toward embedded AI platforms, efficient neural architectures, and edge computing to reduce computational overhead. Adaptive algorithms capable of online recalibration, transfer learning, and user-specific modeling are critical to mitigate the effects of muscle fatigue, electrode shift, and day-to-day physiological variations.

Author Contributions: Conceptualization, J.-H.S. and L.P.; methodology, J.-H.S. and D.M.G.P.; validation, D.M. and S.D.A.; formal analysis, S.D.A.; investigation, D.M. and S.D.A.; resources, A.J.; writing—original draft preparation, J.-H.S. and L.P.; writing—review and editing, G.K., J.-H.S. and L.P.; visualization, J.-H.S., S.D.A. and A.J.; supervision, D.M.G.P. and G.K. All authors have read and agreed to the published version of the manuscript.

Funding: This research received no external funding.

Institutional Review Board Statement: Not applicable.

Informed Consent Statement: Not applicable.

Data Availability Statement: No new data were created or analyzed in this study. Data sharing is not applicable to this article.

Conflicts of Interest: The authors declare no conflict of interest.

References

1. Preethichandra, D.M.G.; Piyathilaka, L.; Sul, J.-H.; Izhar, U.; Samarasinghe, R.; Arachchige, S.D.; and de Silva, L.C. Passive and Active Exoskeleton Solutions: Sensors, Actuators, Applications, and Recent Trends. *Sensors* **2024**, *24*, 7095. [CrossRef]
2. Arachchige, S.D.; Piyathilaka, L.; Sul, J.-H.; Preethichandra, D.M.G. A Review of Potential Exoskeletons for the Prevention of Work-Related Musculoskeletal Disorders in Agriculture. *Sensors* **2024**, *24*, 7026. [CrossRef] [PubMed]
3. Carvalho, C.R.; Fernández, J.M.; Del-Ama, A.J.; Oliveira Barroso, F.; Moreno, J.C. Review of electromyography onset detection methods for real-time control of robotic exoskeletons. *J. Neuroeng. Rehabil.* **2023**, *20*, 141. [CrossRef] [PubMed]

4. Sadikoglu, F.; Kavalcioglu, C.; Dagman, B. Electromyogram (EMG) signal detection, classification of EMG signals and diagnosis of neuropathy muscle disease. *Procedia Comput. Sci.* **2017**, *120*, 422–429. [CrossRef]
5. Nazari, F.; Mohajer, N.; Nahavandi, D.; Khosravi, A.; Nahavandi, S. Applied Exoskeleton Technology: A Comprehensive Review of Physical and Cognitive Human–Robot Interaction. *IEEE Trans. Cogn. Dev. Syst.* **2023**, *15*, 1102–1122. [CrossRef]
6. da Silva, L.D.L.; Pereira, T.F.; Leithardt, V.R.Q.; Seman, L.O.; Zeferino, C.A. Hybrid Impedance-Admittance Control for Upper Limb Exoskeleton Using Electromyography. *Appl. Sci.* **2020**, *10*, 7146. [CrossRef]
7. Zieliński, G.; Gawda, P. Surface Electromyography in Dentistry-Past, Present and Future. *J. Clin. Med.* **2024**, *13*, 1328. [CrossRef]
8. Zhang, X.; Qu, Y.; Zhang, G.; Wang, Z.; Chen, C.; Xu, X. Review of sEMG for Exoskeleton Robots: Motion Intention Recognition Techniques and Applications. *Sensors* **2025**, *25*, 2448. [CrossRef]
9. Yin, G.; Zhang, X.; Chen, D.; Li, H.; Chen, J.; Chen, C.; Lemos, S. Processing Surface EMG Signals for Exoskeleton Motion Control. *Front. Neurorobot.* **2020**, *14*, 40. [CrossRef]
10. Hamtaei Pour Shirazi, F.; Parsaei, H.; Ashraf, A. A clinical decision support system for diagnosis and severity quantification of lumbosacral radiculopathy using intramuscular electromyography signals. *Med. Biol. Eng. Comput.* **2025**, *63*, 239–249. [CrossRef]
11. Crouch, D.L.; Pan, L.; Filer, W.; Stallings, J.W.; Huang, H. Comparing Surface and Intramuscular Electromyography for Simultaneous and Proportional Control Based on a Musculoskeletal Model: A Pilot Study. *IEEE Trans. Neural Syst. Rehabil. Eng* **2018**, *26*, 1735–1744. [CrossRef] [PubMed]
12. Grison, A.; Mendez Guerra, I.; Clarke, A.K.; Muceli, S.; Ibáñez, J.; Farina, D. Unlocking the full potential of high-density surface EMG: Novel non-invasive high-yield motor unit decomposition. *J. Physiol.* **2025**, *603*, 2281–2300. [CrossRef] [PubMed]
13. Montazerin, M.; Zabihi, S.; Rahimian, E.; Mohammadi, A.; Naderkhani, F. ViT-HGR: Vision Transformer-based Hand Gesture Recognition from High Density Surface EMG Signals. In Proceedings of the 44th Annual International Conference of the IEEE Engineering in Medicine & Biology Society (EMBC), Glasgow, UK, 11–15 July 2022.
14. Pei, Y.-C.; Chen, T.-Y.; Hsu, P.-C.; Lin, C.-H.; Huang, J.-J. An electroneurography-based assay for identifying injured nerve segment during surgery: Design and in vivo application in the rat. *J. Neural Eng.* **2019**, *16*, 026027. [CrossRef] [PubMed]
15. Trigili, E.; Grazi, L.; Crea, S.; Accogli, A.; Carpaneto, J.; Micera, S.; Vitiello, N.; Panarese, A. Detection of movement onset using EMG signals for upper-limb exoskeletons in reaching tasks. *J. Neuroeng. Rehabil.* **2019**, *16*, 45. [CrossRef]
16. Thilahar, R.; Manoharan, M.; Sudalai, P.; Sadayan, R.B.; Kaliaraj, G.S. Electromyography (EMG) Signal Acquisition for Exoskeleton Control: Enhancing Precision in Human-Machine Interaction. In Proceedings of the International Conference on Smart Electronics and Communication Systems (ISENSE), Kerala, India, 6–7 December 2024.
17. Karimi, M.; Ahmadi, M. iLeAD: An EMG-Based Adaptive Shared Control Framework for Exoskeleton Assistance via Deep Reinforcement Learning. *IEEE Trans. Artif. Intell.* **2025**. *early access*. [CrossRef]
18. De Luca, C.J. *Surface Electromyography: Detection and Recording*; DelSys Incorporated: Natick, MA, USA, 2002.
19. Galbert, A.; Buis, A. Active, Actuated, and Assistive: A Scoping Review of Exoskeletons for the Hands and Wrists. *Can. Prosthet. Orthot. J.* **2024**, *7*, 43827. [CrossRef]
20. Sousa, A.S.P.; Noites, A.; Vilarinho, R.; Santos, R. Long-Term Electrode–Skin Impedance Variation for Electromyographic Measurements. *Sensors* **2023**, *23*, 8582. [CrossRef]
21. Yang, L.; Gan, L.; Zhang, Z.; Zhang, Z.; Yang, H.; Zhang, Y.; Wu, J. Insight into the Contact Impedance between the Electrode and the Skin Surface for Electrophysical Recordings. *ACS Omega* **2022**, *7*, 13906–13912. [CrossRef]
22. Etana, B.B.; Malengier, B.; Krishnamoorthy, J.; Van Langenhove, L. Types of EMG Textile Electrodes: A Comparative Study Using PCA. *Eng. Proc.* **2023**, *35*, 6. [CrossRef]
23. Kankula, R. Real-Life Skin Impedance Variations with Dry and Wet Electrodes for Bio-Potential Signal Acquisition. *Int. J. Sci. Technol.* **2025**, *16*, 1–17.
24. Perego, P.; Sironi, R.; Gruppioni, E.; Andreoni, G. TWINMED T-SHIRT, a Smart Wearable System for ECG and EMG Monitoring for Rehabilitation with Exoskeletons. In Proceedings of the International Conference on Human-Computer Interaction, Copenhagen, Denmark, 23–28 July 2023.
25. Euler, L.; Guo, L.; Persson, N.-K. A review of textile-based electrodes developed for electrostimulation. *Text. Res. J.* **2022**, *92*, 1300–1320. [CrossRef]
26. Ali, B.; Cheraghi Bidsorkhi, H.; D'Aloia, A.G.; Laracca, M.; Sarto, M.S. Wearable graphene-based fabric electrodes for enhanced and long-term biosignal detection. *Sensors Actuators Rep.* **2023**, *5*, 100161. [CrossRef]
27. Belbasis, A.; Fuss, F.K. Muscle Performance Investigated With a Novel Smart Compression Garment Based on Pressure Sensor Force Myography and Its Validation Against EMG. *Front Physiol.* **2018**, *9*, 408. [CrossRef]
28. Lam, E.; Alizadeh-Meghrazi, M.; Schlums, A.; Eskandarian, L.; Mahnam, A.; Moineau, B.; Popovic, M.R. Exploring textile-based electrode materials for electromyography smart garments. *J. Rehabil. Assist. Technol. Eng.* **2022**, *9*, 20556683211061995. [CrossRef] [PubMed]

29. Kim, H.; Lee, J.; Heo, U.; Jayashankar, D.K.; Agno, K.-C.; Kim, Y.; Kim, C.Y.; Oh, Y.; Byun, S.-H.; Choi, B.; et al. Skin preparation–free, stretchable microneedle adhesive patches for reliable electrophysiological sensing and exoskeleton robot control. *Sci. Adv.* **2024**, *10*, eadk5260. [CrossRef]
30. Molinaro, D.D.; Kang, I.; Young, A.J. Estimating human joint moments unifies exoskeleton control, reducing user effort. *Sci. Robot.* **2024**, *9*, 8852. [CrossRef]
31. Pitzalis, R.F.; Cartocci, N.; Natali, C.D.; Caldwell, D.G.; Berselli, G.; Ortiz, J. Development of a ML-Control Strategy for a Wrist Exoskeleton Based on EMG and Force Measurements with Sensor Strategy Optimisation. In Proceedings of the 10th IEEE RAS/EMBS International Conference for Biomedical Robotics and Biomechatronics (BioRob), Heidelberg, Germany, 1–4 September 2024.
32. Kabiri Ameri, S.; Ho, R.; Jang, H.; Tao, L.; Wang, Y.; Wang, L.; Schnyer, D.M.; Akinwande, D.; Lu, N. Graphene Electronic Tattoo Sensors. *ACS Nano* **2017**, *11*, 7634–7641. [CrossRef]
33. Zhu, C.; Maurya, S.; Yi, J.; Dutta, A. Brain Computer Interface (BCI)-Enhanced Knee Exoskeleton Control for Assisted Sit-to-Stand Movement. In Proceedings of the IEEE International Conference on Advanced Intelligent Mechatronics (AIM), Boston, MA, USA, 15–19 July 2024.
34. Kusche, R.; Ryschka, M. Combining Bioimpedance and EMG Measurements for Reliable Muscle Contraction Detection. *IEEE Sens. J.* **2019**, *19*, 11687–11696. [CrossRef]
35. Farina, D.; Jiang, N.; Rehbaum, H.; Holobar, A.; Graimann, B.; Dietl, H.; Aszmann, O.C. The extraction of neural information from the surface EMG for the control of upper-limb prostheses: Emerging avenues and challenges. *IEEE Trans. Neural Syst. Rehabil. Eng.* **2014**, *22*, 797–809. [CrossRef]
36. Boyer, M.; Bouyer, L.; Roy, J.-S.; Campeau-Lecours, A. Reducing Noise, Artifacts and Interference in Single-Channel EMG Signals: A Review. *Sensors* **2023**, *23*, 2927. [CrossRef]
37. Piskorowski, J. Powerline interference rejection from sEMG signal using notch filter with transient suppression. In Proceedings of the IEEE International Instrumentation and Measurement Technology Conference Proceedings, Graz, Austria, 13–16 May 2012.
38. Stoykov, N.S.; Lowery, M.M.; Kuiken, T.A. A finite-element analysis of the effect of muscle insulation and shielding on the surface EMG signal. *IEEE Trans. Biomed. Eng.* **2005**, *52*, 117–121. [CrossRef]
39. Kauppi, J.P.; Hahne, J.; Müller, K.R.; Hyvärinen, A. Three-way analysis of spectrospatial electromyography data: Classification and interpretation. *PLoS ONE* **2015**, *10*, e0127231. [CrossRef] [PubMed]
40. Wen, Y.; Kim, S.J.; Avrillon, S.; Levine, J.T.; Hug, F.; Pons, J.L. A Deep CNN Framework for Neural Drive Estimation From HD-EMG Across Contraction Intensities and Joint Angles. *IEEE Trans. Neural Syst. Rehabil. Eng.* **2022**, *30*, 2950–2959. [CrossRef]
41. De Luca, C.J.; Donald Gilmore, L.; Kuznetsov, M.; Roy, S.H. Filtering the surface EMG signal: Movement artifact and baseline noise contamination. *J. Biomech.* **2010**, *43*, 1573–1579. [CrossRef] [PubMed]
42. Ladrova, M.; Martinek, R.; Nedoma, J.; Fajkus, M. Methods of Power Line Interference Elimination in EMG Signal. *J. Biomim. Biomater. Biomed. Eng.* **2019**, *40*, 64–70. [CrossRef]
43. Chen, J.; Sun, Y.; Sun, S.; Yao, Z. Reducing Power Line Interference from sEMG Signals Based on Synchrosqueezed Wavelet Transform. *Sensors* **2023**, *23*, 5182. [CrossRef] [PubMed]
44. Abbaspour, S.; Fallah, A.; Lindén, M.; Gholamhosseini, H. A novel approach for removing ECG interferences from surface EMG signals using a combined ANFIS and wavelet. *J. Electromyogr. Kinesiol.* **2016**, *26*, 52–59. [CrossRef]
45. Andrade, A.O.; Nasuto, S.; Kyberd, P.; Sweeney-Reed, C.M.; Van Kanijn, F.R. EMG signal filtering based on Empirical Mode Decomposition. *Biomed. Signal Process. Control* **2006**, *1*, 44–55. [CrossRef]
46. Mishra, V.K.; Bajaj, V.; Kumar, A.; Sharma, D.; Singh, G.K. An efficient method for analysis of EMG signals using improved empirical mode decomposition. *AEU-Int. J. Electron. C.* **2017**, *72*, 200–209. [CrossRef]
47. Menegaldo, L.L. Real-time muscle state estimation from EMG signals during isometric contractions using Kalman filters. *Biol. Cybern.* **2017**, *111*, 335–346. [CrossRef]
48. Limem, M.; Hamdi, M.A.; Maaref, M.A. Denoising uterine EMG signals using LMS and RLS adaptive algorithms. In Proceedings of the 2nd International Conference on Advanced Technologies for Signal and Image Processing (ATSIP), Monastir, Tunisia, 21–23 March 2016.
49. Lu, G.; Brittain, J.-S.; Holland, P.; Yianni, J.; Green, A.L.; Stein, J.F.; Aziz, T.Z.; Wang, S. Removing ECG noise from surface EMG signals using adaptive filtering. *Neurosci. Lett.* **2009**, *462*, 14–19. [CrossRef] [PubMed]
50. Nieto, R.; Fernández, P.R.; Murano, S.; Navarro, V.M.; del-Ama, A.J.; Borromeo, S. Conception of a System-on-Chip (SoC) Platform to Enable EMG-Guided Robotic Neurorehabilitation. *Appl. Sci.* **2025**, *15*, 1699. [CrossRef]
51. Ritzmann, R.; Karacan, I.; Türker, K.S. Electromyographical Recordings During Vibration. In *Manual of Vibration Exercise and Vibration Therapy*; Rittweger, J., Ed.; Springer International Publishing: Cham, Switzerland, 2020; pp. 109–120.

52. Jia, Z.; Chen, G.; Weng, Y.; Su, D. Manipulation of Analog Sensors through Electromagnetic Interference Attacks. In Proceedings of the 2023 IEEE 7th International Symposium on Electromagnetic Compatibility (ISEMC), Hangzhou, China, 20–23 October 2023.
53. Tamburella, F.; Masciullo, M.; Pisotta, I.; Tagliamonte, N.L.; Molinari, M. Lower Limb Wearable Systems for Mobility and Rehabilitation Challenges: Clinical Focus. In Proceedings of the 2nd International Symposium on Wearable Robotics, WeRob2016, Segovia, Spain, 18–21 October 2016.
54. Wang, Z.-Y.; Xiang, Z.-R.; Zhi, J.-Y.; Ding, T.-C.; Zou, R. A novel physiological signal denoising method coupled with multispectral adaptive wavelet denoising(MAWD) and unsupervised source counting algorithm(USCA). *J. Eng. Res.* **2024**, *12*, 175–189. [CrossRef]
55. Jaarsveldt, C.V.; Peters, G.W.; Ames, M.; Chantler, M. Tutorial on Empirical Mode Decomposition: Basis Decomposition and Frequency Adaptive Graduation in Non-Stationary Time Series. *IEEE Access* **2023**, *11*, 94442–94478. [CrossRef]
56. Zhang, L.; Long, J.; Zhao, R.; Cao, H.; Zhang, K. Estimation of the Continuous Pronation–Supination Movement by Using Multichannel EMG Signal Features and Kalman Filter: Application to Control an Exoskeleton. *Front. Bioeng. Biotechnol.* **2022**, *9*, 771255. [CrossRef] [PubMed]
57. Ni, S.; Al-qaness, M.A.A.; Hawbani, A.; Al-Alimi, D.; Abd Elaziz, M.; Ewees, A.A. A survey on hand gesture recognition based on surface electromyography: Fundamentals, methods, applications, challenges and future trends. *Appl. Soft Comput.* **2024**, *166*, 112235. [CrossRef]
58. Tkach, D.; Huang, H.; Kuiken, T.A. Study of stability of time-domain features for electromyographic pattern recognition. *J. Neuroeng. Rehabil.* **2010**, *7*, 21. [CrossRef]
59. Muceli, S.; Merletti, R. Tutorial. Frequency analysis of the surface EMG signal: Best practices. *J. Electromyogr. Kinesiol.* **2024**, *79*, 102937. [CrossRef]
60. Spiewak, C.; Islam, M.; Zaman, M.A.-U.; Rahman, M.H. A Comprehensive Study on EMG Feature Extraction and Classifiers. *Open J. Biomed. Eng. Biosci.* **2018**, *1*, 17–26. [CrossRef]
61. Nazmi, N.; Abdul Rahman, M.A.; Yamamoto, S.-I.; Ahmad, S.A.; Zamzuri, H.; Mazlan, S.A. A Review of Classification Techniques of EMG Signals during Isotonic and Isometric Contractions. *Sensors* **2016**, *16*, 1304. [CrossRef]
62. Bawa, A.; Banitsas, K. Design Validation of a Low-Cost EMG Sensor Compared to a Commercial-Based System for Measuring Muscle Activity and Fatigue. *Sensors* **2022**, *22*, 5799. [CrossRef]
63. González-Izal, M.; Malanda, A.; Gorostiaga, E.; Izquierdo, M. Electromyographic models to assess muscle fatigue. *J. Electromyogr. Kinesiol.* **2012**, *22*, 501–512. [CrossRef] [PubMed]
64. Corvini, G.; Conforto, S. A Simulation Study to Assess the Factors of Influence on Mean and Median Frequency of sEMG Signals during Muscle Fatigue. *Sensors* **2022**, *22*, 6360. [CrossRef]
65. Ozdemir, M.A.; Kisa, D.H.; Guren, O.; Akan, A. Hand gesture classification using time–frequency images and transfer learning based on CNN. *Biomed. Signal Process. Control* **2022**, *77*, 103787. [CrossRef]
66. Vannozzi, G.; Conforto, S.; D'Alessio, T. Automatic detection of surface EMG activation timing using a wavelet transform based method. *J. Electromyogr. Kinesiol.* **2010**, *20*, 767–772. [CrossRef] [PubMed]
67. Gültekin, E.; Ceylan, C.; Kaynak, H.K.; Çelik, H.İ.; Özbay, S.; Erdem, E.U. Analysis and Comparison of Fast Fourier and Wavelet Transform Techniques on Raw sEMG Data From Textile-Based Electrodes. In Proceedings of the Medical Technologies Congress (TIPTEKNO), Famagusta, Cyprus, 10–12 November 2023.
68. Yousefi, J.; Hamilton-Wright, A. Characterizing EMG data using machine-learning tools. *Comput. Biol. Med.* **2014**, *51*, 1–13. [CrossRef] [PubMed]
69. Malik, S.N.A.; Senin, S.F. Automated system for concrete damage classification identification using Naïve-Bayesian classifier. *AIP Conf. Proc.* **2022**, *2532*, 040014.
70. Li, G.; Yu, Z.; Yang, K.; Lin, M.; Chen, C.L.P. Exploring Feature Selection With Limited Labels: A Comprehensive Survey of Semi-Supervised and Unsupervised Approaches. *IEEE Trans. Knowl. Data Eng.* **2024**, *36*, 6124–6144. [CrossRef]
71. Gu, Y.; Yang, D.; Huang, Q.; Yang, W.; Liu, H. Robust EMG pattern recognition in the presence of confounding factors: Features, classifiers and adaptive learning. *Expert Syst. Appl.* **2018**, *96*, 208–217. [CrossRef]
72. Liu, J.; Ying, D.; Rymer, W.Z.; Zhou, P. Robust muscle activity onset detection using an unsupervised electromyogram learning framework. *PLoS ONE* **2015**, *10*, e0127990. [CrossRef]
73. Jiang, Y.; Chen, C.; Zhang, X.; Chen, C.; Zhou, Y.; Ni, G.; Muh, S.; Lemos, S. Shoulder muscle activation pattern recognition based on sEMG and machine learning algorithms. *Comput. Methods Programs Biomed.* **2020**, *197*, 105721. [CrossRef] [PubMed]
74. Parajuli, N.; Sreenivasan, N.; Bifulco, P.; Cesarelli, M.; Savino, S.; Niola, V.; Esposito, D.; Hamilton, T.J.; Naik, G.R.; Gunawardana, U.; et al. Real-Time EMG Based Pattern Recognition Control for Hand Prostheses: A Review on Existing Methods, Challenges and Future Implementation. *Sensors* **2019**, *19*, 4596. [CrossRef] [PubMed]

75. Kok, C.L.; Ho, C.K.; Tan, F.K.; Koh, Y.Y. Machine Learning-Based Feature Extraction and Classification of EMG Signals for Intuitive Prosthetic Control. *Appl. Sci.* **2024**, *14*, 5784. [CrossRef]
76. Ketykó, I.; Kovács, F.; Varga, K.Z. Domain Adaptation for sEMG-based Gesture Recognition with Recurrent Neural Networks. In Proceedings of the International Joint Conference on Neural Networks (IJCNN), Budapest, Hungary, 14–19 July 2019.
77. Gallón, V.M.; Vélez, S.M.; Ramírez, J.; Bolaños, F. Comparison of machine learning algorithms and feature extraction techniques for the automatic detection of surface EMG activation timing. *Biomed. Signal Process. Control* **2024**, *94*, 106266. [CrossRef]
78. Zhang, Z.; Beck, M.W.; Winkler, D.A.; Huang, B.; Sibanda, W.; Goyal, H. Opening the black box of neural networks: Methods for interpreting neural network models in clinical applications. *Ann. Transl. Med.* **2018**, *6*, 216. [CrossRef] [PubMed]
79. Sun, S.; Cao, Z.; Zhu, H.; Zhao, J. A Survey of Optimization Methods From a Machine Learning Perspective. *IEEE Trans. Cybern.* **2019**, *50*, 3668–3681. [CrossRef]
80. Tepe, C.; Demir, M.C. Real-Time Classification of EMG Myo Armband Data Using Support Vector Machine. *IRBM* **2022**, *43*, 300–308. [CrossRef]
81. Laganà, F.; Pratticò, D.; Angiulli, G.; Oliva, G.; Pullano, S.A.; Versaci, M.; La Foresta, F. Development of an Integrated System of sEMG Signal Acquisition, Processing, and Analysis with AI Techniques. *Signals* **2024**, *5*, 476–493. [CrossRef]
82. Li, C.; Chen, X.; Zhang, X.; Wu, D. Research on the electromyography-based pattern recognition for inter-limb coordination in human crawling motion. *Front. Neurosci.* **2024**, *18*, 1349347. [CrossRef]
83. Abdullah, A.A.; Subasi, A.; Qaisar, S.M. Surface EMG Signal Classification by Using WPD and Ensemble Tree Classifiers. In Proceedings of the International Conference on Medical and Biological Engineering, Sarajevo, Bosnia and Herzegovina, 16–18 March 2017.
84. Biau, G.; Scornet, E. A random forest guided tour. *TEST* **2016**, *25*, 197–227. [CrossRef]
85. Cai, S.; Chen, Y.; Huang, S.; Wu, Y.; Zheng, H.; Li, X.; Xie, L. SVM-Based Classification of sEMG Signals for Upper-Limb Self-Rehabilitation Training. *Front. Neurorobot.* **2019**, *13*, 31. [CrossRef]
86. Gao, X.; Bai, W.; Dang, Q.; Yang, S.; Zhang, G. Learnable self-supervised support vector machine based individual selection strategy for multimodal multi-objective optimization. *Inf. Sci.* **2025**, *690*, 121553. [CrossRef]
87. Beltrame, G.; Scano, A.; Marino, G.; Peccati, A.; Molinari Tosatti, L.; Portinaro, N. Recent developments in muscle synergy analysis in young people with neurodevelopmental diseases: A Systematic Review. *Front. Bioeng. Biotechnol.* **2023**, *11*, 1145937. [CrossRef] [PubMed]
88. Borzelli, D.; De Marchis, C.; Quercia, A.; De Pasquale, P.; Casile, A.; Quartarone, A.; Calabrò, R.S.; d'Avella, A. Muscle Synergy Analysis as a Tool for Assessing the Effectiveness of Gait Rehabilitation Therapies: A Methodological Review and Perspective. *Bioengineering* **2024**, *11*, 793. [CrossRef] [PubMed]
89. d'Avella, A.; Bizzi, E. Shared and specific muscle synergies in natural motor behaviors. *Proc. Natl. Acad. Sci. USA* **2005**, *102*, 3076–3081. [CrossRef]
90. Ma, Y.; Liu, D.; Yan, Z.; Yu, L.; Gui, L.; Yang, C.; Yang, W. Optimizing Exoskeleton Assistance: Muscle Synergy-Based Actuation for Personalized Hip Exoskeleton Control. *Actuators* **2024**, *13*, 54. [CrossRef]
91. Afzal, T.; Zhu, F.; Tseng, S.C.; Lincoln, J.A.; Francisco, G.E.; Su, H.; Chang, S.H. Evaluation of Muscle Synergy During Exoskeleton-Assisted Walking in Persons With Multiple Sclerosis. *IEEE Trans. Biomed. Eng.* **2022**, *69*, 3265–3274. [CrossRef]
92. Alibeji, N.A.; Molazadeh, V.; Moore-Clingenpeel, F.; Sharma, N. A Muscle Synergy-Inspired Control Design to Coordinate Functional Electrical Stimulation and a Powered Exoskeleton: Artificial Generation of Synergies to Reduce Input Dimensionality. *IEEE Contr. Syst. Mag.* **2018**, *38*, 35–60. [CrossRef]
93. Hassan, M.; Kadone, H.; Ueno, T.; Hada, Y.; Sankai, Y.; Suzuki, K. Feasibility of Synergy-Based Exoskeleton Robot Control in Hemiplegia. *IEEE Trans. Neural. Syst. Rehabil. Eng.* **2018**, *26*, 1233–1242. [CrossRef]
94. Ma, Y.; Cui, B.; Jiang, C.; Gu, H.; Zhang, H.; Zhong, Q. Extracting Muscle Synergies Using Constrained Non-Negative Matrix Factorization for Motion Intention in Rehabilitation Robotics. In Proceedings of the IEEE International Conference on Robotics and Biomimetics (ROBIO), Bangkok, Thailand, 10–14 December 2024.
95. Ge, W.; She, J.; Guo, S.; Wang, F.; Zhao, J.; Kawata, S. The Analysis of Muscle-Synergy Similarity between Walking and Pedaling Based on Variational Mode Decomposition and Non-Negative Matrix Factorization. In Proceedings of the IEEE International Conference on Engineering, Technology, and Innovation (ICE/ITMC), Madeira, Portugal, 24–28 June 2024.
96. Ao, D.; Vega, M.M.; Shourijeh, M.S.; Patten, C.; Fregly, B.J. EMG-driven musculoskeletal model calibration with estimation of unmeasured muscle excitations via synergy extrapolation. *Front. Bioeng. Biotechnol.* **2022**, *10*, 962959. [CrossRef]
97. Kim, Y.; Stapornchaisit, S.; Miyakoshi, M.; Yoshimura, N.; Koike, Y. The Effect of ICA and Non-negative Matrix Factorization Analysis for EMG Signals Recorded From Multi-Channel EMG Sensors. *Front. Neurosci.* **2020**, *14*, 600804. [CrossRef]

98. Wojtara, T.; Alnajjar, F.; Shimoda, S.; Kimura, H. Muscle synergy stability and human balance maintenance. *J. Neuroeng. Rehabil.* **2014**, *11*, 129. [CrossRef] [PubMed]
99. Lee, J. Characteristics of muscle synergy extracted using an autoencoder in patients with stroke during the curved walking in comparison with healthy controls. *Gait Posture* **2024**, *107*, 225–232. [CrossRef]
100. Fang, C.; He, B.; Wang, Y.; Cao, J.; Gao, S. EMG-Centered Multisensory Based Technologies for Pattern Recognition in Rehabilitation: State of the Art and Challenges. *Biosensors* **2020**, *10*, 85. [CrossRef]
101. De Luca, C.J.; Erim, Z. Common drive in motor units of a synergistic muscle pair. *J. Neurophysiol.* **2002**, *87*, 2200–2204. [CrossRef] [PubMed]
102. Chowdhury, R.H.; Reaz, M.B.I.; Ali, M.A.B.M.; Bakar, A.A.A.; Chellappan, K.; Chang, T.G. Surface Electromyography Signal Processing and Classification Techniques. *Sensors* **2013**, *13*, 12431–12466. [CrossRef]
103. Mewett, D.T.; Reynolds, K.J.; Nazeran, H. Reducing power line interference in digitised electromyogram recordings by spectrum interpolation. *Med. Biol. Eng. Comput.* **2004**, *42*, 524–531. [CrossRef] [PubMed]
104. Asghari Oskoei, M.; Hu, H. Myoelectric control systems—A survey. *Biomed. Signal Process. Control* **2007**, *2*, 275–294. [CrossRef]
105. Kiguchi, K.; Hayashi, Y. An EMG-Based Control for an Upper-Limb Power-Assist Exoskeleton Robot. *IEEE Trans. Syst. Man Cybern.* **2012**, *42*, 1064–1071. [CrossRef]
106. Fu, J.; Choudhury, R.; Hosseini, S.M.; Simpson, R.; Park, J.-H. Myoelectric Control Systems for Upper Limb Wearable Robotic Exoskeletons and Exosuits—A Systematic Review. *Sensors* **2022**, *22*, 8134. [CrossRef]
107. Khushaba, R.N.; Kodagoda, S.; Takruri, M.; Dissanayake, G. Toward improved control of prosthetic fingers using surface electromyogram (EMG) signals. *Expert Syst. Appl.* **2012**, *39*, 10731–10738. [CrossRef]
108. Phinyomark, A.; Quaine, F.; Charbonnier, S.; Serviere, C.; Tarpin-Bernard, F.; Laurillau, Y. EMG feature evaluation for improving myoelectric pattern recognition robustness. *Expert Syst. Appl.* **2013**, *40*, 4832–4840. [CrossRef]
109. Englehart, K.; Hudgins, B.; Chan, A.D.C. Continuous multifunction myoelectric control using pattern recognition. *Technol. Disab.* **2003**, *15*, 95–103. [CrossRef]
110. Boostani, R.; Moradi, M.H. Evaluation of the forearm EMG signal features for the control of a prosthetic hand. *Physiol. Meas.* **2003**, *24*, 309–319. [CrossRef] [PubMed]
111. Zecca, M.; Micera, S.; Carrozza, M.C.; Dario, P. Control of multifunctional prosthetic hands by processing the electromyographic signal. *Crit. Rev. Biomed. Eng.* **2002**, *30*, 459–485. [CrossRef]
112. Xia, P.; Hu, J.; Peng, Y. EMG-Based Estimation of Limb Movement Using Deep Learning with Recurrent Convolutional Neural Networks. *Artif. Organs.* **2018**, *42*, E67–E77. [CrossRef]
113. Scheme, E.; Englehart, K. Electromyogram pattern recognition for control of powered upper-limb prostheses: State of the art and challenges for clinical use. *J. Rehabil. Res. Dev.* **2011**, *48*, 643–659. [CrossRef]
114. Wang, X.; Ao, D.; Li, L. Robust myoelectric pattern recognition methods for reducing users' calibration burden: Challenges and future. *Front. Bioeng. Biotechnol.* **2024**, *12*, 1329209. [CrossRef]
115. Young, A.J.; Hargrove, L.J.; Kuiken, T.A. The effects of electrode size and orientation on the sensitivity of myoelectric pattern recognition systems to electrode shift. *IEEE Trans. Biomed. Eng.* **2011**, *58*, 2537–2544. [CrossRef]
116. Georgi, M.; Amma, C.; Schultz, T. Fusion and Comparison of IMU and EMG Signals for Wearable Gesture Recognition. In Proceedings of the International Joint Conference on Biomedical Engineering Systems and Technologies, Lisbon, Portugal, 12–15 January 2015.
117. Gordleeva, S.Y.; Lobov, S.A.; Grigorev, N.A.; Savosenkov, A.O.; Shamshin, M.O.; Lukoyanov, M.V.; Khoruzhko, M.A.; Kazantsev, V.B. Real-Time EEG–EMG Human–Machine Interface-Based Control System for a Lower-Limb Exoskeleton. *IEEE Access* **2020**, *8*, 84070–84081. [CrossRef]
118. Atzori, M.; Gijsberts, A.; Castellini, C.; Caputo, B.; Hager, A.G.; Elsig, S.; Giatsidis, G.; Bassetto, F.; Müller, H. Electromyography data for non-invasive naturally-controlled robotic hand prostheses. *Sci. Data* **2014**, *1*, 140053. [CrossRef]
119. Prasanth, H.; Caban, M.; Keller, U.; Courtine, G.; Ijspeert, A.; Vallery, H.; von Zitzewitz, J. Wearable Sensor-Based Real-Time Gait Detection: A Systematic Review. *Sensors* **2021**, *21*, 2727. [CrossRef]
120. Phinyomark, A.; Phukpattaranont, P.; Limsakul, C. Feature reduction and selection for EMG signal classification. *Expert Syst. Appl.* **2012**, *39*, 7420–7431. [CrossRef]
121. Krasoulis, A.; Kyranou, I.; Erden, M.S.; Nazarpour, K.; Vijayakumar, S. Improved prosthetic hand control with concurrent use of myoelectric and inertial measurements. *J. Neuroeng. Rehabil.* **2017**, *14*, 71. [CrossRef] [PubMed]
122. Luo, S.; Androwis, G.; Adamovich, S.; Su, H.; Nunez, E.; Zhou, X. Reinforcement Learning and Control of a Lower Extremity Exoskeleton for Squat Assistance. *Front. Robot. AI* **2021**, *8*, 702845. [CrossRef] [PubMed]

123. Tu, X.; Li, M.; Liu, M.; Si, J.; Huang, H.H. A Data-Driven Reinforcement Learning Solution Framework for Optimal and Adaptive Personalization of a Hip Exoskeleton. In Proceedings of the IEEE International Conference on Robotics and Automation (ICRA), Xi'an, China, 30 May–5 June 2021.
124. Valdivieso Caraguay, Á.L.; Vásconez, J.P.; Barona López, L.I.; Benalcázar, M.E. Recognition of Hand Gestures Based on EMG Signals with Deep and Double-Deep Q-Networks. *Sensors* **2023**, *23*, 3905. [CrossRef]
125. Huang, L.; Zheng, J.; Gao, Y.; Song, Q.; Liu, Y. A Lower Limb Exoskeleton Adaptive Control Method Based on Model-free Reinforcement Learning and Improved Dynamic Movement Primitives. *J. Intell. Robot. Syst.* **2025**, *111*, 24. [CrossRef]
126. Geng, Y.; Zhou, P.; Li, G. Toward attenuating the impact of arm positions on electromyography pattern-recognition based motion classification in transradial amputees. *J. Neuroeng. Rehabil.* **2012**, *9*, 74. [CrossRef]
127. Echeveste, S.; Bhounsule, P.A. Electromyography-Based Human-in-the-Loop Bayesian Optimization to Assist Free Leg Swinging. *Biomech.* **2025**, *5*, 21. [CrossRef]
128. Cifrek, M.; Medved, V.; Tonković, S.; Ostojić, S. Surface EMG based muscle fatigue evaluation in biomechanics. *Clin. Biomech.* **2009**, *24*, 327–340. [CrossRef]
129. Turpin, N.A.; Guével, A.; Durand, S.; Hug, F. Fatigue-related adaptations in muscle coordination during a cyclic exercise in humans. *J. Exp. Biol.* **2011**, *214*, 3305–3314. [CrossRef] [PubMed]
130. Lalitharatne, T.D.; Teramoto, K.; Hayashi, Y.; Nanayakkara, T.; Kiguchi, K. Evaluation of Fuzzy-Neuro Modifiers for Compensation of the Effects of Muscle Fatigue on EMG-Based Control to be Used in Upper-Limb Power-Assist Exoskeletons. *J. Adv. Mech. Des. Syst. Manuf.* **2013**, *7*, 736–751. [CrossRef]
131. Zheng, Z.; Wu, Z.; Zhao, R.; Ni, Y.; Jing, X.; Gao, S. A Review of EMG-, FMG-, and EIT-Based Biosensors and Relevant Human-Machine Interactivities and Biomedical Applications. *Biosensors* **2022**, *12*, 516. [CrossRef] [PubMed]
132. Nazari, V.; Zheng, Y.-P. Controlling Upper Limb Prostheses Using Sonomyography (SMG): A Review. *Sensors* **2023**, *23*, 1885. [CrossRef]
133. Zandigohar, M.; Han, M.; Sharif, M.; Günay, S.Y.; Furmanek, M.P.; Yarossi, M.; Bonato, P.; Onal, C.; Padır, T.; Erdoğmuş, D.; et al. Multimodal fusion of EMG and vision for human grasp intent inference in prosthetic hand control. *Front. Robot. AI.* **2024**, *11*, 1312554. [CrossRef]
134. Al-Quraishi, M.S.; Elamvazuthi, I.; Tang, T.B.; Al-Qurishi, M.; Parasuraman, S.; Borboni, A. Multimodal Fusion Approach Based on EEG and EMG Signals for Lower Limb Movement Recognition. *IEEE Sens. J.* **2021**, *21*, 27640–27650. [CrossRef]
135. Zeng, J.; Zhou, Y.; Yang, Y.; Xu, Z.; Zhang, H.; Liu, H. Robustness of Combined sEMG and Ultrasound Modalities Against Muscle Fatigue in Force Estimation. In Proceedings of the 14th International Conference, ICIRA 2021, Yantai, China, 22–25 October 2021.
136. Covi, E.; Donati, E.; Liang, X.; Kappel, D.; Heidari, H.; Payvand, M.; Wang, W. Adaptive Extreme Edge Computing for Wearable Devices. *Front. Neurosci.* **2021**, *15*, 611300. [CrossRef]
137. Jeong, J.-W.; Lee, W.; Kim, Y.-J. A Real-Time Wearable Physiological Monitoring System for Home-Based Healthcare Applications. *Sensors* **2022**, *22*, 104. [CrossRef]
138. Li, J.; Bhuiyan, M.; Huang, X.; McDonald, B.; Farrell, T.; Clancy, E.A. Reducing Electric Power Consumption When Transmitting ECG/EMG/EEG Using a Bluetooth Low Energy Microcontroller. In Proceedings of the 2018 IEEE Signal Processing in Medicine and Biology Symposium (SPMB), Philadelphia, PA, USA, 1 December 2018.
139. Salkic, S.; Ustundag, B.C.; Uzunovic, T.; Golubovic, E. Edge Computing Framework for Wearable Sensor-Based Human Activity Recognition. In Proceedings of the International Symposium on Innovative and Interdisciplinary Applications of Advanced Technologies (IAT 2019), Sarajevo, Bosnia and Herzegovina, 20–23 June 2020.
140. Hazar, Y. and Faruk Ertuğrul, Ö.; Developing a real-time hand exoskeleton system that controlled by a hand gesture recognition system via wireless sensors. *Biomed. Signal Process. Control* **2025**, *99*, 106886. [CrossRef]
141. Vescio, G.; Rosell, J.; Nescolarde, L.; Giovinazzo, G. Muscle Fatigue Monitoring Using a Multifrequency Bioimpedance Technique. In Proceedings of the 5th European Conference of the International Federation for Medical and Biological Engineering, Budapest, Hungary, 14–18 September 2012.
142. Huang, L.K.; Huang, L.N.; Gao, Y.M.; Lučev, V.Ž.; Cifrek, M.; Du, M. Electrical Impedance Myography Applied to Monitoring of Muscle Fatigue During Dynamic Contractions. *IEEE Access* **2020**, *8*, 13056–13065. [CrossRef]
143. Jaiswal, A.; Zadeh, M.Z.; Hebri, A.; Makedon, F. Assessing fatigue with multimodal wearable sensors and machine learning. *arXiv* **2022**, arXiv:2205.00287.
144. Peternel, L.; Noda, T.; Petrič, T.; Ude, A.; Morimoto, J.; Babič, J. Adaptive Control of Exoskeleton Robots for Periodic Assistive Behaviours Based on EMG Feedback Minimisation. *PLoS ONE* **2016**, *11*, 0148942. [CrossRef] [PubMed]
145. De Angelis, S.; Princi, A.A.; Dal Farra, F.; Morone, G.; Caltagirone, C.; Tramontano, M. Vibrotactile-Based Rehabilitation on Balance and Gait in Patients with Neurological Diseases: A Systematic Review and Metanalysis. *Brain Sci.* **2021**, *11*, 518. [CrossRef] [PubMed]

146. Kawase, T.; Sakurada, T.; Koike, Y.; Kansaku, K. A hybrid BMI-based exoskeleton for paresis: EMG control for assisting arm movements. *J. Neural Eng.* **2017**, *14*, 016015. [CrossRef]
147. Wei, W.; Ren, L. From Unimodal to Multimodal: Improving sEMG-Based Pattern Recognition via deep generative models. *arXiv* **2023**, arXiv:2308.04091.

MDPI AG
Grosspeteranlage 5
4052 Basel
Switzerland
Tel.: +41 61 683 77 34

Sensors Editorial Office
E-mail: sensors@mdpi.com
www.mdpi.com/journal/sensors

www.ingramcontent.com/pod-product-compliance
Lightning Source LLC
Chambersburg PA
CBHW061602210926
51850CB00009B/2188